Neuroendocri

T0249768

Editors

JENNIFER A. CHAN
MATTHEW H. KULKE

HEMATOLOGY/ONCOLOGY
CLINICS OF NORTH AMERICA

www.hemonc.theclinics.com

Consulting Editors
GEORGE P. CANELLOS
H. FRANKLIN BUNN

February 2016 • Volume 30 • Number 1

ELSEVIER

1600 John F. Kennedy Boulevard ● Suite 1800 ● Philadelphia, Pennsylvania, 19103-2899

http://www.theclinics.com

HEMATOLOGY/ONCOLOGY CLINICS OF NORTH AMERICA Volume 30, Number 1
February 2016 ISSN 0889-8588, ISBN 13: 978-0-323-41692-4

Editor: Jennifer Flynn-Briggs
Developmental Editor: Kristen Helm

Hematology/Oncology Clinics (ISSN 0889-8588) is published bimonthly by Elsevier Inc., 360 Park Avenue South, New York, NY 10010-1710. Months of issue are February, April, June, August, October, and December. Business and Editorial Offices: 1600 John F. Kennedy Blvd., Ste. 1800, Philadelphia, PA 19103–2899. Customer Service Office: 3251 Riverport Lane, Maryland Heights, MO 63043. Periodicals postage paid at New York, NY and at additional mailing offices. Subscription prices are $385.00 per year (domestic individuals), $707.00 per year (domestic institutions), $100.00 per year (domestic students/residents), $440.00 per year (Canadian individuals), $875.00 per year (Canadian institutions) $520.00 per year (international individuals), $875.00 per year (international institutions), and $255.00 per year (international and Canadian students/residents). International air speed delivery is included in all *Clinics* subscription prices. All prices are subject to change without notice. **POSTMASTER:** Send address changes to *Hematology/Oncology Clinics of North America*, Elsevier Health Sciences Division, Subscription Customer Service, 3251 Riverport Lane, Maryland Heights, MO 63043. Customer Service (orders, claims, online, change of address): Elsevier Health Sciences Division, Subscription **Customer Service, 3251 Riverport Lane, Maryland Heights, MO 63043. Tel: 1-800-654-2452 (U.S. and Canada); 314-447-8871 (outside U.S. and Canada). Fax: 314-447-8029. E-mail: journalscustomerservice-usa@elsevier.com (for print support); journalsonlinesupport-usa@elsevier.com (for online support).**

Reprints. For copies of 100 or more, of articles in this publication, please contact the Commercial Reprints Department, Elsevier Inc., 360 Park Avenue South, New York, New York 10010-1710; Tel.: 212-633-3874, Fax: 212-633-3820, E-mail: reprints@elsevier.com.

Hematology/Oncology Clinics of North America is covered in *MEDLINE/PubMed (Index Medicus), EMBASE/ Excerpta Medica, and BIOSIS.*

Contributors

CONSULTING EDITORS

GEORGE P. CANELLOS, MD
William Rosenberg Professor of Medicine, Department of Medical Oncology, Dana-Farber Cancer Institute, Boston, Massachusetts

H. FRANKLIN BUNN, MD
Professor of Medicine, Division of Hematology, Brigham and Women's Hospital, Harvard Medical School, Boston, Massachusetts

EDITORS

JENNIFER A. CHAN, MD, MPH
Assistant Professor of Medicine, Harvard Medical School, Department of Medical Oncology, Dana-Farber Cancer Institute, Boston, Massachusetts

MATTHEW H. KULKE, MD, MMSc
Associate Professor of Medicine, Harvard Medical School, Department of Medical Oncology, Dana-Farber Cancer Institute, Boston, Massachusetts

AUTHORS

EMILY K. BERGSLAND, MD
Professor, Division of Hematology/Oncology, Department of Medicine, University of California, San Francisco, San Francisco, California

CELINE CHAYA, MD
Fellow, Division of Endocrinology and Metabolism, Department of Medicine, Strelitz Diabetes and Neuroendocrine Center, Eastern Virginia Medical School, Norfolk, Virginia

THOMAS E. CLANCY, MD
Division of Surgical Oncology, Brigham and Women's Hospital, Dana-Farber Cancer Institute, Harvard Medical School, Boston, Massachusetts

JENNIFER R. EADS, MD
Assistant Professor of Medicine, Division of Hematology and Oncology, University Hospitals Seidman Cancer Center, Case Western Reserve University, Case Comprehensive Cancer, Cleveland, Ohio

HEATHER A. FARLEY, MD
Department of Surgery, Oregon Health and Science University, Portland, Oregon

LAUREN FISHBEIN, MD, PhD, MTR
Instructor of Medicine, Division of Endocrinology, Diabetes and Metabolism, Department of Medicine, Perelman School of Medicine, University of Pennsylvania, Philadelphia, Pennsylvania

DANIEL M. HALPERIN, MD
Assistant Professor, Department of Gastrointestinal Medical Oncology, The University of Texas MD Anderson Cancer Center, Houston, Texas

ANDREW S. KENNEDY, MD, FACRO
Physician in Chief; Director, Radiation Oncology Research, Sarah Cannon Research Institute, Nashville, Tennessee; Adjunct Associate Professor, Department of Biomedical Engineering, Department of Mechanical and Aerospace Engineering, North Carolina State University, Raleigh, North Carolina

DAVID S. KLIMSTRA, MD
Professor of Pathology and Laboratory Medicine, Weill Cornell Medical College; Attending Pathologist and Chairman, James Ewing Alumni Chair in Pathology, Department of Pathology, Memorial Sloan Kettering Cancer Center, New York, New York

ERIC P. KRENNING, MD, PhD
Department of Nuclear Medicine, Erasmus MC, University Medical Center, Rotterdam, The Netherlands

PAMELA L. KUNZ, MD
Assistant Professor, Medicine/Oncology, Stanford University School of Medicine, Stanford, California

DIK J. KWEKKEBOOM, MD, PhD
Department of Nuclear Medicine, Erasmus MC, University Medical Center, Rotterdam, The Netherlands

ANYA LITVAK, MD
Fellow, Thoracic Oncology Service, Division of Solid Tumor Oncology, Department of Medicine, Memorial Sloan Kettering Cancer Center, New York, New York

CLAIRE K. MULVEY, MD
Resident, Department of Medicine, University of California, San Francisco, San Francisco, California

SUJATA NARAYANAN, MD
Instructor, Medicine/Oncology, Stanford University School of Medicine, Stanford, California

M. CATHERINE PIETANZA, MD
Assistant Member, Thoracic Oncology Service, Division of Solid Tumor Oncology, Department of Medicine; Assistant Professor of Medicine, Memorial Sloan Kettering Cancer Center, Weill Cornell Medical College, New York, New York

RODNEY F. POMMIER, MD
Professor of Surgery, Division of Surgical Oncology, Oregon Health and Science University, Portland, Oregon

NITYA RAJ, MD
Medical Oncology Fellow, Gastrointestinal Oncology Service, Division of Solid Tumor Oncology, Department of Medicine, Memorial Sloan Kettering Cancer Center, New York, New York

DIANE REIDY-LAGUNES, MD, MS
Assistant Attending, Gastrointestinal Oncology Service, Division of Solid Tumor Oncology, Department of Medicine, Memorial Sloan Kettering Cancer Center, New York, New York

AARON I. VINIK, MD, PhD, FCP, MACP, FACE
Division of Endocrinology and Metabolism, Department of Medicine, Strelitz Diabetes and Neuroendocrine Center, Eastern Virginia Medical School, Norfolk, Virginia

JAMES C. YAO, MD
Professor and Chair, Department of Gastrointestinal Medical Oncology, The University of Texas MD Anderson Cancer Center, Houston, Texas

Contents

The pathologic classification of neuroendocrine neoplasms has evolved over the past decades, as new understanding of the biological behavior, histologic characteristics, and genetic features have emerged. Nonetheless, many aspects of the classification systems remain confusing or controversial. Despite these difficulties, much progress has been made in determining the features predicting behavior. Genetic findings have helped establish relationships among different types of neuroendocrine neoplasms and revealed potential therapeutic targets. This review summarizes the current approach to the diagnosis, classification, grading, and therapeutic stratification of neuroendocrine neoplasms, with a focus on those arising in the lung and thymus, pancreas, and intestines.

Neuroendocrine tumors (NETs) are slow-growing neoplasms capable of storing and secreting different peptides and neuroamines. Some of these substances cause specific symptom complexes, whereas others are silent. They usually have episodic expression, and the diagnosis is often made at a late stage. Although considered rare, the incidence of NETs is increasing. For these reasons, a high index of suspicion is needed. In this article, the different clinical syndromes and the pathophysiology of each tumor as well as the new and emerging biochemical markers and imaging techniques that should be used to facilitate an early diagnosis, follow-up, and prognosis are reviewed.

Neuroendocrine tumors of the small bowel are rare, slow-growing malignancies that commonly metastasize to nodes at the root of the mesentery and the liver. Liver metastases are associated with carcinoid syndrome. Mesenteric nodal masses can cause bowel obstruction, intestinal angina, or variceal hemorrhage. Patients die of liver failure or bowel obstruction. Primary resection is associated with improved survival rates. Selected patients may benefit from liver debulking operations. Liver resection has excellent survival rates even in the event of an incomplete resection, as well as improvement in hormonal symptoms. Radiofrequency ablation can help to preserve hepatic parenchyma during resection.

neuroendocrine tumors patients. Most studies report objective response rates in 15% to 35% of patients. Progression-free (PFS) and overall survival (OS) compare favorably with that for somatostatin analogues, chemotherapy, or newer, "targeted" therapies. Prospective, randomized data regarding the potential PFS and OS benefit of PRRT compared with standard therapies is anticipated.

Neuroendocrine tumors (NETs) of the gastrointestinal (GI) tract have a propensity for producing hepatic metastases. Most GI NETs arise from the foregut or midgut, are malignant, and can cause severe debilitating symptoms adversely affecting quality of life. Aggressive treatments to reduce symptoms have an important role in therapy. Patients with GI NETs usually present with inoperable metastatic disease and severe symptoms from a variety of hormones and biogenic amines. This article describes intra-arterial hepatic-directed therapies for metastases from NETs, a group of treatments in which the therapeutic and/or embolic agents are released intra-arterially in specific hepatic vessels to target tumors.

Neuroendocrine tumors (NETs) present tremendous opportunities for productive clinical investigation, but substantial challenges as well. Investigators must be aware of common pitfalls in study design, informed by an understanding of the history of trials in the field, to make the best use of available data and our patient volunteers. We believe the salient issues in clinical trial design and interpretation in the NET field are patient homogeneity, standardized response assessment, and rigorous design and execution. Whether designing or interpreting a study in patients with NETs, these principles should drive assessment.

HEMATOLOGY/ONCOLOGY CLINICS OF NORTH AMERICA

THE CLINICS ARE AVAILABLE ONLINE!
Access your subscription at:
www.theclinics.com

Preface

Neuroendocrine Tumors—Current and Future Clinical Advances

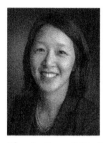 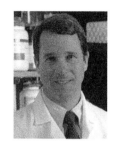

Jennifer A. Chan, MD, MPH   Matthew H. Kulke, MD, MMSc
Editors

Remarkable progress has been made over the last several years in our understanding of the biology and treatment of neuroendocrine tumors. The field has been transformed from one where patients have limited treatment options to one characterized by an increasing number of clinical trials and approved therapeutic agents. Recent studies have also revealed that we can no longer view neuroendocrine tumors as a single disease entity. Biological differences based on primary site, histologic grade, and ability to secrete hormones and other peptides influence clinical presentation, prognosis, and response to treatment; these factors must be taken into account when formulating treatment plans for individual patients and when designing clinical trials. This issue of *Hematology/Oncology Clinics of North America* brings together a multidisciplinary team of experts to discuss our current understanding of neuroendocrine tumors and to provide perspective on future clinical advances.

The issue begins with a comprehensive overview of the evolving histologic classification of neuroendocrine tumors by Dr Klimstra. Drs Vinik and Chaya next describe the clinical presentation and diagnosis of neuroendocrine tumors, with a focus on imaging and biomarkers. The subsequent articles focus on the management of neuroendocrine tumors and are divided according to primary site. The surgical management of gastrointestinal neuroendocrine tumors is discussed by Drs Farley and Pommier, and systemic treatment options are covered by Drs Mulvey and Bergsland. Drs Litvak and Pietanza provide a comprehensive discussion of the biology and management of lung and thymic neuroendocrine tumors. Dr Clancy provides an overview of surgical management of pancreatic neuroendocrine tumors, and Drs Raj and Reidy-Lagunes examine systemic therapy of this disease. Dr Fishbein reviews the diagnostic approach, genetics, and management of pheochromocytoma and paraganglioma. In the following article, Dr Eads discusses the management of poorly differentiated neuroendocrine tumors.

Hematol Oncol Clin N Am 30 (2016) xiii–xiv
http://dx.doi.org/10.1016/j.hoc.2015.09.012
0889-8588/16/$ – see front matter © 2016 Published by Elsevier Inc.

In addition to providing disease-specific reviews, this issue also includes specific articles focused on evolving classes of therapy of particular importance for patients with neuroendocrine tumors. Drs Narayanan and Kunz provide an overview of existing and novel somatostatin analogues and their role in controlling both hormone secretion and tumor growth. Drs Kwekkeboom and Krenning provide an in-depth discussion of the use of peptide receptor radiotherapy using radiolabeled somatostatin analogues for the treatment of neuroendocrine tumors. Dr Kennedy discusses hepatic-directed therapies, including various hepatic artery embolization approaches, for neuroendocrine tumor liver metastases. The final article of the issue by Drs Halperin and Yao focuses on the unique challenges that must be taken into consideration when designing clinical trials for neuroendocrine tumors, including patient heterogeneity and appropriate response and endpoint assessment.

It is our hope that this issue of *Hematology/Oncology Clinics of North America* provides readers with an overview of the current treatment landscape for neuroendocrine tumors and serves as a useful reference as we continue to advance our understanding of this disease.

Jennifer A. Chan, MD, MPH
Department of Medical Oncology
Dana-Farber Cancer Institute
Harvard Medical School
450 Brookline Avenue
Boston, MA 02115, USA

Matthew H. Kulke, MD, MMSc
Department of Medical Oncology
Dana-Farber Cancer Institute
Harvard Medical School
450 Brookline Avenue
Boston, MA 02115, USA

E-mail addresses:
jang@partners.org (J.A. Chan)
Matthew_Kulke@dfci.harvard.edu (M.H. Kulke)

Pathologic Classification of Neuroendocrine Neoplasms

David S. Klimstra, MD[a,b]

KEYWORDS

- Pathological classification • Neuroendocrine • Lung • Thymus • Pancreas
- Intestines

KEY POINTS

- Neuroendocrine neoplasms arise throughout the body. They are recognized pathologically based on characteristic morphologic patterns and immunoexpression of neuroendocrine differentiation markers.
- The pathologic classification of neuroendocrine neoplasms has evolved over the past decades, as new understanding of the biological behavior, histologic characteristics, and genetic features of these neoplasms has emerged.
- Many aspects of the classification systems remain confusing or controversial. The reasons for the lack of uniformity in approach include the diversity of neuroendocrine neoplasms, the functional status of some neuroendocrine neoplasms, and the organ-specific differences.
- Recent efforts to standardize the classification of gastroenteropancreatic neuroendocrine neoplasms have been reasonably successful; but other organ systems, such as the lung and thymus, use different terminology and classification criteria.
- Genetic findings have not only helped establish relationships among different types of neuroendocrine neoplasms but they have also revealed potential therapeutic targets. Thus, the pathologic approach to neuroendocrine neoplasms is becoming more consistent and clinically relevant.

INTRODUCTION

Neuroendocrine neoplasms arise throughout the body. They are recognized pathologically based on characteristic morphologic patterns and immunoexpression of neuroendocrine differentiation markers. The pathologic classification of neuroendocrine neoplasms has evolved over the past decades, as new understanding of the biological behavior, histologic characteristics, and genetic features of these neoplasms has

[a] Weill Cornell Medical College, 1305 York Avenue, New York, NY 10021, USA; [b] Department of Pathology, Memorial Sloan Kettering Cancer Center, 1275 York Avenue, New York, NY 10065, USA
E-mail address: klimstrd@mskcc.org

Hematol Oncol Clin N Am 30 (2016) 1–19
http://dx.doi.org/10.1016/j.hoc.2015.08.005
0889-8588/16/$ – see front matter © 2016 Elsevier Inc. All rights reserved.
hemonc.theclinics.com

emerged. Nonetheless, many aspects of the classification systems remain confusing or controversial. The reasons for the lack of uniformity in approach include the diversity of neuroendocrine neoplasms. Although their shared neuroendocrine differentiation suggests a closely related family, it is now clear that several distinct types of neuroendocrine neoplasms exist. Most importantly, the well-differentiated neuroendocrine tumor (WD-NET) and poorly-differentiated neuroendocrine carcinoma (PD-NEC) families are increasingly recognized to be very different and, in all likelihood, not closely related. Other variables include the functional status of some neuroendocrine neoplasms, which can drive their clinical manifestations and treatment, relative to the nonfunctional counterparts. Finally, there are organ-specific differences.

Recent efforts to standardize the classification of gastroenteropancreatic neuroendocrine neoplasms, first proposed by the European Neuroendocrine Tumor Society (ENETS) and then adopted by the World Health Organization (WHO), have been reasonably successful; but other organ systems, such as the lung and thymus, use different terminology and classification criteria; even within the gastroenteropancreatic group there exists biological heterogeneity that is partially obscured by the standardization of classification criteria. Despite these difficulties, much progress has been made in determining the features predicting behavior. In particular, recently implemented grading schemes can effectively stratify the indolent, moderately aggressive, and highly aggressive groups of neuroendocrine neoplasms. Genetic findings have not only helped establish relationships among different types of neuroendocrine neoplasms but they have also revealed potential therapeutic targets. Thus, the pathologic approach to neuroendocrine neoplasms is becoming more consistent and clinically relevant. This review summarizes the current approach to the diagnosis, classification, grading, and therapeutic stratification of neuroendocrine neoplasms, with a focus on those arising in the lung and thymus, pancreas, and intestines. The array of rare neuroendocrine neoplasms affecting other epithelial organs and the skin (Merkel cell carcinoma) is beyond the scope of this review.

GENERAL FEATURES OF NEUROENDOCRINE NEOPLASMS

Neuroendocrine differentiation in tumors is conceptually defined as the secretion by the neoplastic cells of bioactive substances, usually bioamines or peptide hormones, into the bloodstream. Non-neoplastic neuroendocrine cells, which are dispersed within the epithelium of most organs and clustered in islets of Langerhans in the pancreas, produce similar substances; their morphologic appearance is shared by the cells of neuroendocrine neoplasms, WD-NETs in particular. The origin of neuroendocrine neoplasms from normal neuroendocrine cells has, thus, been postulated, although the concept that neoplasms arise from their mature non-neoplastic cellular counterparts is likely overly simplistic. Potentially, it is more primitive cells with stem cell features that give rise to these neoplasms, and it is the differentiation, rather than the cell of origin, of the neoplasm that allows its classification. Pathologically, neuroendocrine differentiation is defined as architectural and cytologic patterns reminiscent of non-neoplastic neuroendocrine cells (such as a nesting or trabecular growth pattern and coarsely stippled nuclear chromatin (**Fig. 1**)) and the production of characteristic neurosecretory proteins that can be detected by immunohistochemistry. A wide array of peptide hormones and bioamines can be produced as well; but for the purposes of pathologic diagnosis, it is the so-called general neuroendocrine markers that are detected. The most specific general neuroendocrine markers in wide use are chromogranin A and synaptophysin. Staining for one or both of these can be detected in essentially all WD-NETs. Other general neuroendocrine markers

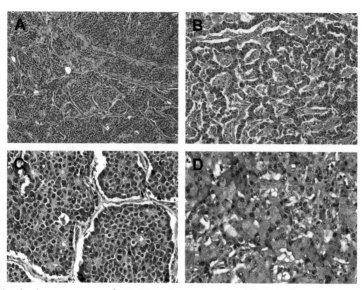

Fig. 1. Histologic appearance of WD-NETs. An organoid architecture is present, usually with a nesting (*A*) or trabecular (hematoxylin-eosin, original magnification ×100) (*B*) pattern (hematoxylin-eosin, original magnification ×100). High power of an ileal WD-NET (*C*) reveals nests of cells with granular eosinophilic cytoplasm (hematoxylin-eosin, original magnification ×200). The nuclei have coarsely granular (salt and pepper) chromatin. Mitoses and necrosis are not present. A pancreatic WD-NET (*D*) exhibits similar nuclear features; but there are prominent nucleoli, and the cytoplasm is more abundant. Again, mitotic activity is essentially nil (hematoxylin-eosin, original magnification ×200).

are available, such as CD56 (neural cell adhesion molecule) and neuron-specific enolase; but these label other types of neoplasms without known neuroendocrine differentiation and are, therefore, considered less reliable.[1–3] In many cases typical examples of WD-NETs are readily recognizable as having neuroendocrine differentiation based on their routine histologic features, and immunolabeling for chromogranin A and synaptophysin is not absolutely required for their diagnosis.[1]

Although WD-NETs closely resemble non-neoplastic neuroendocrine cells, PD-NECs are high-grade carcinomas that exhibit neuroendocrine differentiation. These neoplasms share some histologic features with WD-NETs, but they are obviously less differentiated. Although PD-NECs typically express the same general neuroendocrine markers described earlier, the staining may be less intense and more focal. PD-NECs are usually classified as a small cell carcinoma or large cell neuroendocrine carcinoma (LCNEC), variants that are distinguished based on the cell size and nuclear morphology.[4] Small cell carcinomas have round to fusiform cells with very little cytoplasm and hyperchromatic nuclei with a finely granular chromatin pattern and inconspicuous or absent nucleoli. The cells are often arranged in sheets, although a nested pattern can occur; there is usually single cell or geographic necrosis and a very high mitotic rate (**Fig. 2**). The histologic features of small cell carcinoma are sufficiently distinctive that the entity can be diagnosed without the need to demonstrate neuroendocrine differentiation by immunohistochemistry, although most cases (85%) do express chromogranin or synaptophysin. LCNECs more typically demonstrate a nested architecture and are composed of larger cells with moderate cytoplasm and round or oval nuclei with more open chromatin and prominent nucleoli

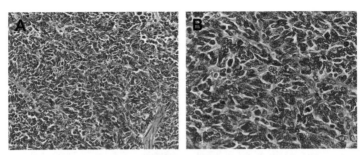

Fig. 2. Histologic appearance of a PD-NEC, small cell type (small cell carcinoma). The neoplastic cells form only vague nests (A) (hematoxylin-eosin, original magnification ×100). The cells are closely packed and have minimal cytoplasm. At high power (B), the nuclei are fusiform and have finely granular chromatin and no nucleoli. Abundant mitotic figures are present (hematoxylin-eosin, original magnification ×200).

(**Fig. 3**). The necrosis and high mitotic rate of small cell carcinomas is also present in LCNECs. This histologic pattern is not entity defining, however. LCNECs must demonstrate immunoexpression of at least one neuroendocrine marker to be distinguished from poorly-differentiated carcinomas of an exocrine type, such as poorly-differentiated adenocarcinoma or large cell undifferentiated carcinoma. PD-NECs are primarily distinguished from WD-NETs by having a substantially higher proliferative rate, although there are many other differences.

The relationship between WD-NETs and PD-NECs is becoming clearer. Although classification systems that include both entities seem to suggest that they represent the opposite ends of a spectrum of neuroendocrine neoplasms, and they do share neuroendocrine differentiation and histologic features associated with the neuroendocrine phenotype, accumulating evidence demonstrates that WD-NETs and PD-NECs are in fact two very different families of neoplasms.[4] Several lines of evidence support this distinction. WD-NETs are generally relatively indolent and may be surgically curable if detected early, and their evolution can take years to decades when they recur; PD-NECs are highly aggressive, usually progressing rapidly even when detected at an early stage.[5] WD-NETs and PD-NECs are etiologically different in some organs, such as the lung where small cell carcinomas and LCNECs have a close association with smoking that is lacking in carcinoid tumors (WD-NETs). Also, it is usually only

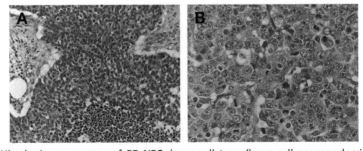

Fig. 3. Histologic appearance of PD-NEC, large cell type (large cell neuroendocrine carcinoma). The neoplastic cells form large nests with central necrosis (A) (hematoxylin-eosin, original magnification ×100). The cells have moderate cytoplasm and round to oval nuclei. At high power (B), the chromatin is open and coarsely granular and there are prominent nucleoli (hematoxylin-eosin, original magnification ×200). Numerous mitoses are present.

WD-NETs that arise in patients with neuroendocrine neoplasia syndromes (eg, multiple endocrine neoplasia 1 [MEN1] or von Hippel Lindau syndromes). PD-NECs, at least small cell carcinomas, exhibit marked but transient sensitivity to platinum-based chemotherapy; but WD-NETs are usually resistant to platinum and other cytotoxic chemotherapies.[6,7] PD-NECs often arise in association with exocrine-type precursor lesions, such as adenomas in the large intestine or ampulla of Vater, or they may be combined with adenocarcinoma or squamous cell carcinoma components, as in mixed adenocarcinoma neuroendocrine carcinoma (MANEC). WD-NETs rarely have exocrine components. Also, individual tumors containing both WD-NET and PD-NEC components are exceedingly rare. Finally, there are distinct molecular alterations in these two families of neuroendocrine neoplasms. Although some alterations are specific to the site of origin (see later discussion), WD-NETs lack alterations in genes, such as *RB1* and *TP53*, that are commonly found in PD-NECs.

Thus, the evidence is strong that WD-NETs and PD-NECs must be distinguished whenever possible. The distinction can be challenging in some instances, such as when only biopsy samples are available; but a pathologic diagnosis that only indicates a neuroendocrine neoplasm with specifying the differentiation is considered inadequate to direct therapy. It should also be noted that the concept of differentiation differs from that of grade, because it signifies a specific category of neuroendocrine neoplasm rather than a degree of aggressiveness. Although most classification schemes use 3 grades, current thinking is that only 2 categories of neuroendocrine tumors exist (WD-NETs and PD-NECs); there is no longer a definable group of moderately differentiated neoplasms.

The terminology for neuroendocrine neoplasms has been problematic for various reasons. Even following significant recent efforts to standardize the terminology, different terms are used in different organs to describe the same category of neoplasm. Historically, the term *carcinoid tumor*, coined by Oberndorfer[8] in 1907, has been used for WD-NETs; in the pancreas, *islet cell tumor* was used. Currently, in the gastroenteropancreatic system, these terms have been replaced with *NET* to emphasize that a carcinoid tumor is a not benign neoplasm.[1–3] However, this concept is not used for neuroendocrine neoplasms of the lung and thymus; also, in other rare sites (gallbladder, kidney, larynx, and so forth), the term *carcinoid tumor* persists. Although terminology systems vary by organ (http://meetinglibrary.asco.org/content/115000092-156; **Table 1**), the distinction between the well and poorly-differentiated categories applies throughout the body.[2,9]

A major objective of pathologic classification is to stratify neuroendocrine neoplasms by prognosis. Many different pathologic findings have been shown to correlate with outcomes, and some are incorporated in staging systems that were developed for the first time in the most recent American Joint Committee on Cancer's (AJCC) staging system (2009), some neuroendocrine neoplasms being staged using the same parameters as exocrine carcinomas of the same organ, others having unique NET-specific staging systems.[10] In some organs, immunohistochemical labeling for various markers has prognostic significance, and even cytogenetic or molecular features can predict outcomes in certain circumstances. But apart from staging, the emphasis has been on grading neuroendocrine neoplasms, and grading systems based largely on the proliferative rate have been developed for thoracic and gastroenteropancreatic neuroendocrine neoplasms.[11] Proliferative rate can be determined by counting mitotic figures (usually expressed as the number of mitoses in 10 high power microscopic fields or 2 mm^2) or, in the gastroenteropancreatic organs, by measuring the percentage of tumor cells immunolabeling for the proliferation marker Ki67 (the Ki67 index). The thoracic system does not use the Ki67 index, but the presence of necrosis is included. In both of these major grading schemes, neuroendocrine neoplasms are divided into 3 grades, with the low

Table 1
Classification of neuroendocrine neoplasms of the lung, gastrointestinal tract, and pancreas

Differentiation	Grade	Lung	Gastrointestinal Tract and Pancreas
Well differentiated	Low grade	Carcinoid tumor	WD-NET, grade 1
	Intermediate grade	Atypical carcinoid tumor	WD-NET, grade 2
Poorly differentiated	High grade	Small cell carcinoma	PD-NEC, grade 3; small cell carcinoma
		Large cell neuroendocrine carcinoma	PD-NEC, grade 3; large cell neuroendocrine carcinoma
Combined	High grade	Combined small cell carcinoma (with adenocarcinoma or squamous cell carcinoma)	Mixed adenocarcinoma neuroendocrine carcinoma (small cell carcinoma)
		Combined large cell neuroendocrine carcinoma (with adenocarcinoma or squamous cell carcinoma)	Mixed adenocarcinoma neuroendocrine carcinoma (large cell neuroendocrine carcinoma)

Data from Klimstra DS, Modlin IR, Coppola D, et al. The pathologic classification of neuroendocrine tumors: a review of nomenclature, grading, and staging systems. Pancreas 2010;39(6):707–12; and Basturk O, Tang L, Hruban RH, et al. Poorly differentiated neuroendocrine carcinomas of the pancreas: a clinicopathologic analysis of 44 cases. Am J Surg Pathol 2014;38(4):437–47.

and intermediate grades (grade 1 and 2) being WD-NETs, and the high-grade (grade 3) group generally consisting of PD-NECs.[2]

The grading parameters for neuroendocrine neoplasms of the entire gastroentero-pancreatic system have been unified, such that a single system proposed by ENETS[12,13] and endorsed by the WHO[14,15] is now widely used for these primaries (http://meetinglibrary.asco.org/content/115000092-156; **Table 2**). In the lung and thymus, a different WHO-accepted system has been in place for many years (http://meetinglibrary.asco.org/content/115000092-156; **Table 3**).[16] For organs outside of these sites, no formal systems exist; but individual proposals have been based on the thoracic or gastroenteropancreatic systems. The major differences between the thoracic and gastroenteropancreatic systems are as follows:

1. The use of necrosis to separate low- from intermediate-grade WD-NETs in the thorax
2. The requirement for Ki67 staining in the gastroenteropancreatic system
3. The different mitotic rate cut point that defines high grade (10 mitoses per 10 high power fields in the thorax; 20 mitoses per 10 high power fields in gastroentero-pancreatic organs)

Table 2
ENETS/WHO grading system for gastroenteropancreatic neuroendocrine neoplasms

Tumor Grade	Definition
Low grade (grade 1)	<2 mitoses per 10 HPF *and* Ki67 index <3%
Intermediate grade (grade 2)	2–20 mitoses per 10 HPF *or* Ki67 index 3%–20%
High grade (grade 3)	>20 mitoses per 10 HPF *or* Ki67 index >20%

Abbreviation: HPF, high power field.
Data from Refs.[12–15]

Table 3
IASLC/WHO grading system for pulmonary neuroendocrine neoplasms

Neoplasm	Morphology	Mitoses	Necrosis	Immunohistochemistry
Typical carcinoid tumor	Polygonal cells arranged in nested or trabecular patterns	<2 per 10 HPF	Absent	Chromogranin, synaptophysin, CD56 (supportive but not required)
Atypical carcinoid tumor	Polygonal cells arranged in nested or trabecular patterns	2–10 per 10 HPF	Present, usually punctate	Chromogranin, synaptophysin, CD56 (supportive but not required)
Large cell neuroendocrine carcinoma	Large cells, moderate cytoplasm, round nuclei, frequent nucleoli	>10 per HPF	Present, usually extensive	Chromogranin, synaptophysin, CD56 (at least one required)
Small cell carcinoma	Small cells, scant cytoplasm, fusiform nuclei, no nuclei	>10 per HPF	Present, usually extensive	Chromogranin, synaptophysin, CD56 (supportive, but not required)

Abbreviations: HPF, high power field; IASLC, International Association for the Study of Lung Cancer.
From Travis WD. The concept of pulmonary neuroendocrine tumors. In: Travis WD, Brambilla E, Muller-Hermelink KH, et al, editors. Pathology and genetics of tumours of the lung, pleura, thymus, and heart. Lyon (France): IARC Press; 2004. p. 20; with permission.

The ability of these systems to stratify the outcome of neuroendocrine neoplasms has been convincingly demonstrated for multiple anatomic sites. Interestingly, the outcome difference between low grade and intermediate grade is striking, even though the proliferative rate that distinguishes these groups is very modest (0–1 mitoses per 10 high power fields vs 2 or more). To some extent, the grade correlates with stage; but these prognostic parameters are independently predictive of outcome. Even among patients with stage IV disease, the grade stratifies the length of survival. Thus, the importance of accurate grading is now well accepted for neuroendocrine neoplasms, even though there may not presently be major management differences between low- and intermediate-grade NETs. It should be emphasized that the initial proposed grading parameters were chosen based on the experience and intuition of the individuals who proposed the systems, rather than on rigorous review of outcome data. The specific cut points of mitotic rate and Ki67 index chosen to separate the grades are continually reevaluated and may require adjustment as data accumulate. Also, the attempts to unify the grading parameters for many anatomic sites are laudable; but it is clear that distinctive features specific to each site of origin exist, and organ-specific grading systems may prove necessary for optimal stratification.

Grading neuroendocrine neoplasms requires precise determination of mitotic rate and Ki67 index. These assessments have proven more challenging than they might seem. The mitotic rate is expressed as a number per unit area (10 high power fields), but in fact the diameter of a high power microscopic field varies among microscopes.[17] In an effort to render this more reproducible, some investigators have used an actual area (2 mm^2), which corresponds to the size of 10 fields on one of the most standard microscopes in current use. But this means that pathologists using other microscopes would need to adjust their counting based on measuring the field area, a correction that is not often performed.

Another obvious issue is that within the family of WD-NETs, there is considerable variation in cell size and stromal content, both of which affect the number of cells within a given area. There has been no proposal to correct for these variables; but in theory a tumor composed of large cells with more abundant stroma would have fewer mitotic figures identified than a densely cellular tumor with minimal cytoplasm, even though the actual proportion of cells undergoing division were the same. These vagaries settle out when examining the outcome of a large patient cohort; but for the individual case, they can lead to underestimation of grade.

The use of the Ki67 index corrects for these issues because the index is expressed as a percentage of positive-labeling nuclei, rather than a number per unit area. In order to calculate the Ki67 index, it was originally recommended to count the regions with the greatest proportion of positive nuclei (hot spots). Heterogeneity of labeling is common, and data comparing the average labeling rate with that of the hot spots confirm that the more proliferative regions more accurately predict the outcome.[18] Nonetheless, the exact size of a hot spot is uncertain (one 200 × microscopic field has been proposed). Furthermore, the identification of hot spots requires that a large sample of the tumor be stained for Ki67.

When biopsy samples are evaluated, this is not possible. The theoretic risk that biopsies may, therefore, underestimate the grade of WD-NETs has been proven, using virtual randomly oriented biopsies of resected hepatic metastases.[18] A single core biopsy from a G2 WD-NET has only a 35% chance of accurately identifying the higher proliferative rate; 3 core biopsies identify the G2 focus in 48%, and it would take 31 core biopsies to identify 90% of G2 cases.[19] Conversely, an apparent G1 WD-NET graded on a core biopsy has only a 59% chance of truly being low grade. The phenomenon of grade heterogeneity exists within the primary WD-NET, between the primary and metastases, and also between different foci of metastatic disease.[20] A higher-grade component can also emerge during the course of disease progression. Targeting a metastasis that shows radiographic evidence of growth may be a more reliable way to ensure that the highest-grade focus is detected.

Another consideration, for gastroenteropancreatic NETs, is that the mitotic rate and Ki67 index may point to different grades. In one study of pancreatic WD-NETs, 107 of 297 tumors (36%) had discordance between these two proliferation indices.[21] Usually it is the Ki67 index that suggests the higher grade, and the original grading system proposed by ENETS recommended relying on whichever measure defined the higher grade.[12,15,16] This suggestion has also been supported by data showing that WD-NETs with discordant mitotic rate and Ki67 index (G1 by mitoses, G2 by Ki67) behave more like cases whereby both indices point to the higher grade.[21]

A final consideration regarding Ki67 is the means to assess the index itself. The ENETS and WHO recommend counting 2000 cells (or at least 500 cells) to accurately determine the Ki67 index. It is very challenging to undertake this count while reviewing the actual glass slide, and many pathologists have been simply estimating the percentage by casual observation (eyeballed estimate). Although eyeballing is simple and fast, the degree of interobserver and intraobserver variability using eyeballing is unacceptably high.[22]

Digital image analysis can be used to determine a highly accurate percentage, provided that the instrument is calibrated to recognize truly positive cells and non-neoplastic cells, whether positive or negative, are excluded from analysis. Digital image analysis has been shown to correlate almost perfectly with manual counting, but it is not in routine use and requires considerable time to perform properly. Therefore, many experts suggest manual counting based on a printed photomicrograph of the hot-spot regions (**Fig. 4**).[23] All of these issues have called into question the entire concept of measuring proliferation to grade NETs, but the practice is now well established; the resulting grades have strong prognostic implications, even with all of the challenges.

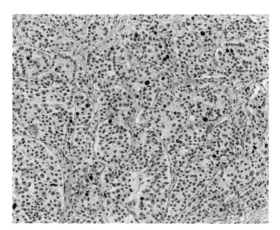

Fig. 4. Method to determine the Ki67 index. The most intensely labeling region of the Ki67 immunohistochemical stain (hot spot) is printed. Each positive (*brown staining*) neoplastic nucleus is counted, and then the negative (*blue*) nuclei are individually marked to ensure accurate counting. In this case, 61 of 1421 tumor nuclei are labeled, giving a Ki67 index of 4.3% (ENETS/WHO grade G2).

One potentially promising addition to the assessment of proliferation is the antibody against phosphohistone H3 (PHH3), which can be used immunohistochemically to detect mitotic figures. PHH3 staining is more sensitive and specific for detecting mitoses than hematoxylin-eosin (H&E) staining, in which hyperchromatic nuclei or poor-quality histology can render recognition of true mitotic figures challenging. Immunolabeling mitoses also has the potential to detect hot spots of mitotic activity, which may more accurately reflect tumor biology. Additionally, there is the theoretical possibility to express the mitotic rate as a percentage of neoplastic cells, rather than a number per unit area, circumventing the issues raised earlier regarding mitotic counting. Because somewhat different counts are obtained with PHH3 compared with H&E, more experience is needed to determine whether grading cut points using this stain are the same as for mitoses detected routinely. Early data are promising.[24]

Just as the mitotic rate and Ki67 index discordance can occur between the low and intermediate grade groups of WD-NETs, there are some gastroenteropancreatic neuroendocrine neoplasms with a mitotic rate in the G2 range but a Ki67 index greater than 20%. These cases would be assigned to the G3 (high grade) category, which has been regarded as synonymous with PD-NEC. However, several studies have suggested that a subset of such cases remain well differentiated morphologically, have a prognosis better than bona fide PD-NECs, and do not respond well to platinum-based chemotherapy.[6,18,25] These uncommon tumors are increasingly regarded as G3 WD-NETs rather than PD-NECs, and emerging genomic data also suggest they are part of the well-differentiated spectrum, as they lack mutations in *TP53* and *RB1* and, in the case of pancreatic primaries, instead have abnormalities in genes involved in other pancreatic WD-NETs, such as *DAXX*, *ATRX*, and *MEN1*.[9] Although the prognosis of G3 WD-NETs is not as poor as that of small cell carcinomas and LCNECs, these are aggressive tumors, perhaps somewhat more so than G2 WD-NETs.[25] This group has yet to be formally recognized in the WHO classification, and there are cases in which the distinction between a G3 WD-NET and an LCNEC is very difficult; thus, additional data must be obtained to definitively characterize these cases. Interestingly, it is rarely difficult to distinguish a small cell carcinoma from a WD-NET.

Another aspect of neuroendocrine neoplasm classification is related to the functional status of the neoplasm. In both the WD-NET and PD-NEC families, some cases exhibit inappropriate secretion of peptide hormones or bioamines, resulting in highly characteristic paraneoplastic syndromes, such as carcinoid syndrome, Cushing syndrome, insulinoma syndrome, and Zollinger-Ellison syndrome.[15] The frequency of clinical functional neuroendocrine tumors varies by organ and, to some extent, by stage of disease because some bioactive substances are cleared by the liver until hepatic metastases develop and the burden of disease increases. An even greater proportion of neuroendocrine tumors can be shown to produce bioactive substances if serologic or immunohistochemical assays are performed, but it is the clinical manifestation of the syndrome that defines a tumor as functional. The one exception to this rule is for pancreatic WD-NETs producing pancreatic polypeptide. Although excess levels of this hormone do not generally produce symptoms, WD-NETs associated with significant pancreatic polypeptide production have been designated "PPomas."[26] Because only clinical findings define all other neuroendocrine neoplasms to be functional, searching for the expression of specific hormones by immunohistochemistry is rarely necessary in the pathologic characterization of neuroendocrine tumors.[1] The clinical picture of patients with functional neuroendocrine tumors can be dominated by the paraneoplastic symptoms, which create management challenges unique to each tumor type. Also, some functional tumors have a characteristic prognosis, such as the low rate of malignant behavior in pancreatic insulinomas. Pathologically, the primary diagnosis of functional neuroendocrine neoplasms is the same as for their nonfunctional counterparts (WD-NET, PD-NEC, and so forth), but the further characterization as a specific functional type (eg, consistent with gastrinoma) is often appended to the primary diagnosis.

NEUROENDOCRINE NEOPLASMS OF SPECIFIC ANATOMIC SITES
Thoracic Neuroendocrine Neoplasms

The classification of neuroendocrine neoplasms in the lung was established many years ago and has persisted unchanged, now being applied for thymic primaries as well.[16] The classification system combines the grading system with the terminology. As shown in **Table 3**, the name of each entity corresponds to the grade. The low- and intermediate-grade NETs (typical carcinoid tumor and atypical carcinoid tumor) are well differentiated, and the high-grade NECs (small cell carcinoma and large cell neuroendocrine carcinoma) are poorly-differentiated.[27–29] Atypical carcinoid tumors were first recognized by Arrigoni and colleagues[30] in 1972, and LCNEC is the most recently described entity (1991) in the group.[17] The morphologic appearance of LCNEC is typically neuroendocrine (nesting or trabecular pattern, rosettes, and so forth), but the cells are larger than in small cell carcinoma and have more abundant cytoplasm and prominent nucleoli. In contrast to small cell carcinoma, immunohistochemical labeling for chromogranin, synaptophysin, or CD56 is required for the diagnosis of LCNEC (see http://meetinglibrary.asco.org/content/115000092-156 and **Table 3**). Not all solid carcinomas with the morphologic appearance of LCNEC prove to have neuroendocrine differentiation, however. The term *large cell carcinoma with neuroendocrine morphology* is used for carcinomas with neuroendocrine morphology but no labeling for neuroendocrine markers. Conversely, some large cell carcinomas without characteristic neuroendocrine morphology nonetheless express neuroendocrine markers; the term *large cell carcinoma with neuroendocrine differentiation* is used for these cases.[16] The clinical implications of these diagnoses are unclear, and both of these entities are usually approached clinically as a non–small cell lung cancer, as opposed to LCNEC, which is managed with similar chemotherapy to small cell carcinoma.

Although only mitotic rate and not Ki67 is not used in the formal classification, there are several new studies evaluating the significance of the Ki67 index; one formal proposal to incorporate the Ki67 index into a new grading scheme has been published.[31] Ki67 is useful to distinguish small cell carcinoma from carcinoid tumors when examining small specimens, such as biopsies or cytology, because the difference in labeling between these two entities is extreme (>50% vs <5%, respectively) and can readily be appreciated even when insufficient cells are present for formal counting.[32,33]

As in other anatomic sites, pulmonary neuroendocrine neoplasms actually constitute two families that may not be closely related.[33] Carcinoid tumors, which can be central or peripheral in the lung, usually arise in nonsmokers and can occur in patients with MEN1. They may also be associated with hyperplasia of pulmonary neuroendocrine cells (diffuse idiopathic pulmonary neuroendocrine cell hyperplasia),[34] and they usually are not combined with adenocarcinoma or squamous cell carcinoma.[35] The PD-NECs, in contrast, are closely linked to tobacco use and commonly (up to 30%) contain elements of adenocarcinoma or squamous cell carcinoma. Such tumors in the lung are designated as combined neuroendocrine carcinomas. Finally, individual neoplasms containing both carcinoid tumor and PD-NEC are almost nonexistent.

Molecular data further support the separation of carcinoids from PD-NECs. PD-NECs, especially small cell carcinomas, commonly exhibit *TP53* and *RB1* mutations,[36,37] whereas carcinoid tumors lack these alterations and instead have abnormalities in chromatin remodeling genes, such as *MEN1*, *PSIP1*, and *ARID1A*.[38]

Neuroendocrine neoplasms of the thymus are classified using the same criteria as those in the lung. However, a somewhat different spectrum of tumors occurs in the thymus. Typical carcinoid is uncommon; most WD-NETs represent atypical carcinoid tumors and have an aggressive clinical course.[39] The associations of thymic carcinoid tumors with MEN1 syndrome and with Cushing syndrome are well documented and much more common than with lung carcinoids.[40] PD-NECs occur in the thymus but are very rare, and a metastasis from the lung must always be considered when a small cell carcinoma or LCNEC is found in the mediastinum.

Pancreatic Neuroendocrine Neoplasms

WD-NETs arising within the pancreas, previously designated islet cell tumors, are referred to as *pancreatic neuroendocrine tumors* (PanNETs). PanNETs include an array of functional entities (insulinoma, glucagonoma, gastrinoma, VIPoma, somatostatinoma, and so forth) as well as nonfunctional PanNETs, which are now the most prevalent type[41] because of their more frequent incidental detection by cross-sectional imaging. PD-NECs (small cell carcinoma and LCNEC) also arise in the pancreas but are rare.[9,38] PanNETs range from small (0.5 cm, by definition the size separating a PanNET from a neuroendocrine microadenoma), circumscribed, organ-confined tumors with a very low risk for aggressive behavior to large, necrotic, highly infiltrative malignancies[42] (http://meetinglibrary.asco.org/content/115000092-156-bibr17-EdBookAM20153592). Among the organs commonly giving rise to WD-NETs, the pancreas produces the largest variety of histologic patterns. PanNETs with clear cell, oncocytic, glandular, pleomorphic, and rhabdoid morphologies have been described[43–45]; although these features by themselves have limited clinical significance (clear cell PanNETs may be more prevalent in patients with von Hippel–Lindau syndrome[46]), these unusual morphologies can lead to confusion for other neoplasms. Immunolabeling for chromogranin and synaptophysin will usually resolve diagnostic uncertainties, although some neoplasms in the differential diagnosis can also label with one or both of these markers, such as solid pseudopapillary neoplasm (synaptophysin) and mixed acinar neuroendocrine carcinoma (both).[47]

PanNETs are now classified using the WHO system for all gastroenteropancreatic neuroendocrine neoplasms (see http://meetinglibrary.asco.org/content/115000092-156 and **Table 2**), which relies exclusively on the proliferative rate to separate G1, G2, and G3 neoplasms,[15] the last group largely representing the PD-NECs.[9,18,48] Several studies have validated the prognostic significance of this classification, even for metastatic disease; the difference in outcome between G1 and G2 is quite dramatic.[30,32,49] As previously mentioned, the highest grade identified drives the prognosis,[21,50] an important consideration because there can be grade heterogeneity within well-differentiated PanNETs, between the primary and metastases, and even among different metastatic sites.[51,52] Compared with other anatomic sites, the pancreas gives rise to more cases that straddle the G2/G3 boundary; many of the reported cases of neuroendocrine tumors with a G2 mitotic rate but a G3 Ki67 index are of pancreatic origin.[25] Thus, the concept of G3 WD-NETs as distinct from PD-NECs has been principally developed with data from pancreatic primaries. For patients with distant metastases, tumor growth rate observed on cross-sectional imaging is also helpful to predict the prognosis, especially for cases in which inadequate biopsy material may be available for definitive grading. Many other potential prognostic markers for PanNETs have been evaluated, such as immunohistochemical staining for CD117, cytokeratin 19, CD99, CD44, p27, progesterone receptor, and PTEN; but none of these has achieved sufficient independent predictive value to be incorporated into routine practice.[53]

The molecular alterations in PanNETs have been better characterized recently as a result of the completion of whole-exome sequencing studies.[43] Well-differentiated PanNETs differ genetically from pancreatic ductal adenocarcinomas. PanNETs lack frequent alterations in the genes involved in ductal neoplasia, such as *KRAS, TP53, CDKN2A*, and *SMAD4*. Instead, PanNETs often have alterations in chromatin remodeling genes, such as *MEN1, DAXX*, and *ATRX*.[54] Also, alterations in members of the mammalian target of rapamycin (mTOR) pathway are found. Both *MEN1* and mTOR pathway alterations may be expected, given that PanNETs arise in patients with MEN1, von Hippel–Lindau syndrome, neurofibromatosis-1, and tuberous sclerosis syndromes. Involvement of the mTOR pathway also provides a rationale for targeted therapy, and clinical trials using the mTOR inhibitor everolimus have shown promise.[55] Pancreatic PD-NECs have different molecular alterations from PanNETs, including common *TP53* and *RB1* mutations and, less frequently, alterations in *KRAS* and *CDKN2A*.[56] These results demonstrate the genetic distinction between the well-differentiated and poorly-differentiated families of pancreatic neuroendocrine neoplasms.

In terms of predicting response to specific therapy, there are few well-established biomarkers. Loss of expression of O^6-methylguanine DNA methyltransferase (MGMT) or methylation of its promoter can predict sensitivity to temozolomide.[57] In theory, inactivation of the mTOR pathway should also correlate in the response to mTOR inhibitor therapy; but this is a complex pathway with multiple positive and negative regulators, and a simple biomarker of pathway activation status has not been developed.[58,59]

Intestinal Neuroendocrine Neoplasms

The spectrum of neuroendocrine neoplasms varies considerably through the course of the small and large intestines; the appendix gives rise to unique neoplasms, goblet cell carcinoid tumors, that differ substantially from the neoplasms of the rest of the intestinal tract.[60] A historical distinction that has faded in recent years is among WD-NETs of the foregut, midgut, and hindgut.[61–63] Differences in morphology and biology among primaries of these various sites were not thought sufficient to justify separate classification systems. However, it is true that the spectrum of neoplasms varies with the region of the intestines, and some features are sufficiently distinctive to suggest the likely origin. The upper small intestine (predominantly the duodenum) gives rise to both WD-NETs and PD-NECs, the latter being particularly centered on the ampulla of Vater.[64–66] The duodenal WD-NETs include conventional carcinoid tumors, which are usually nonfunctional,[67] as well as gastrinomas (particularly in MEN1 syndrome) and highly distinctive glandular WD-NETs that occur in patients with neurofibromatosis, type 1 and are variably termed *glandular duodenal carcinoid, ampullary somatostatinomas*, and *psammomatous somatostatinomas*.[68–70] These synonyms reflect the distinctive features of these NETs, including gland formation, psammoma body production, and somatostatin expression. However, somatostatinoma syndrome is very rare in duodenal primaries, so these tumors are considered nonfunctional. Prognostic studies of duodenal and ampullary neuroendocrine neoplasms are hampered by the rarity and diversity of these entities; but as in other locations, the PD-NECs are highly aggressive[65] and the WD-NETs are relatively indolent. Within the latter group, tumor size (and therefore stage) and grade predict survival.[67]

In the remainder of the small bowel, terminal ileum in particular, most of the neuroendocrine neoplasms are WD-NETs—the classic midgut carcinoid tumor composed of enterochromaffin (EC) cells that produce serotonin.[15] This is the most common site of origin for WD-NETs associated with carcinoid syndrome. PD-NECs are extremely rare, as are other carcinomas, with the exception of cases arising in the terminal ileum in the setting of Crohn disease.[71] Ileal WD-NETs are staged and graded like other neuroendocrine neoplasms of the gastroenteropancreatic system. Perhaps because they are asymptomatic when localized, they commonly present with advanced disease, which can be in the form of regional lymph node metastases, mesenteric involvement, or liver metastases. In the mesentery in particular, ileal WD-NETs often produce abundant fibrosis,[72] which can constitute the majority of the tumor mass. Ileal WD-NETs are also more commonly multicentric than in other anatomic sites; conflicting data exist about whether multicentric tumors represent intramural metastases[73] or truly multiple independent primaries.[74] Most ileal WD-NETs are low or intermediate grade; the phenomenon of G3 WD-NET has been rarely observed in this location. The histologic pattern of ileal WD-NETs is highly characteristic, including a nesting architecture, peripheral nuclear palisading, eosinophilic granular cytoplasm, and lumen formation (see **Fig. 1**C). Metastatic WD-NETs with this morphology can often be recognized as originating in the midgut purely by morphology.

The large intestine proximal to the rectum most commonly gives rise to PD-NECs, which can be small cell carcinomas but more commonly are LCNECs or carcinomas with features intermediate between these two PD-NEC entities.[75–77] They commonly arise in association with adenomas or have components of adenocarcinoma (MANEC), further demonstrating that these neoplasms are more closely related to the exocrine cell lineage rather than to WD-NETs.[78] Platinum-based chemotherapy, commonly used for PD-NECs of the colon, has not been shown to be more effective than other treatments in a randomized clinical trial; but it is widely thought that PD-NECs should be treated more like small cell carcinoma than colonic adenocarcinoma. The outcome is poor unless they are detected at a very early stage. WD-NETs occur in the cecum, where they are identical to the midgut-type EC cell WD-NETs of the terminal ileum.[79] Otherwise, WD-NETs are usually limited to the rectum, where they exhibit L-cell differentiation and express enteroglucagons.[80] Rectal WD-NETs are often detected incidentally by colonoscopy when they are quite small, and the prognosis of those less than 1 cm is excellent. With increasing size (especially >2 cm) and proliferative activity, the potential for aggressive behavior increases; prognostic models in addition to the AJCC staging and WHO grading systems have been proposed.[81]

PRIMARY SITE DETERMINATION IN NEUROENDOCRINE NEOPLASMS

Some patients present with metastatic neuroendocrine neoplasms that have an occult primary, despite attempts at radiographic localization. For PD-NECs, small cell carcinomas in particular, it is generally not possible to identify the primary site pathologically. Thyroid transcription factor-1 (TTF1) expression occurs in most pulmonary small cell carcinomas, but primaries from many other sites also express this marker. For WD-NETs there are several transcription factors that can point to a particular primary, but they must be used in combination because no individual marker is perfectly specific or sensitive.[53] TTF1 labels pulmonary carcinoid tumors and is a helpful but insensitive marker if a medullary thyroid carcinoma can be excluded. CDX2 is an intestinal lineage marker and generally stains only small bowel WD-NETs. Isl1 and PAX8 are positive in pancreatic WD-NETs and also are expressed in rectal WD-NETs. A combination of these stains can supplement data from imaging studies in an attempt to identify the primary site.

REFERENCES

1. Klimstra DS, Modlin IR, Adsay NV, et al. Pathology reporting of neuroendocrine tumors: application of the Delphic consensus process to the development of a minimum pathology data set. Am J Surg Pathol 2010;34(3):300–13.
2. Klimstra DS, Modlin IR, Coppola D, et al. The pathologic classification of neuroendocrine tumors: a review of nomenclature, grading, and staging systems. Pancreas 2010;39(6):707–12.
3. Yang Z, Tang LH, Klimstra DS. Gastroenteropancreatic neuroendocrine neoplasms: historical context and current issues. Semin Diagn Pathol 2013;30(3): 186–96.
4. Sorbye H, Strosberg J, Baudin E, et al. Gastroenteropancreatic high-grade neuroendocrine carcinoma. Cancer 2014;120(18):2814–23.
5. Strosberg J, Nasir A, Coppola D, et al. Correlation between grade and prognosis in metastatic gastroenteropancreatic neuroendocrine tumors. Hum Pathol 2009; 40(9):1262–8.
6. Sorbye H, Welin S, Langer SW, et al. Predictive and prognostic factors for treatment and survival in 305 patients with advanced gastrointestinal neuroendocrine carcinoma (WHO G3): the NORDIC NEC study. Ann Oncol 2013;24(1): 152–60.
7. Kunz PL, Reidy-Lagunes D, Anthony LB, et al. Consensus guidelines for the management and treatment of neuroendocrine tumors. Pancreas 2013;42(4):557–77.
8. Oberndorfer S. Karzinoide Tumoren des Dünndarms. Frankf Z Pathol 1907;1: 425–32.
9. Basturk O, Tang L, Hruban RH, et al. Poorly differentiated neuroendocrine carcinomas of the pancreas: a clinicopathologic analysis of 44 cases. Am J Surg Pathol 2014;38(4):437–47.
10. Edge S, Byrd DR, Compton CC, et al. AJCC cancer staging manual. New York: Springer; 2009.
11. Panzuto F, Boninsegna L, Fazio N, et al. Metastatic and locally advanced pancreatic endocrine carcinomas: analysis of factors associated with disease progression. J Clin Oncol 2011;29(17):2372–7.
12. Rindi G, Klöppel G, Alhman H, et al. TNM staging of foregut (neuro)endocrine tumors: a consensus proposal including a grading system. Virchows Arch 2006; 449(4):395–401.
13. Rindi G, Klöppel G, Couvelard A, et al. TNM staging of midgut and hindgut (neuro) endocrine tumors: a consensus proposal including a grading system. Virchows Arch 2007;451(4):757–62.
14. Rindi G, Petrone G, Inzani F. The 2010 WHO classification of digestive neuroendocrine neoplasms: a critical appraisal four years after its introduction. Endocr Pathol 2014;25(2):186–92.
15. Bosman FC, Carneiro F, Hruban RH. World Health Organization (WHO) classification of tumours of the digestive system. Geneva (United Kingdom): WHO Press; 2010.
16. Travis WD. The concept of pulmonary neuroendocrine tumors. In: Travis WD, Brambilla E, Muller-Hermelink KH, et al, editors. Pathology and genetics of tumours of the lung, pleura, thymus, and heart. Lyon (France): IARC Press; 2004. p. 19–20.
17. Thunnissen FB, Ambergen AW, Koss M, et al. Mitotic counting in surgical pathology: sampling bias, heterogeneity and statistical uncertainty. Histopathology 2001;39(1):1–8.

18. Velayoudom-Cephise FL, Duvillard P, Foucan L, et al. Are G3 ENETS neuroendocrine neoplasms heterogeneous? Endocr Relat Cancer 2013;20(5):649–57.
19. Yang Z, Tang LH, Klimstra DS. How many needle core biopsies are needed to comfortably predict the histologic grade of metastatic well differentiated neuroendocrine tumors to the liver? Mod Pathol 2012;25:426A.
20. Shi C, Gonzalez RS, Zhao Z, et al. Liver metastases of small intestine neuroendocrine tumors: Ki-67 heterogeneity and World Health Organization grade discordance with primary tumors. Am J Clin Pathol 2015;143(3):398–404.
21. McCall CM, Shi C, Cornish TC, et al. Grading of well-differentiated pancreatic neuroendocrine tumors is improved by the inclusion of both Ki67 proliferative index and mitotic rate. Am J Surg Pathol 2013;37(11):1671–7.
22. Tang LH, Gonen M, Hedvat C, et al. Objective quantification of the Ki67 proliferative index in neuroendocrine tumors of the gastroenteropancreatic system: a comparison of digital image analysis with manual methods. Am J Surg Pathol 2012;36(12):1761–70.
23. Reid MD, Bagci P, Ohike N, et al. Calculation of the Ki67 index in pancreatic neuroendocrine tumors: a comparative analysis of four counting methodologies. Mod Pathol 2015;28(5):686–94.
24. Voss SM, Riley MP, Lokhandwala PM, et al. Mitotic count by phosphohistone H3 immunohistochemical staining predicts survival and improves interobserver reproducibility in well-differentiated neuroendocrine tumors of the pancreas. Am J Surg Pathol 2015;39(1):13–24.
25. Basturk O, Yang Z, Tang LH, et al. The high-grade (WHO G3) pancreatic neuroendocrine tumor category is morphologically and biologically heterogeneous and includes both well differentiated and poorly differentiated neoplasms. Am J Surg Pathol 2015;39(5):683–90.
26. Kuo SC, Gananadha S, Scarlett CJ, et al. Sporadic pancreatic polypeptide secreting tumors (PPomas) of the pancreas. World J Surg 2008;32(8):1815–22.
27. Travis WD, Linnoila RI, Tsokos MG, et al. Neuroendocrine tumors of the lung with proposed criteria for large-cell neuroendocrine carcinoma. An ultrastructural, immunohistochemical, and flow cytometric study of 35 cases. Am J Surg Pathol 1991;15(6):529–53.
28. Travis WD, Rush W, Flieder DB, et al. Survival analysis of 200 pulmonary neuroendocrine tumors with clarification of criteria for atypical carcinoid and its separation from typical carcinoid. Am J Surg Pathol 1998;22(8):934–44.
29. Skov BG, Krasnik M, Lantuejoul S, et al. Reclassification of neuroendocrine tumors improves the separation of carcinoids and the prediction of survival. J Thorac Oncol 2008;3(12):1410–5.
30. Arrigoni MG, Woolner LB, Bernatz PE. Atypical carcinoid tumors of the lung. J Thorac Cardiovasc Surg 1972;64(3):413–21.
31. Rindi G, Klersy C, Inzani F, et al. Grading the neuroendocrine tumors of the lung: an evidence-based proposal. Endocr Relat Cancer 2014;21(1):1–16.
32. Pelosi G, Rodriguez J, Viale G, et al. Typical and atypical pulmonary carcinoid tumor overdiagnosed as small-cell carcinoma on biopsy specimens: a major pitfall in the management of lung cancer patients. Am J Surg Pathol 2005;29(2):179–87.
33. Travis WD. Pathology and diagnosis of neuroendocrine tumors: lung neuroendocrine. Thorac Surg Clin 2014;24(3):257–66.
34. Gosney JR, Williams IJ, Dodson AR, et al. Morphology and antigen expression profile of pulmonary neuroendocrine cells in reactive proliferations and diffuse

idiopathic pulmonary neuroendocrine cell hyperplasia (DIPNECH). Histopathology 2011;59(4):751–62.

35. Oba H, Nishida K, Takeuchi S, et al. Diffuse idiopathic pulmonary neuroendocrine cell hyperplasia with a central and peripheral carcinoid and multiple tumorlets: a case report emphasizing the role of neuropeptide hormones and human gonadotropin-alpha. Endocr Pathol 2013;24(4):220–8.

36. Yokota J, Akiyama T, Fung YK, et al. Altered expression of the retinoblastoma (RB) gene in small-cell carcinoma of the lung. Oncogene 1988;3(4):471–5.

37. Rusch VW, Klimstra DS, Venkatraman ES. Molecular markers help characterize neuroendocrine lung tumors. Ann Thorac Surg 1996;62(3):798–809 [discussion: 809–10].

38. Fernandez-Cuesta L, Peifer M, Lu X, et al. Frequent mutations in chromatin-remodelling genes in pulmonary carcinoids. Nat Commun 2014;5:3518.

39. Filosso PL, Yao X, Ahmad U, et al. Outcome of primary neuroendocrine tumors of the thymus: a joint analysis of the International Thymic Malignancy Interest Group and the European Society of Thoracic Surgeons databases. J Thorac Cardiovasc Surg 2015;149(1):103–9.e2.

40. Hasani-Ranjbar S, Rahmanian M, Ebrahim-Habibi A, et al. Ectopic Cushing syndrome associated with thymic carcinoid tumor as the first presentation of MEN1 syndrome-report of a family with MEN1 gene mutation. Fam Cancer 2014;13(2): 267–72.

41. Pu H, Komminoth P, Perren A, et al. Pancreatic endocrine tumours: introduction, in pathology and genetics of tumours of endocrine organs. Lyon (France): IARC Press; 2004. p. 177–82.

42. Yao JC, Eisner MP, Leary C, et al. Population-based study of islet cell carcinoma. Ann Surg Oncol 2007;14(12):3492–500.

43. Shi C, Klimstra DS. Pancreatic neuroendocrine tumors: pathologic and molecular characteristics. Semin Diagn Pathol 2014;31(6):498–511.

44. Klimstra DS, Perren A, Oberg K, et al. Pancreatic endocrine tumours: non-functioning tumours and microadenomas. Pathology and genetics of tumours of endocrine organs. IARC Press; 2004.

45. Hruban RH, Pitman MB, Klimstra DS. Tumors of the pancreas. Atlas of tumor pathology. Washington, DC: American Registry of Pathology; 2007.

46. Hoang MP, Hruban RH, Albores-Saavedra J. Clear cell endocrine pancreatic tumor mimicking renal cell carcinoma: a distinctive neoplasm of von Hippel-Lindau disease. Am J Surg Pathol 2001;25(5):602–9.

47. Klimstra DS, Pitman MB, Hruban RH. An algorithmic approach to the diagnosis of pancreatic neoplasms. Arch Pathol Lab Med 2009;133(3):454–64.

48. Hochwald SN, Zee S, Conlon KC, et al. Prognostic factors in pancreatic endocrine neoplasms: an analysis of 136 cases with a proposal for low-grade and intermediate-grade groups. J Clin Oncol 2002;20(11):2633–42.

49. Rindi G, Falconi M, Klersy C, et al. TNM staging of neoplasms of the endocrine pancreas: results from a large international cohort study. J Natl Cancer Inst 2012;104(10):764–77.

50. Khan MS, Luong TV, Watkins J, et al. A comparison of Ki-67 and mitotic count as prognostic markers for metastatic pancreatic and midgut neuroendocrine neoplasms. Br J Cancer 2013;108(9):1838–45.

51. Yang Z, Tang LH, Klimstra DS. Effect of tumor heterogeneity on the assessment of Ki67 labeling index in well-differentiated neuroendocrine tumors metastatic to the liver: implications for prognostic stratification. Am J Surg Pathol 2011;35(6): 853–60.

52. Singh S, Hallet J, Rowsell C, et al. Variability of Ki67 labeling index in multiple neuroendocrine tumors specimens over the course of the disease. Eur J Surg Oncol 2014;40(11):1517–22.

53. Klimstra DS. Pathology reporting of neuroendocrine tumors: essential elements for accurate diagnosis, classification, and staging. Semin Oncol 2013;40(1): 23–36.

54. Jiao Y, Shi C, Edil BH, et al. DAXX/ATRX, MEN1, and mTOR pathway genes are frequently altered in pancreatic neuroendocrine tumors. Science 2011;331(6021): 1199–203.

55. Yao JC, Phan AT, Chang DZ, et al. Efficacy of RAD001 (everolimus) and octreotide LAR in advanced low- to intermediate-grade neuroendocrine tumors: results of a phase II study. J Clin Oncol 2008;26(26):4311–8.

56. Yachida S, Vakiani E, White CM, et al. Small cell and large cell neuroendocrine carcinomas of the pancreas are genetically similar and distinct from well-differentiated pancreatic neuroendocrine tumors. Am J Surg Pathol 2012;36(2): 173–84.

57. Kulke MH, Hornick JL, Frauenhoffer C, et al. O6-methylguanine DNA methyltransferase deficiency and response to temozolomide-based therapy in patients with neuroendocrine tumors. Clin Cancer Res 2009;15(1):338–45.

58. Yao JC, Shah MH, Ito T, et al. Everolimus for advanced pancreatic neuroendocrine tumors. N Engl J Med 2011;364(6):514–23.

59. Han X, Ji Y, Zhao J, et al. Expression of PTEN and mTOR in pancreatic neuroendocrine tumors. Tumour Biol 2013;34(5):2871–9.

60. Tang LH, Shia J, Soslow RA, et al. Pathologic classification and clinical behavior of the spectrum of goblet cell carcinoid tumors of the appendix. Am J Surg Pathol 2008;32(10):1429–43.

61. Pavel M, Baudin E, Couvelard A, et al. ENETS consensus guidelines for the management of patients with liver and other distant metastases from neuroendocrine neoplasms of foregut, midgut, hindgut, and unknown primary. Neuroendocrinology 2012;95(2):157–76.

62. Kirshbom PM, Kherani AR, Onaitis MW, et al. Carcinoids of unknown origin: comparative analysis with foregut, midgut, and hindgut carcinoids. Surgery 1998;124(6):1063–70.

63. Chejfec G, Falkmer S, Askensten U, et al. Neuroendocrine tumors of the gastrointestinal tract. Pathol Res Pract 1988;183(2):143–54.

64. Stamm B, Hedinger CE, Saremaslani P. Duodenal and ampullary carcinoid tumors. A report of 12 cases with pathological characteristics, polypeptide content and relation to the MEN I syndrome and von Recklinghausen's disease (neurofibromatosis). Virchows Arch A Pathol Anat Histopathol 1986; 408(5):475–89.

65. Nassar H, Albores-Saavedra J, Klimstra DS. High-grade neuroendocrine carcinoma of the ampulla of Vater: a clinicopathologic and immunohistochemical analysis of 14 cases. Am J Surg Pathol 2005;29(5):588–94.

66. Capella C, Riva C, Rindi G, et al. Endocrine tumors of the duodenum and upper jejunum. A study of 33 cases with clinico-pathological characteristics and hormone content. Hepatogastroenterology 1990;37(2):247–52.

67. Untch BR, Bonner KP, Roggin KK, et al. Pathologic grade and tumor size are associated with recurrence-free survival in patients with duodenal neuroendocrine tumors. J Gastrointest Surg 2014;18(3):457–62 [discussion: 462–3].

68. Dayal Y, Doos WG, O'Brien MJ, et al. Psammomatous somatostatinomas of the duodenum. Am J Surg Pathol 1983;7(7):653–65.

69. Taccagni GL, Carlucci M, Sironi M, et al. Duodenal somatostatinoma with psammoma bodies: an immunohistochemical and ultrastructural study. Am J Gastroenterol 1986;81(1):33–7.

70. Tanaka S, Yamasaki S, Matsushita H, et al. Duodenal somatostatinoma: a case report and review of 31 cases with special reference to the relationship between tumor size and metastasis. Pathol Int 2000;50(2):146–52.

71. Bassi D, Ruffolo C, Scarpa M, et al. Ileal neuroendocrine carcinoma following restorative proctocolectomy for colonic adenocarcinoma in Crohn's disease. Int J Colorectal Dis 2011;26(2):253–4.

72. Druce M, Rockall A, Grossman AB. Fibrosis and carcinoid syndrome: from causation to future therapy. Nat Rev Endocrinol 2009;5(5):276–83.

73. Guo Z, Li Q, Wilander E, et al. Clonality analysis of multifocal carcinoid tumours of the small intestine by X-chromosome inactivation analysis. J Pathol 2000;190(1): 76–9.

74. Katona TM, Jones TD, Wang M, et al. Molecular evidence for independent origin of multifocal neuroendocrine tumors of the enteropancreatic axis. Cancer Res 2006;66(9):4936–42.

75. Bernick PE, Klimstra DS, Shia J, et al. Neuroendocrine carcinomas of the colon and rectum. Dis Colon Rectum 2004;47(2):163–9.

76. Mills SE, Allen MS Jr, Cohen AR. Small-cell undifferentiated carcinoma of the colon. A clinicopathological study of five cases and their association with colonic adenomas. Am J Surg Pathol 1983;7(7):643–51.

77. Shia J, Tang LH, Weiser MR, et al. Is nonsmall cell type high-grade neuroendocrine carcinoma of the tubular gastrointestinal tract a distinct disease entity? Am J Surg Pathol 2008;32(5):719–31.

78. La Rosa S, Marando A, Furlan D, et al. Colorectal poorly differentiated neuroendocrine carcinomas and mixed adenoneuroendocrine carcinomas: insights into the diagnostic immunophenotype, assessment of methylation profile, and search for prognostic markers. Am J Surg Pathol 2012;36(4):601–11.

79. Berardi RS. Carcinoid tumors of the colon (exclusive of the rectum): review of the literature. Dis Colon Rectum 1972;15(5):383–91.

80. Fiocca R, Rindi G, Capella C, et al. Glucagon, glicentin, proglucagon, PYY, PP and proPP-icosapeptide immunoreactivities of rectal carcinoid tumors and related non-tumor cells. Regul Pept 1987;17(1):9–29.

81. Fahy BN, Tang LH, Klimstra D, et al. Carcinoid of the rectum risk stratification (CaRRs): a strategy for preoperative outcome assessment. Ann Surg Oncol 2007;14(5):1735–43.

Clinical Presentation and Diagnosis of Neuroendocrine Tumors

Aaron I. Vinik, MD, PhD, FCP, MACP*, Celine Chaya, MD

KEYWORDS

- GEP-NETs • PNETs • Biomarkers • Syndromes and their tumors • Diagnosis

KEY POINTS

- Neuroendocrine gastroenteropancreatic tumors are a heterogeneous group of tumors that arise from the diffuse endocrine system.
- They derive from the embryologic endocrine system predominantly in the gut in the gastric mucosa, the small and large intestine, and the rectum but are also found in the pancreas, lung, ovaries, C cells of thyroid, and autonomic nervous system.
- They are slow-growing and capable of storing and secreting different peptides and neuroamines.
- Some of these substances cause specific clinical syndromes, whereas others do not.
- Biomarkers can be used for diagnosis, following the patient's prognosis.

INTRODUCTION

Neuroendocrine tumors (NETs) are tumors that arise from the diffuse endocrine system. They are slow-growing and capable of storing and secreting different peptides and neuroamines.[1] Some of these substances cause specific clinical syndromes; others do not.[2]

Although considered rare, the annual incidence of NETs has risen to 40 to 50 cases per million due to the availability of improved techniques for tumor detection.[3] A review of the Surveillance, Epidemiology, and End Results (SEER) database showed a 5-fold increase in the incidence of NETs from 1.09 per 100,000 in 1973 to 5.25 per 100,000 in 2004. In the United States, the prevalence is estimated to be 103,312 cases, which is twice the prevalence of gastric and pancreatic cancers combined.[4]

There are impediments to the diagnosis of NETs. They are not first in the differential because they comprise less than 2% of the gastrointestinal (GI) malignancies. Symptoms are often nonspecific, and the manifestations mimic a variety of disorders. A

Division of Endocrinology and Metabolism, Department of Medicine, Strelitz Diabetes and Neuroendocrine Center, Eastern Virginia Medical School, 855 West Brambleton Avenue, Norfolk, VA 23510, USA
* Corresponding author.
E-mail address: vinikai@evms.edu

Hematol Oncol Clin N Am 30 (2016) 21–48
http://dx.doi.org/10.1016/j.hoc.2015.08.006
0889-8588/16/$ – see front matter © 2016 Elsevier Inc. All rights reserved.

hemonc.theclinics.com

delay in diagnosis can also occur when the biopsy material is not examined for secretory peptides. Tumors may then be labeled erroneously as adenocarcinoma, affecting the management and underestimating prospects for survival.[5] There is typically a delay of many years before the right diagnosis is made, by which time metastases have occurred and survival has directly been affected, as shown in **Fig. 1**. Learning to recognize the symptoms is very important for early diagnosis. Clinically suspicious symptoms necessitate biochemical testing.

The biochemical markers are hormones or amines secreted by the neuroendocrine cells. Some are secreted by most NETs; others are specific to a type of tumor and lead to the diagnosis. NETs can also be nonfunctional and present with signs and symptoms due to the mechanical complications (pain, obstruction, bleeding), but those silent tumors can at any point in time start producing hormones and become syndromic.[3] The substance secreted by one tumor may change with time and yield an entirely different clinical syndrome. Indeed, metastases are known to each secrete different hormones than the parent tumor. NETs can also secrete other substances not related to their original cell properties, like cytokines, autoantibodies, and so on, which result in paraneoplastic syndromes.[6]

In general, NETs are named according to the hormone they produce (eg, gastrinoma if gastrin secreting, vasoactive intestinal polypeptide [VIP]-oma if VIP secreting).

The authors suggest an approach to diagnosing an NET based on the clinical presentation and the biochemical markers, as summarized in **Table 1**.

NETs are classified based on the embryologic origins and the vascular supply of the digestive tract into foregut (lung, stomach, liver, biliary tract, pancreas, the first portion of the duodenum, and the ovaries), midgut (the distal duodenum, small intestines, appendix, right colon, and the proximal transverse colon), and hindgut (the distal transverse colon, left colon, and the rectum) tumors.

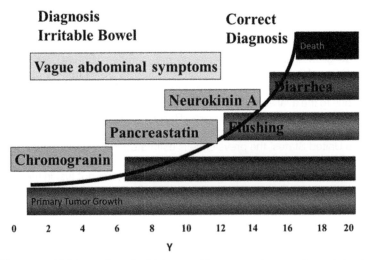

Fig. 1. The natural history of carcinoid tumors. Vague symptoms such as abdominal pain precede the diagnosis by a median of 9.2 years, and flushing and diarrhea, the major manifestations of carcinoid NETs, occur after the tumor has metastasized. Also shown is the relationship between tumor extent and when the biochemical markers are positive when measured in blood. Pancreastatin and neurokinin are both important, because they correlated with mortality, metastases, and survival, respectively. (*Data from* Vinik A. Biochemical testing for neuroendocrine tumors. Pancreas 2009;38:876–89.)

Table 1
An approach to diagnosing a neuroendocrine tumor based on the clinical presentation and the biochemical markers

Clinical Presentation	Syndrome	Tumor Type	Sites	Hormones
Flushing	Carcinoid Medullary carcinoma of thyroid PHEO	Carcinoid C-cell tumor Tumor of chromaffin cells	Mid/foregut Gastric Thyroid C cells Adrenal and sympathetic nervous system	Serotonin, CGRP, calcitonin Metanephrine and Normetanephrine
Diarrhea, abdominal pain, and dyspepsia	Carcinoid, WDHHA, ZE, PP, MCT	Carcinoid, VIPoma, Gastrinoma, PPoma, medullary carcinoma thyroid thyroid, mastocytoma	As above, pancreas, mast cells, thyroid	As above, VIP, gastrin, PP, calcitonin
Diarrhea/steatorrhea	Somatostatin Bleeding GI tract	Somatostatinoma, neurofibromatosis	Pancreas Duodenum	Somatostatin
Wheezing	Carcinoid	Carcinoid	Gut/pancreas/lung	SP, CGRP, serotonin
Ulcer/dyspepsia	Zollinger Ellison	Gastrinoma	Pancreas/duodenum	Gastrin
Hypoglycemia	Whipple's triad	Insulinoma, sarcoma, hepatoma	Pancreas, retroperitoneal liver	Insulin, IGF1, IGF11
Dermatitis	Sweet syndrome Pellagra	Glucagonoma Carcinoid	Pancreas Midgut	Glucagon Serotonin
Dementia	Sweet syndrome	Glucagonoma	Pancreas	Glucagon
Diabetes	Glucagonoma Somatostatin	Glucagonoma Somatostatinoma	Pancreas Pancreas	Glucagon Somatostatin
DVT, steatorrhea, cholelithiasis Neurofibromatosis	Somatostatin	Somatostatinoma	Pancreas Duodenum	Somatostatin
Silent, liver metastases	Silent	PPoma	Pancreas	PP
Fever	With weight loss cachexia	Any	Any	Cytokines (IL-6, NF-κβ, TNF-α)
Bone metastasis	Pain/fracture/spinal compression	Any	Any	Bone Alk phos N-telopeptide
Paraneoplastic syndromes	Peripheral neuropathy, myopathy, mysthenia, CIDP, Lambert Eaton, cerebellar ataxia	Any	Any	Antibodies to calcium channels, acetylocholine receptors, C-ANCA, P-ANCA, Hu

Abbreviations: Alk phos, alkaline phosphatase; C-ANCA, cytoplasmic anti-neutrophil cytoplasmic antibodies; CGRP, calcitonin gene-related peptide; CIDP, chronic inflammatory demyelinating polyneuropathy; IL-6, interleukin-6; MCT, medullary carcinoma of thyroid; NF-κβ, nuclear factor-κβ; P-ANCA, perinuclear anti-neutrophil cytoplasmic antibodies; TNF-α, tumor necrosis factor-α.

Data from Vinik A, O'Dorisio TM, Woltering EA, et al. Neuroendocrine tumors: a comprehensive guide to diagnosis and management. 1st edition. Inglewood (CA): Interscience Institute; 2006.

CLINICAL PRESENTATION
The Classic Carcinoid Syndrome

Classic carcinoid syndrome is the result of hypersecretion of vasoactive amines (eg, serotonin, histamine, tachykinins, and prostaglandins). It is common with small intestine NETs but also occurs with bronchial, ovarian, and other foregut carcinoids.[7] Because the liver can inactivate these substances, carcinoid syndrome typically presents after hepatic metastasis has occurred. However, this is not essential in foregut NETs.

The clinical manifestations are flushing (which occurs in 84% of patients), diarrhea (70%), and heart disease (37%), but symptoms could also be widespread to include bronchospasm (17%) and myopathy (7%).[3,8] Other recently recognized associated symptoms include abnormal increase in skin pigmentation, which is a pellagra-like eruption (5%), arthropathy, paraneoplastic neuropathy, and edema.[9] Mesenteric fibrosis is associated with midgut carcinoids even in the absence of a visible mass and could compress the vessels, which leads to bowel ischemia and malabsorption.

The specific etiologic substances of each of the manifestations are not known. Serotonin, prostaglandin, 5-hydroxytryptophan (5-HTP), substance P (SP), kallikrein, histamine, dopamine, and neuropeptide K are thought to be involved. Pancreatic polypeptide (PP) and motilin levels are often elevated.

Flushing

Although flushing is a cardinal manifestation of carcinoid syndrome, it occurs in other conditions like menopause, panic attacks, medullary thyroid cancer, autonomic neuropathy, mastocytosis, and simultaneous ingestion of chlorpropamide and alcohol. **Table 2** lists tests suggested to help with the differential.

When the flushing is dry, it is due to a carcinoid tumor until proven otherwise.

The flush in foregut tumors tends to be of protracted duration, is often a purplish or violaceous hue, and frequently results in telangiectasia and hypertrophy of the skin of the face and upper neck. The face may assume a "leonine" characteristic, resembling that seen in leprosy or acromegaly.

The flush in midgut tumors is of a faint pink to red color and involves the face and upper trunk down to the nipple line. It is initially provoked by alcohol and tyramine-containing food, like blue cheese, chocolate, red wine, and red sausage. With time, it becomes spontaneous. It usually lasts for a few minutes and occurs many times a day. It generally does not lead to permanent discoloration of the skin.

Table 2
Tests to identify causes of flushing

Clinical Condition	Tests
Carcinoid	5-HIAA, 5-HTP, SP, CGRP, CgA
Medullary carcinoma of the thyroid	Calcitonin, *RET* proto-oncogene
PHEO/paraganglioma	Plasma fractionated metanephrines and catecholamines
Autonomic neuropathy	Heart rate variability, 2H postprandial glucose
Menopause	Follicle stimulating hormone
Epilepsy	Electroencephalogram
Panic	Pentagastrin/ACTH
Mastocytosis	Plasma histamine, urine tryptase
Hypomastia, mitral valve prolapse	Cardiac echo

Abbreviation: CGRP, calcitonin gene-related peptide.

It is ascribed to several neurohumor: prostaglandins, kinins, serotonin, dopamine, histamine, 5-hydroxyindole acetic acid (5-HIAA), kallikrein, SP, neurotensin, motilin, somatostatin release inhibitory factor, VIP, neuropeptide K, and gastrin-releasing peptide (GRP). Feldman and O'Dorisio[10] have reported a further increase in SP and neurotensin levels during ethanol-induced facial flushing. These neuropeptide abnormalities also frequently occur in patients with other forms of flushing and may be pathogenic.[11]

Pentagastrin provocation has improved reliability compared with the calcium infusion stimulation test. It has occasional false negative results in patients with subclinical disease.[12] In the authors' experience, pentagastrin uniformly induced flushing in 11 patients with gastric NET (GNET), and serum SP levels increased in 80%.[13]

Diarrhea

Diarrhea is secretory in nature like all endocrine diarrheas. As opposed to osmotic diarrhea, it generates a large amount of stool with no osmotic gap, and the key is that it persists with fasting. It occurs in other syndromes like watery diarrhea hypokalemia, hypochlorhydria, acidosis (WDHHA syndrome), Verner-Morrison syndrome (VIPoma), Zollinger-Ellison syndrome (ZES; gastrinoma), calcitonin-secreting tumors (medullary carcinoma of the thyroid or C-cell hyperplasia), PNET-secreting pancreatic polypeptide (PPoma), and SP-secreting tumors.

In the gastrinoma syndrome, the diarrhea is associated with steatorrhea, and it improves with administration of a proton pump inhibitor (PPI) or histamine 2 (H2) blockers. The acidity in the duodenum and small intestine inactivates lipase, amylase, and trypsin, damages the mucosa of the small intestine, and precipitates the succus entericus, thereby causing malabsorption and steatorrhea.

In VIPoma, the diarrhea is associated with hypercalcemia. VIP stimulates GI secretions and increases the rate of fluid delivery from the proximal to the distal small bowel so it exceeds its absorptive capacity. The diarrhea is watery, and there is great loss of bicarbonate and potassium.

C-cell hyperplasia syndrome is a more recently described cause of secretory diarrhea and flushing. Total thyroidectomy is the treatment of choice.

The different mechanisms involved in the generation of the diarrhea are illustrated in **Fig. 2**.

Carcinoid Heart Disease

Carcinoid heart disease is characterized by fibrous endocardial thickening that mainly involves the right side of the heart. This fibrous tissue characteristically devoid of elastic fibers is known as carcinoid plaque. It causes retraction and fixation of the tricuspid and pulmonary valves, which leads to valvular regurgitation, but pulmonary and tricuspid stenosis may also occur.[14] The cause is unclear but direct actions of serotonin and bradykinin have been implicated in animal studies.[15] The clinical presentation is that of right-sided heart failure with fatigue, dyspnea, ascites, edema, and cardiac cachexia. Left-heart disease is uncommon.

Bronchoconstriction

Bronchoconstriction is clinically apparent as wheezing. The differential diagnosis includes asthma and chronic obstructive pulmonary disease. The bronchospasm is usually caused by SP, histamine, or serotonin.[5]

Pellagra

Pellagra occurs when niacin becomes deficient as its precursor tryptophan is shunted toward serotonin production.

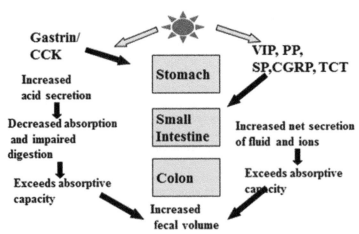

Fig. 2. Pathogenesis of endocrine diarrhea. CGRP, calcitonin gene related peptide; TCT, calcitonin. (*From* Vinik AI, Feliberti E, Perry RR, et al. Chapter 2—carcinoid tumors. In: DeGroot L, editor. Diffuse hormonal systems and endocrine syndromes. South Dartmouth (MA): 2014. Available at: www.endotext.org; with permission.)

BLOOD AND URINE BIOMARKERS POTENTIALLY USEFUL FOR DIAGNOSIS AND FOLLOW-UP

Several circulating tumor markers have been evaluated for the diagnosis and follow-up of NETs; however, a tissue confirmation is needed to make the diagnosis. Measurement of specific hormones may be helpful and is used in conjunction with imaging to follow clinical status and treatment response. There is controversy over the need for biomarkers and the frequency with which they should be sampled in following progress and response to intervention. In some instances, the relationship between the clinical syndrome and the hormone implicated is clear, in which case the specific hormone causing the clinical syndrome should be measured and followed over time, for example, gastrin in gastrinoma syndrome. Other markers may also be secreted by less well-differentiated tumors and nonfunctioning ones.[2] The key is to identify few biomarkers in a particular patient and follow them over time in conjunction with symptoms and measurements of tumor bulk.

Potential Diagnostic Markers

Potential diagnostic markers include chromogranin A (CgA), chromogranin B (CgB), chromogranin C, 5-HIAA, pancreastatin, and PP.

Markers Useful in Follow-Up

Markers that may be useful in follow-up include pancreastatin, which helps monitor response to surgery and predict tumor growth. Neurokinin A is a prognosticating marker when followed during treatment. Neuron-specific enolase (NSE) has a very low false negative rate, which makes it a good marker for follow-up.

Chromogranin A

CgA is a most important marker. It is a 49-kDa acidic polypeptide present in the secretory granules of all neuroendocrine cells. Its sensitivity varies between 53% and 68%, and the specificity varies between 84% and 98%.[16–20] A recent meta-analysis of 13 studies has shown a high sensitivity of 73% and specificity of 95% for the diagnosis of NETs.[21] CgA level should be measured while fasting, and exercise should be avoided before the testing because both eating and exercise lead to increased levels.[20] Somatostatin analogues affect the CgA level so the serial measurements should be done at the same interval from the injections.

There are caveats to the use of CgA as a universal tumor marker for NETs. First, the level of CgA correlates with tumor volume[22]; hence, small tumors may be associated with a normal level. Second, false positive measurements are reported in common conditions, including decreased renal function, liver or heart failure, chronic gastritis, inflammatory bowel disease, hyperthyroidism, PPI use, and even benign essential hypertension and exercise-induced physical stress.[23,24] Also, elevations of CgA are reported in malignant non-NETs like breast cancer and hepatocellular carcinoma.[20] These problems are not seen with CgB or pancreastatin.[23]

The "pearls" and pitfalls" on the use of CgA are shown in **Box 1**.

CgA also has a prognostic role in well-differentiated tumors. In midgut NETs, an increase in CgA level greater than 5000 µg/L is an independent predictor of shorter survival of 33 months compared with 57 months.[25] A reduction of the level by more than 80% after surgery predicts symptom relief and better outcome even after incomplete cytoreduction.[26]

Urinary 5-Hydroxyindole Acetic Acid (24-hour Collection) as a Biomarker for Neuroendocrine Tumors

5-HIAA, a serotonin degradation product, is a useful laboratory marker for serotonin-secreting NETs. It is more useful than the serum serotonin level because the latter varies during the day depending on the level of activity and stress. This test has 88% specificity.[14] It is used for diagnosis and follow-up. The reference range varies between laboratories, but is approximately 2 to 8 mg per day.

Certain foods and medications should be avoided during the collection because they increase the level of urinary 5-HIAA: bananas, kiwis, pineapple, plantains, plums, and tomatoes. Also, moderate elevations are seen with ingestion of avocado, black olives, spinach, broccoli, cauliflower, eggplant, cantaloupe, dates, figs, grapefruit, and honeydew melon. Drugs that can increase 5-HIAA include acetanalid, phenacetin,

---

Box 1
Pearls and pitfalls on use of chromogranin A as a biomarker

- Try and stay with the same laboratory
  - Very different levels, for example, less than 30 ng/mL to less than 5 pmol/L
- Is very helpful when you know you have an NET
- May be elevated when there is no actual NET
  - Severe hypertension
  - Gastric acid suppression (PPIs)
  - Renal insufficiency
- May be a good marker of response to therapy
- Does not correlate with symptoms

From Woltering EA, Hilton RS, Zolfoghary CM, et al. Validation of serum versus plasma measurements of chromogranin a levels in patients with carcinoid tumors: lack of correlation between absolute chromogranin a levels and symptom frequency. Pancreas 2006;33:250–4; with permission.

reserpine, glyceryl guiacolate (found in cough syrups), and methocarbamol. Drugs that decrease the level are chlorpromazine, heparin, imipramine, isoniazid, levodopa, monoamine oxidase inhibitors, methenamine, methyldopa, phenothiazines, promethazine, and tricyclic antidepressants.

It is presumed that foregut carcinoids are deficient in dopa-decarboxylase, so they poorly convert 5-HTP to 5-hydroxytryptamine (serotonin), which explains the only modest increase in 5-HIAA in those patients.

Plasma 5-Hydroxyindole Acetic Acid as a Biomarker for Neuroendocrine Tumors

Measuring a single fasting plasma 5-HIAA level is much more convenient than the 24-hour urine collection. A recent study compared the 2 assays in a group of 115 individuals with all types of NETs (among which 72 had midgut tumors) and 47 patients with midgut tumors metastatic to the liver. They found a statistically significant correlation between the urine and plasma assays, indicating that these are equivalent.[27] A prospective study is needed to determine its sensitivity and specificity to detect primary tumors, recurrence, or progression of the disease over time.

Overall, CgA seems a better tumor marker than 5-HIAA despite its limitations. **Fig. 3** shows the percent positivity of CgA versus 5-HIAA.

Pancreastatin as a Biomarker for Neuroendocrine Tumors

Pancreastatin is a posttranslational processing product of CgA. It has been proposed as an alternative biomarker to CgA, because the level is less susceptible to nonspecific effects and the assay is more standardized. When elevated at diagnosis, it has a negative prognostic value. It correlates with the number of liver metastases, so it is also useful for follow-up. It has been shown to be a better predictor of tumor growth than CgA.[28] Increasing levels during somatostatin analogue therapy is associated with poor survival.[29] An increase in level even if the tumor seems to respond to tyrosine kinase inhibitors predicts mortality.[30] A level higher than 5000 pg/mL is associated with periprocedure mortality in patients who underwent hepatic artery chemoembolization.[31] Pancreastatin may also monitor response to surgery, and less than 30% debulking is associated with an increase in levels.[32] Higher levels are associated with worse progression-free and overall survival in midgut and pancreatic NETs independent of age, site, and presence of metastases. It also may identify surgical patients at high risk of recurrence.[33] These observations suggest that pancreastatin is

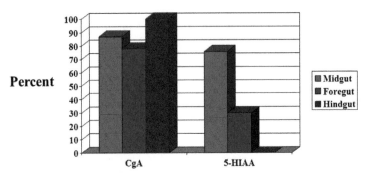

Fig. 3. CgA versus 5-HIAA in NETs. (*From* Vinik AI, Feliberti E, Perry RR, et al. Chapter 2—carcinoid tumors. In: DeGroot L, editor. Diffuse hormonal systems and endocrine syndromes. South Dartmouth (MA): 2014. Available at: www.endotext.org; with permission.)

potentially a very useful marker not only for diagnosis but also, more importantly, for monitoring treatment response.

Neurokinin A as a Biomarker for Neuroendocrine Tumors

Neurokinin A (NKA) is a tachykinin that has a highly sensitive and specific radioimmunoassay. It may be an important marker for prognosis. When NKA levels continue to increase despite treatment with somatostatin analogues, patients have poorer prognosis: 1-year survival decreases from 87% to 40%.[34]

Neuron-specific Enolase as a Biomarker for Neuroendocrine Tumors

NSE is a dimer of the glycolytic enzyme enolase. It is mainly present in the cytoplasm of cells of neuronal and neuroectodermal origin. NSE is elevated in only 30% to 50% of patients with NETs, especially the poorly differentiated ones.[35] It is a 100% sensitive but has a very low specificity of 32.9%,[19] which makes it a useful marker for follow-up of patients with a known diagnosis of NET but is not very useful as a diagnostic tool.

Other secreted molecules can be measured: CgB and chromogranin C, neuropeptide K, PP, and SP, but there are insufficient data to evaluate their usefulness as biomarkers in NETs.

PANCREATIC NEUROENDOCRINE TUMORS
Classification

Pancreatic neuroendocrine tumors (PNETs) are divided into 2 groups: those associated with a functional syndrome due to the secretion of a biologically active substance and those that are nonfunctional (NF-PNETs).[36–39] Approximately 10% to 30% of PNETs are functional.[40] PNETs represent 1.3% of all pancreatic neoplasms.[36] However, the number of patients diagnosed with PNETs has been increasing. An epidemiologic survey in Japan showed a 1.7 times higher incidence of NF-PNETs in 2010 compared with 2005.[41]

With all pancreatic NETs, one should always screen for multiple endocrine neoplasia type I (MEN-1) syndrome by measuring ionized calcium, serum parathyroid hormone (PTH), and prolactin.[30]

NF-PNETs have an annual incidence of 1.8 in female patients and 2.6 in male patients per million, according to the SEER.[4,42] They usually become clinically apparent when they reach a size that causes compression. In the past, 70% were more than 5 cm in size. However, the mean tumor diameter decreased in the last decades, mainly because of the widespread use of cross-sectional imaging technique.[43] They are malignant in 60% to 90% of cases, and 60% to 85% have metastasized to the liver at the time of diagnosis.[44] Although they do not secrete a hormone responsible for a syndrome, they do release substances that aid in their diagnosis: CgA (70%–100%) and PP (50%–100%).[44,45] NF-PNETs have a 5-year survival rate of 43%.[43]

Functional PNETs include insulinomas, which are the most common, followed in order of frequency by gastrinomas, glucagonomas, VIPomas, and somatostatinomas. Other rare functioning PNETs include those secreting adrenocorticotropic hormone (ACTH; ACTHomas), growth-hormone releasing factor (GRFomas), PTH-related peptide (PTHrp-omas), and those causing the carcinoid syndrome. Very rarely, PNETs secrete luteinizing hormone, renin, insulin-like growth factor (IGF)-II, glucagon-like peptide-1 (GLP-1), cholecystokinin (CCK), ghrelin, calcitonin-related peptide, or erythropoietin.[36,46–56]

Clinical Presentation of Pancreatic Neuroendocrine Tumors

PNETs can have quite different clinical presentations, secretory products, and histochemistry (**Table 3**).[41]

Table 3
Different clinical presentations, secretory products, and histochemistry

Syndrome/Tumor Type	Location	Signs and Symptoms	Circulating Biomarkers	Malignant, %
Insulinoma/nesidioblastosis	Pancreas (>99%)	Hypoglycemia, dizziness, sweating, tachycardia, tremulousness, confusion, seizure	CgA and CgB, insulin inappropriate for blood glucose level, proinsulin, C-peptide	<10
ZES (gastrinoma)	Duodenum (70%); pancreas (25%); other sites (5%)	Gastric acid hypersecretion, peptic ulcer, diarrhea, esophagitis, epigastric pain	CgA, gastrin, PP (35%)	60–90
WDHA (VIPoma)	Pancreas (90%, adult); other (10%, neural, adrenal, periganglionic)	Watery diarrhea, hypokalemia, achlorhydria (or acidosis)	CgA, VIP	40–70
Sweet syndrome (glucagonoma)	Pancreas (100%)	Diabetes (hyperglycemia), necrolytic migratory erythema, stomatitis, glossitis, angular cheilitis	CgA, glucagon, glycentin	50–80
Somatostatinoma	Pancreas (55%); duodenum/jejunum (44%)	Gallstones, diabetes (hyperglycemia), steatorrhea	CgA, somatostatin	>70
PPoma	Head of pancreas	Diarrhea	CgA, PP	50
GRHoma	Pancreas (30%); lung (54%); jejunum (7%); other (13%)	Acromegaly	GRH	>60
ACTHoma	Lung, thymus, pheos pancreas (4%–16%)	Cushing syndrome	ACTH	>95
PTHrp-oma	Lung, thymus, pancreas	Symptoms due to hypercalcemia	PTH-rp	84
Carcinoid syndrome	Small intestines, bronchi/lungs Duodenum Stomach Pancreas <1%	Flushing, diarrhea, abdominal pain, wheezing, dermatitis, heart disease	Serotonin tachychinins	60–90

			Calcitonin-like substance	>80
CGRP-oma	Pancreas	Flushing, diarrhea		
CCKoma	Biliary tract, pancreas	Peptic ulcer, diarrhea	CCK	Unknown
Ghrelinoma	Stomach, Pancreas	Gastroparesis	Ghrelin	Unknown
Renin-oma	Pancreas	Hypertension	Renin	Unknown
LH-oma	Pancreas	Anovulation, virilization (female): reduced libido (male)	LH	Unknown
Erythropoietinoma	Pancreas	Polycythemia	Erythropoietin	100
GLP-1 secreting NEET	Reported in ovary and pancreas	Hypoglycemia	GLP-1	Unknown
IGF-II-oma	Pancreas	Hypoglycemia	IGF-II	Unknown

Abbreviations: CGRP, calcitonin gene-related peptide; pheos, pheochromocytomas; LH, luteinizing hormone.

Modified from Vinik A, Woltering EA, O'Dorisio TM, et al. Neuroendocrine tumors: a comprehensive guide to diagnosis and management. 5th edition. Inglewood (CA): InterScience Institute; 2012; with permission.

Insulinoma

Patients usually present with the Whipple triad and fail to appropriately suppress insulin in the presence of hypoglycemia. Insulinomas have an estimated annual incidence of 1 to 4 per million. They are usually single (except in MEN-1), generally less than 1 cm in size, and almost always are intrapancreatic. They are benign in 85% to 90% of patients.[57–60]

Noninsulinoma Pancreatogenous Hypoglycemia Syndrome (or Nesidioblastosis)

Noninsulinoma pancreatogenous hypoglycemia syndrome is most commonly seen after gastric bypass. It usually presents with postprandial neuroglycopenic symptoms (within 4 hours of meal ingestion) with a negative 72-hour fasting test and nonrevealing tumor localization studies.[61,62]

Glucagonoma (the Sweet Syndrome)

Glucagonoma (the Sweet syndrome) clinically presents with diabetes accompanied by the 4D syndrome (dermatosis/necrolytic migratory erythema, depression, deep vein thrombosis, diarrhea). Patients are frequently initially diagnosed by a dermatologist when evaluated for the rash. This dermatosis is characterized by raised erythematous patches beginning in the perineum and subsequently involving the trunk and extremities. Glucagon levels can also be elevated in other conditions like diabetes mellitus (DM), burn injury, acute trauma, bacteremia, cirrhosis, renal failure, or Cushing syndrome (but <500 pg/mL). Glucagonomas are generally single and large in size (mean 6 cm). They are almost always intrapancreatic and associated with liver metastases in more than 60% of cases at diagnosis.[36,45,63–65]

Verner-Morrison Syndrome

VIPoma is also called pancreatic cholera or WDHA syndrome (watery diarrhea, hypokalemia, and achlorhydria). Patients clinically present with profound large-volume diarrhea (>700 mL/d). VIPomas are single, intrapancreatic in more than 95% of cases, and metastatic at diagnosis in 70% to 80% of cases.[45,66]

Somatostatinoma

Somatostatin is a tetradecapeptide that inhibits the secretion of numerous other hormones and peptides of endocrine and exocrine function; this leads, for example, to decreased gastric acid secretion, slowing of the GI transit time, and malabsorption of fat and calcium. The clinical syndrome includes diabetes, diarrhea, steatorrhea, gallbladder disease, hypochlorhydria, and weight loss. Somatostatinomas are usually diagnosed incidentally. Increased physician awareness of the syndrome and more readily available somatostatin assays will help suspect the diagnosis based on signs and symptoms in the future. The authors suggest measuring plasma somatostatin-like immunoreactivity concentrations during routine workup for postprandial dyspepsia due to gallbladder disorder, and in patients with diabetes without a family history, and for unexplained steatorrhea. The tumors tend to be large and located in the pancreas (60%) or duodenum/small intestine (40%); other locations were also reported in the hypothalamus and brain, C cells of the thyroid gland, sympathetic ganglia, and small-cell lung cancer. Metastatic disease is present at diagnosis in 70% of cases.[67,68] Most recently reported is a new syndrome found in young women that includes multiple paragangliomas, somatostatinomas, and polycythemia. It is associated with gain-of-function mutation in the gene coding for the hypoxia-inducible factor (*HIF2alpha*), which is known to upregulate the erythropoietin gene, hence the polycythemia.[69,70]

Ghrelinoma

Ghrelin is a 28-amino-acid peptide, primarily produced by neuroendocrine cells in the stomach. This hormone is also found in the small intestine, hypothalamus, pituitary gland, pancreas, heart, adipose tissue, and immune system. It has an important role in the physiologic regulation of appetite, response to hunger, and starvation. It also regulates metabolic and endocrine functions like energy expenditure, gastric motility and acid secretion, insulin secretion, and glucose homeostasis.[71] Only a few cases of NET associated with hyperghrelinemia have been reported: in the first, the tumor was located in the stomach, and the patient had no signs or symptom of acromegaly. In the second, the tumor was in the pancreas, and the patient was obese with diabetes. The most recent case initially had diabetes, but the tumor switched to secreting insulin; it was a metastatic pancreatic NET.[72–74]

POTENTIAL BIOCHEMICAL MARKERS OF PANCREATIC NEUROENDOCRINE TUMORS
Chromogranin A

CgA can be used as a marker in patients with both functional and nonfunctional pancreatic endocrine tumors.

Chromogranin B

As is CgA, CgB is part of the granin family, stored and secreted from vesicles present in the neuroendocrine cells.[75] CgA is the best studied.[76] The authors suggest complementary measurement of CgB because it does not have the problem of false positivity like CgA.[23]

Pancreatic Polypeptide

PP is a hormone secreted by islet cells of the ventral pancreas. It is another nonspecific biochemical marker. Its sensitivity is shown to be 54% in functioning tumors, 57% in nonfunctioning tumors, 63% in pancreatic tumors, and 53% in GI tumors. Also shown in the same study in 2004 by Panzuto and colleagues,[77] PP specificity was 81% compared with disease-free patients, and 67% compared with nonendocrine tumor patients.

When combined with CgA, the sensitivity is higher compared with either one of the markers alone: for gastroenteropancreatic NETs, the combination has 96% sensitivity; for nonfunctioning tumors, 95%; and for pancreatic tumors, 94%. The combination may be very useful for screening for an NET in a pancreatic mass workup.

Recently, a blunted PP response to a mixed meal has been proposed to distinguish DM secondary to pancreatic disease from type 2 DM.[78]

Specific Diagnostic Hormonal Assays

For insulinomas, an assessment of plasma insulin, proinsulin, and C-peptide is needed at the time of glucose determinations, usually during a fast. For ZES, a fasting serum gastrin is needed either alone or during a secretin provocation test. The following are needed: for VIPomas, a plasma VIP level is needed; for glucagonoma, plasma glucagon level is needed; for GRFomas, plasma growth hormone (GH) and GRF levels are needed; for Cushing syndrome, urinary cortical, plasma ACTH, and appropriate ACTH suppression studies are needed; for hypercalcemia with PET, both serum PTH levels and PTH-related peptide levels are indicated; and for a PNET with carcinoid syndrome, urinary 5-H1AA should be measured. For somatostatinomas and PPomas, the biochemical markers are somatostatin and PP, respectively.[1,79]

Screening

Once a pancreatic NET is diagnosed, one should consider screening for MEN type 1 syndrome by measuring ionized calcium, serum PTH, and prolactin.[30]

In the presence of suspected MEN-1 syndrome, biochemical screening for PNETs includes gastrin, insulin/proinsulin, PP, glucagon, and CgA. Together, they have a sensitivity of approximately 70%.[62]

GASTRIC NEUROENDOCRINE TUMORS

Foregut carcinoids have low serotonin content (5-HT). They often secrete 5-HTP (a serotonin precursor), histamine, and a multitude of hormones.

GNETs are divided into 3 types.

Type 1: Enterochromaffin-like Cell-oma

The fasting hypergastrinemia is secondary to chronic atrophic gastritis and pernicious anemia. They represent 70% to 80% of the gastric carcinoid tumors.[80] These tumors are typically multiple small lesions that arise from the enterochromaffin-like cell (ECL) and are less likely to metastasize. Gastrin production is normally suppressed by an acidic gastric pH. The achlorhydria caused by atrophic gastritis will lead to an elevated gastrin, which is trophic to the ECL cells. At levels higher than 1000 pg/mL, gastrin induces polyps and tumor formation.[13,81] The patients have premature graying of the hair, pernicious anemia, and antibodies against gastric parietal cells and intrinsic factor as well as other autoimmune diseases like chronic thyroiditis. Sampling of the gastric content reveals near neutral pH. In animal models, this clinical condition has been replicated by long-term PPI use. In humans, PPI use raises the fasting gastrin levels but not to a critical level to induce dysplasia.

Type 2: Enterochromaffin-like Cell-omas Associated with Gastrinomas

Clinically, patients present with ZES (peptic ulcerations, diarrhea, and heartburn) with highly acidic gastric pH. ZES should be suspected in cases of recurrent or severe or familial peptic ulcer disease (PUD); ulcers without *Helicobacter pylori* or other risk factors (nonsteroidal anti-inflammatory drugs, aspirin); severe gastroesophageal reflux disease; PUD resistant to treatment; and the presence of complications (perforation, bleeding). Prominent gastric folds are seen on endoscopy in 92% of cases.[82] The diarrhea typically responds to therapy with PPI.

Both hypercalcemia and PPI cause hypergastrinemia. Making the diagnosis of gastrinoma requires switching PPI to H2 receptor antagonists, which could potentially cause complications (worsening PUD, bleeding, perforation, and other complications); hence, it should be done in a specialty unit experienced in diagnosing ZES. The presence of fasting serum gastrin level of 1000 ng/L (pg/mL) or more, gastric pH less than 2, in a normocalcemic patient, free of pyloric obstruction, with normal renal function establishes the diagnosis of gastrinoma.[62] Measuring the gastric acid output will help differentiate a gastrinoma from other causes of secondary hypergastrinemia.

Gastrinomas represent approximately 5% of the gastric carcinoid tumors. They are typically single and localized in the gastrinoma triangle 90% of the time (first part of the duodenum including the bulb and the pancreatic head). Duodenal gastrinomas are usually small (mean 0.93 cm), whereas the pancreatic gastrinomas are generally large in size (mean 3.8 cm).[82] The risk of metastasis of gastrinomas is higher than that of type 1 GNETs.[83] MEN-1 should be explored in all patients with ZES because it is highly frequent, occurring in 20% to 25% of patients. Serum PTH, ionized calcium, and prolactin levels should be checked at diagnosis and yearly thereafter.[82] When associated with MEN-1, gastrinomas can be multiple and present at an earlier age (approximately 1 decade earlier).[41]

Type 3 Enterochromaffin-like Cell-omas

Patients may present with atypical carcinoid syndrome due to histamine secretion: extended episodes of flushing, headache, shortness of breath, and, in rare cases, lacrimation. The flushing can be deep purple and last for hours. It may be followed by increased blood flow to the limbs and trunk (chest, stomach, and back). This flush is not brought on by food.[84] These lesions are typically large and solitary and have the highest risk of metastasis. They represent 20% of the GNETs. Gastrin levels are not elevated.

HINDGUT NEUROENDOCRINE TUMORS

Hindgut neuroendocrine tumors are usually silent and discovered on rectal or endoscopic examination. They rarely contain 5-HT and rarely secrete 5-HTP or other peptides.

GENE STUDIES AS BIOMARKERS OF GASTROENTEROPANCREATIC NEUROENDOCRINE TUMORS

The genetics of neuroendocrine tumorigenesis have yet to be elucidated.

Although small familial clusters of midgut carcinoids have been described, they are not associated with known genetic cancer syndromes. Among sporadic midgut carcinoids, several studies using comparative genomic hybridization or microsatellite markers have shown frequent allelic deletion of chromosome 18.[85,86] On an epigenetic level, midgut NETs have been found to have global hypomethylation.[87]

PNETs, on the other hand, can occur sporadically and in association with various inherited disorders.[36,57] PNETs occur in 80% to 100% of patients with MEN-1; in 10% to 17% of patients with von Hippel-Lindau syndrome (VHL); in up to 10% of patients with von Recklinghausen disease (neurofibromatostis-1); and only occasionally in patients with tuberous sclerosis.[57] In MEN-1, NF-PNETs are small and microscopic. Gastrinomas develop in 54% cases, insulinomas in 18%, and glucagonomas, VIPomas, GRFomas, somatostatinomas in less than 5%. In VHL, 98% of all the PNETs are nonfunctional. In neurofibromatosis-1, they are characteristically duodenal somatostatinomas, which do not cause the clinical syndrome. In tuberous sclerosis, rare functional and NF-PNETs are reported.[57]

Genetic analysis should be performed in suspected cases of MEN-1, VHL, neurofibromatosis-1, and tuberous sclerosis. Genetic counseling should be sought before testing in all patients. Germline DNA testing is recommended in the presence of a positive family history of MEN-1, if there are suspicious clinical findings or if multiple tumors or precursor lesions are present. Somatic (tumor) DNA testing is not recommended.[88–90]

Recent molecular studies looked at the genomic landscape of NETs, which resulted in the discovery of mutations in specific genes and pathways like the PI3K/Akt/mTOR, DAXX/ATRX, and MEN1. This discovery has led to the use of new targeted therapies and may lead to new and better prognostic biomarkers.[91–96]

MULTIPLE ENDOCRINE NEOPLASIA SYNDROMES

MEN syndromes are rare cancer syndromes that are mostly dominantly inherited, but also have sporadic and atypical forms. They are classified as type 1, associated with inactivating mutations of the *MEN1* tumor suppressor gene on chromosome 11q13, or type 2, associated with activating mutation of the *RET* proto-oncogene.[97] Once MEN syndrome is suspected, genetic testing should be performed, and if positive, first-degree relatives should also be tested.

Multiple Endocrine Neoplasia Type 1

The syndrome is characterized by 3 main tumors: parathyroid adenomas (90%), PNETs (60%), and pituitary adenomas (40%). Many other benign and malignant endocrine and nonendocrine tumors have been associated with the syndrome, including other foregut NETs (gastric, thymic, and bronchial carcinoids), adrenal cortex neoplasia (benign and malignant), pheochromocytomas (PHEOs), lipomas, facial angiofibromas, collagenomas, gingival papules, and periungual fibromas.[98] The NETs are usually multifocal and more aggressive, and 60% are functional. They secrete gastrin (60%), insulin (10%–33%), somatostatin, or VIP.[98–100] A point of interest is that if a NET coexists with MEN-1, it would be located in the thymus more than two-thirds of the time in men, whereas in women, it is in the lung more than 75% of the time.

A diagnosis of MEN-1 may be established in an individual by 1 of 3 criteria[88,101]:

- Occurrence of 2 or more primary MEN-1-associated endocrine tumors
- Occurrence of one of the MEN-1-associated tumors in a first-degree relative of a patient with known MEN-1
- Identification of a germline MEN-1 mutation

In 2012, a clinical practice guideline was published by a group of international experts. They recommended annual biochemical screening for PNETs in MEN-1 including gastrin, insulin with an associated fasting glucose level, PP, glucagon, VIP, and CgA.[102] For thymic, bronchopulmonary, and GNETs, biochemical evaluation with urinary 5-HIAA and CgA is deemed not helpful. Instead, they recommend computed tomography (CT) or MRI of the chest every 1 to 2 years and gastroscopic examination (with biopsy) every 3 years in those with hypergastrinemia. Endoscopic ultrasound and somatostatin receptor (SSTR) scintigraphy may aid the diagnosis.[102]

Multiple Endocrine Neoplasia Type 2

MEN type 2 is subclassified into 3 groups:

- MEN2A: Medullary thyroid carcinoma (MTC) associated with PHEO and hyperparathyroidism; some may present in childhood with features of Hirschsprung disease and others with cutaneous lichen amyloidosis.[103,104]
- MEN2B: MTC associated with mucosal neuromas, PHEO, marfanoid body habitus, GI ganglioneuromatosis, and myelinated corneal nerves
- Familial MTC: only MTC is present.[98]

Each subtype is characterized by a specific germline mutation of the *RET* proto-oncogene. Once the genetic mutation is proven, a prophylactic thyroidectomy is mandatory.[105]

The North American Neuroendocrine Tumor Society published guidelines for the management of patients with sporadic and hereditary MTC and recommended timing of early thyroidectomy based on the specific *RET* mutation.[106] The European Society of Endocrine Surgeons and several other professional groups have also developed guidelines for the timing of thyroidectomy based on the perceived clinical behavior of the specific *RET* mutation.[107]

Table 4 shows the recommended surveillance program for PHEO and hyperparathyroidism in patients with a genetic diagnosis of MEN2.[88]

PHEOs occur in 50% of cases of MEN2A and MEN2B. It is important to recognize them, because they should be resected before definitive surgery for MTC.[106]

The PHEOs associated with MEN2A are almost always benign and are usually multicentric, bilateral, confined to the adrenal gland, and associated with adrenal medullary hyperplasia. Patients with MEN2A and a unilateral PHEO usually develop a contralateral PHEO within 10 years.[108]

IMAGING OF NEUROENDOCRINE TUMORS

The goal of imaging is to help make the diagnosis, determine the tumor burden, and assess the potential for surgical resection as well as establish the prognosis and determine the potential for nonconventional therapies especially in inoperable disease. Modalities include standard cross-sectional technique and nuclear functional imaging.

The sensitivity and specificity for some imaging modalities are shown in **Table 5**.

STANDARD CROSS-SECTIONAL IMAGING
Computed Tomography

CT is the most common method of imaging NETs. Its strengths are the wide field of view in the chest, abdomen, and pelvis; accurate measurement of the lesions; and the detail of vascular anatomy. Its weaknesses are the relative insensitivity in detecting small liver lesions and the concern of repeated radiation exposure during long-term follow-up. Metastatic NETs are particularly sensitive to the timing of the administration of the contrast. Liver metastases are most visible on the arterial phase, difficult to visualize on the venous phase, and not visible on noncontrast phases.

MRI

MRI is a powerful tool in the evaluation of NETs. It is the most useful examination for liver metastasis.[109] Liver metastases are uniquely vascular, which makes evaluation of water motion by MRI highly sensitive. Multiple sequences improve the detection of very small lesions. Moreover, with the introduction of hepatocyte-specific contrast agents (eg, gadoxetic acid or gadopentetic acid–based gadolinium), tumors can be seen in great detail and measured accurately; this is very important in patients potentially undergoing liver resection.

Table 4				
Recommended surveillance program for pheochromocytoma and hyperparathyroidism in patients with a genetic diagnosis of multiple endocrine neoplasia type 2				
Tumor Type	MEN Syndrome	Age to Start (y)	Annual Biochemical Screening	Imaging Test
PHEO	MEN2A	5	Plasma metanephrines	MRI every 3 y
	MEN2B	3		
Hyperparathyroidism	MEN2A	10	Calcium profile	—
	MEN2B			

Adapted from Brandi ML, Gagel RF, Angeli A, et al. Guidelines for diagnosis and therapy of MEN type 1 and type 2. J Clin Endocrinol Metab 2001;86:5658–71.

Table 5		
Sensitivity and specificity for some imaging modalities		
Test	Sensitivity, %	Specificity, %
CT	83	76
MRI	93	88
Ultrasound	50–85	76–97
Octreoscan	52–78	93
PET/CT ^{68}Ga-DOTATOC	97	92
PET/CT ^{68}Ga-DOTANOC	78	93
PET/CT ^{18}F-FDG-PET	92	—

Ultrasound

Ultrasonography is an excellent tool especially as an adjunct for biopsy. It is the most common examination done as part of the evaluation of abdominal pain. It is also highly effective in evaluating hepatic lesions intraoperatively. Echocardiography is the most effectively used for the carcinoid heart disease. Screening for valvular disease and heart failure is critical before any surgical procedure.

Endoscopy

Endoscopy is a valuable tool that allows direct visualization of the gastric, duodenal, terminal ileal, colonic, and rectal lesions. To visualize lesions beyond the reach of the standard endoscope, small bowel enteroscopy and pill-cam endoscopy can be used.

Endoscopic ultrasonography is much more effective for localizing intrapancreatic NETs than extrapancreatic ones (eg, duodenal gastrinomas or somatostatinomas). It can identify an intrapancreatic tumor in about 90% of cases.[36]

FUNCTIONAL IMAGING
[111]Indium-OTPA-octreotide Scan (Octreoscan)

[111]Indium-DTPA-octreotide Scan (Octreoscan) is the most sensitive imaging modality for detecting widespread metastatic disease. Octreoscans are extremely useful in confirming the diagnosis and evaluating tumor burden.

Most NETs express SSTR, especially type 2 and type 5. Pentetreotide, the somatostatin analogue most commonly used, is attached to [111]Indium, an isotope that emits single photon emission tomography (SPECT). Other analogues used include In-DOTA Lanreotide, and a newer one, SOM-230, that has potency to bind to SSTR2, SSTR3, and SSTR5. Full-body imaging is performed after the tracer (eg, pentetreotide) binds to the SSTR in the tumor. Those SPECT images can be fused with the CT scans to add functional information to the tumor. The whole body is imaged, which allows detection of distant metastases that were not in the field of view on CT or MRI.[110] However, it will not be helpful if the tumor does not express SSTRs or if the receptor does not have affinity to the tracer. Another major issue is its relative insensitivity for lesions less than 1 cm. Also, physiologic activity in the kidney, spleen, liver, and bowel can obscure the lesion. To improve the sensitivity, the authors recommend a third scan at 96 hours after the injection in addition to the 4-hour and 24-hour scans, but this renders the test more cumbersome to the patient.

Octreotide scanning is useful in predicting response to octreotide treatment. A study by Janson and colleagues[111] showed good response to ocreotide in 22 of 27 patients with carcinoid tumor and positive scans, whereas the 3 patients with negative scans failed treatment.

PET

The PET technique offers greater sensitivity and resolution of the images compared with SPECT, especially for distant metastases and difficult-to-locate abdominal lesions.[112] Positron emitters that are used include [68]Gallium and [11]Carbon. Those could be attached to different tracers like a somatostatin analogue (DOTATOC or DOTA-NOC) or [18]Ffluorodeoxyglucose (FDG). The technique is simple because the patient will only wait approximately 1 hour before a single imaging session.

An emerging new technology is [68]Gallium-somatostatin analogue imaging that requires binding to the SSTR. It is currently only available at a few specialty centers in the United States. It is not used as a screening imaging tool. It has a higher sensitivity showing a known tumor and metastases with better resolution.

11-C-Hydroxytryptophan is another agent that uses the amine precursor uptake machinery to detect serotonin-producing tumors, but it is only available in a few centers worldwide.[113]

FDG-PET has not been very helpful for NETs because of their generally lower proliferative activity, but it is the imaging modality of choice in malignant cases, like in paragangliomas associated with *SDH-B* mutations. Also, its use in undifferentiated tumors or small cell-like lesions of the bronchus or thymus is highly effective.

[123]I Metaiodobenzylguanidine

Metaiodobenzylguanidine (MIBG) is an analogue of the catecholamine norepinephrine, which can be labeled with a radioactive isotope, [123]Iodine, to use clinically for imaging of NETs. Tumors of sympathetic neuronal precursors express the norepinephrine transporter, a transmembrane protein that functions to shuttle norepinephrine across the cell membrane.

MIBG is taken up by a wide verity of NETs as well as normal adrenal tissue; therefore, its specificity depends on the certainty of the clinical and biochemical diagnosis. It is of no value if the metanephrine and catecholamine levels are not elevated. Only in the correct clinical context, the specificity is greater than 95% for PHEO and neuroblastoma,[114] but it is definitely less for carcinoid tumors. Patients with a positive scan may be candidates for future therapy with ^{131}I-MIBG, if the tumor uptake is measured to be at least 2 to 3 times more than that of the background.

Glucagon-like Peptide-1 Agonists Scans

GLP-1 agonists scans are available only in a few centers in the world. They help localize the GLP-1 receptor-expressing insulinomas.

VENOUS SAMPLING

Assessment of hormonal gradients is now rarely used except in occasional patients with insulinomas or gastrinomas not localized by other imaging methods. It is now usually performed at the time of angiography and combined with selective intra-arterial injections of calcium for primary insulinomas or secretin for gastrinoma (primary or metastatic to the liver) with hepatic venous hormonal sampling.[115–117]

In cases where the tumor cannot be identified by imaging techniques, total body venous sampling with measurement of a peptide hormone that is produced and percutaneous transhepatic portal and systemic venous sampling with hormone assay are generally not very useful techniques for localization of NETs. Data must be used cautiously and has proved useful in SP-producing tumors but not in serotonin-secreting ones.[118]

SPECIFIC NEUROENDOCRINE TUMORS IMAGING EVALUATION
Gastric Neuroendocrine Tumors

Most gastric tumors are visualized by endoscopy. Endoscopic ultrasound offers the opportunity to assess the depth of tumor invasion and nearby nodes. The predominant site of metastasis is the liver. Cross-sectional imaging like CT scan or MRI should be done to look for metastasis in cases of type I and type II carcinoids when larger than 2 cm and in all cases of type III carcinoids.[119] Liver metastases are hypervascular and become isodense compared with the liver after intravenous administration; hence, CT scan studies should be done without and with contrast.[120] SSTR scintigraphy is also useful for the detection of metastasis.[120]

Pancreatic Neuroendocrine Tumors

Functional PNETs (especially insulinomas and duodenal gastrinomas) are often small in size, and localization may be difficult. Different conventional imaging studies (CT, MRI, ultrasound, angiography) have been used. They detect greater than 70% of PNETs greater than 3 cm, but less than 50% of PNETs less than 1 cm. CT scanning with contrast is the most frequently used as the first-line imaging modality. PNETs, similar to carcinoid tumors, frequently (>80%, except insulinomas) overexpress SSTRs, which bind various synthetic analogues of somatostatin (octreotide, lanreotide) with high affinity. Octreoscan detects 50% to 70% of primary PNETs (less frequent with insulinomas or duodenal gastrinomas) and greater than 90% of patients with metastatic disease.[121–123]

Bronchial and Thymic Neuroendocrine Tumors

Chest radiograph and CT scan usually suffice to detect bronchial and thymic tumors.

Midgut Neuroendocrine Tumors

The most difficult to localize tumors are the small bowel and the extraintestinal NETs. With more sophisticated CT scanning apparatus, the authors are able to better detect the midgut NETs, but many remain not visible. MRI is not particularly strong in evaluating the small intestines or the mesentery because of movement artifact. Capsule endoscopy and push-pull enteroscopy have been occasionally useful. Other modalities commonly used include (^{111}In-diethylenetriamine pentaacetic acid) octreotide scintigraphy (^{123}I) MIBG scintigraphy, and PET. In the setting of emergent situations, like small bowel obstruction, CT scan remains the examination of choice.

Hindgut Neuroendocrine Tumors

The hindgut tumors as well as the ones located in the right colon and cecum can be demonstrable by lower endoscopy or barium enema examination.

Metastases

According to the SEER database, 49% of NETs were localized, 24% showed regional metastases, and 27% were associated with distant metastases. The median survival in distant metastatic disease was 33 months in patients with grade 1 and 2 NETs, but only 5 months in patients with poorly differentiated carcinomas/grade 3.[4]

Liver metastases are the most common. Extrahepatic metastatic sites include lymph nodes, peritoneal cavity, lung, bone, and rare others (eg, brain, heart, ovaries).[124] The presence of carcinoid heart disease or bone metastases is a negative prognostic factor.[124] A valuable biomarker for carcinoid heart disease is brain natriuretic peptide.[125]

BONE METASTASES

Metastases from NETs can be either osteolytic or osteoblastic.

Bone markers include bone alkaline phosphatase, an indicator of osteoblast function, and urinary N-telopeptide, which reflects osteoclast activity or bone resorption. Only blastic metastases show an increase in both markers.[126]

The higher the N-telopeptide levels at baseline, the higher the skeletal-related event rate and disease progression rate and risk of death.[127]

SUMMARY

NETs are a heterogeneous group of tumors that arise from the diffuse endocrine system. They derive from the embryologic endocrine system predominantly in the gut in the gastric mucosa, the small and large intestine, and the rectum but are also found in the pancreas, lung, and ovaries. They are slow-growing and capable of storing and secreting different peptides and neuroamines. Some of these substances cause specific clinical syndromes, whereas others do not. For convenience, they are separated into functional, in which the consequence is a clinical syndrome derived from the hormone or amine being produced, or nonfunctional, in which case the syndrome derives from the tumor bulk and the impact of metastases usually to liver, lymph nodes, and bone. Although considered rare, the annual incidence of NETs has risen to 40 to 50 cases per million because of the availability of improved techniques for tumor detection. A review of the SEER database showed a 5-fold increase in the incidence of NETs from 1.09 of 100,000 in 1973 to 5.25 of 100,000 in 2004. In the United States, the prevalence is estimated to be 103,312 cases, which is twice the prevalence of gastric and pancreatic cancers combined. Similar estimates have been reported from England and Sweden. These tumors occur predominantly at all ages with the highest incidence in the fifth decade onwards except for appendiceal carcinoid, which occurs at around 40 years, and the genetic syndromes, such as VHL, neurofibromatosis, tuberous sclerosis, MEN-1 and -2, have their onset many years earlier. Life expectancy is determined by the current grading system of tumors based on the KI67 index of cell proliferation and the mitotic index. There are impediments to the diagnosis of NETs. They are not first in the differential because they comprise less than 2% of the GI malignancies. Symptoms are often nonspecific, and the manifestations mimic a variety of disorders. A delay in diagnosis can also occur when the biopsy material is not examined for the secretory peptides. Tumors may then be labeled erroneously as adenocarcinoma, affecting the management and underestimating prospects for survival. Clinically suspicious symptoms necessitate biochemical testing.

Several circulating tumor markers have been evaluated for the diagnosis and follow-up of NETs; however, a tissue confirmation is needed to make the diagnosis. The specific hormone causing the clinical syndrome should be measured, for example, gastrin, insulin, PP, and so on, and followed over time. Potential diagnostic markers include CgA, CgB, chromogranin C, 5-HIAA, pancreastatin, and PP.

Markers useful in follow-up include pancreastatin, which may help monitor response to surgery and predict tumor growth. Neurokinin A is a possible prognosticating marker when followed during treatment. NSE has a very low false negative rate, which makes it a reasonable marker for follow-up. MicroRNA profiling has entered the arena, and when it becomes clearer what is being measured and what this reflects, may remain a prophecy yet to be fulfilled.

As Moertel once said 3 decades ago, "this is an Odyssey in the land of slow growing tumors." The authors present the evolution of this Odyssey and the rapid rate of progress that has been made in earlier and better identification with an increasing awareness and better tools for detection.

REFERENCES

1. Massironi S, Sciola V, Peracchi M, et al. Neuroendocrine tumors of the gastro-entero-pancreatic system. World J Gastroenterol 2008;14:5377–84.
2. Eriksson B, Oberg K, Stridsberg M. Tumor markers in neuroendocrine tumors. Digestion 2000;62(Suppl 1):33–8.
3. Vinik AI, Woltering EA, Warner RR, et al. NANETS consensus guidelines for the diagnosis of neuroendocrine tumor. Pancreas 2010;39:713–34.
4. Yao JC, Hassan M, Phan A, et al. One hundred years after "carcinoid": epidemiology of and prognostic factors for neuroendocrine tumors in 35,825 cases in the United States. J Clin Oncol 2008;26:3063–72.
5. Vinik A, O'Dorisio TM, Woltering EA, et al. Neuroendocrine tumors: a comprehensive guide to diagnosis and management. 1st edition. Los Angeles (CA): Interscience Institute; 2006.
6. Li SC, Khan M, Caplin M, et al. Somatostatin analogs treated small intestinal neuroendocrine tumor patients circulating microRNAs. PLos One 2015;10: e0125553.
7. Davis Z, Moertel CG, McIlrath DC. The malignant carcinoid syndrome. Surg Gynecol Obstet 1973;137:637–44.
8. Creutzfeldt W, Stockmann F. Carcinoids and carcinoid syndrome. Am J Med 1987;82:4–16.
9. Vinik AI, Gonzales MR. New and emerging syndromes due to neuroendocrine tumors. Endocrinol Metab Clin North Am 2011;40:19–63, vii.
10. Feldman JM, O'Dorisio TM. Role of neuropeptides and serotonin in the diagnosis of carcinoid tumors. Am J Med 1986;81:41–8.
11. Aldrich LB, Moattari AR, Vinik AI. Distinguishing features of idiopathic flushing and carcinoid syndrome. Arch Intern Med 1988;148:2614–8.
12. Ahlman H, Dahlstrom A, Gronstad K, et al. The pentagastrin test in the diagnosis of the carcinoid syndrome. Blockade of gastrointestinal symptoms by ketanserin. Ann Surg 1985;201:81–6.
13. Eckhauser FE, Lloyd RV, Thompson NW, et al. Antrectomy for multicentric, argyrophil gastric carcinoids: a preliminary report. Surgery 1988;104:1046–53.
14. Tormey WP, FitzGerald RJ. The clinical and laboratory correlates of an increased urinary 5-hydroxyindoleacetic acid. Postgrad Med J 1995;71:542–5.
15. Fox DJ, Khattar RS. Carcinoid heart disease: presentation, diagnosis, and management. Heart 2004;90:1224–8.
16. Goebel SU, Serrano J, Yu F, et al. Prospective study of the value of serum chromogranin A or serum gastrin levels in the assessment of the presence, extent, or growth of gastrinomas. Cancer 1999;85:1470–83.
17. Bernini GP, Moretti A, Ferdeghini M, et al. A new human chromogranin 'A' immunoradiometric assay for the diagnosis of neuroendocrine tumours. Br J Cancer 2001;84:636–42.
18. Nehar D, Lombard-Bohas C, Olivieri S, et al. Interest of Chromogranin A for diagnosis and follow-up of endocrine tumours. Clin Endocrinol (Oxf) 2004;60: 644–52.
19. Bajetta E, Ferrari L, Martinetti A, et al. Chromogranin A, neuron specific enolase, carcinoembryonic antigen, and hydroxyindole acetic acid evaluation in patients with neuroendocrine tumors. Cancer 1999;86:858–65.

20. Lawrence B, Gustafsson BI, Kidd M, et al. The clinical relevance of chromogranin A as a biomarker for gastroenteropancreatic neuroendocrine tumors. Endocrinol Metab Clin North Am 2011;40:111–34, viii.

21. Yang X, Yang Y, Li Z, et al. Diagnostic value of circulating chromogranin a for neuroendocrine tumors: a systematic review and meta-analysis. PLos One 2015;10:e0124884.

22. Kolby L, Bernhardt P, Sward C, et al. Chromogranin A as a determinant of midgut carcinoid tumour volume. Regul Pept 2004;120:269–73.

23. Stridsberg M, Eriksson B, Fellstrom B, et al. Measurements of chromogranin B can serve as a complement to chromogranin A. Regul Pept 2007;139:80–3.

24. Takiyyuddin MA, Cervenka JH, Hsiao RJ, et al. Storage and release in hypertension. Hypertension 1990;15:237–46.

25. Janson ET, Holmberg L, Stridsberg M, et al. Carcinoid tumors: analysis of prognostic factors and survival in 301 patients from a referral center. Ann Oncol 1997;8:685–90.

26. Jensen EH, Kvols L, McLoughlin JM, et al. Biomarkers predict outcomes following cytoreductive surgery for hepatic metastases from functional carcinoid tumors. Ann Surg Oncol 2007;14:780–5.

27. Tellez MR, Mamikunian G, O'Dorisio TM, et al. A single fasting plasma 5-HIAA value correlates with 24-hour urinary 5-HIAA values and other biomarkers in midgut neuroendocrine tumors (NETs). Pancreas 2013;42:405–10.

28. O'Dorisio TM, Krutzik SR, Woltering EA, et al. Development of a highly sensitive and specific carboxy-terminal human pancreastatin assay to monitor neuroendocrine tumor behavior. Pancreas 2010;39:611–6.

29. Stronge RL, Turner GB, Johnston BT, et al. A rapid rise in circulating pancreastatin in response to somatostatin analogue therapy is associated with poor survival in patients with neuroendocrine tumours. Ann Clin Biochem 2008;45:560–6.

30. Vinik AI, Silva MP, Woltering EA, et al. Biochemical testing for neuroendocrine tumors. Pancreas 2009;38:876–89.

31. Bloomston M, Al-Saif O, Klemanski D, et al. Hepatic artery chemoembolization in 122 patients with metastatic carcinoid tumor: lessons learned. J Gastrointest Surg 2007;11:264–71.

32. Calhoun K, Toth-Fejel S, Cheek J, et al. Serum peptide profiles in patients with carcinoid tumors. Am J Surg 2003;186:28–31.

33. Sherman SK, Maxwell JE, O'Dorisio MS, et al. Pancreastatin predicts survival in neuroendocrine tumors. Ann Surg Oncol 2014;21:2971–80.

34. Turner GB, Johnston BT, McCance DR, et al. Circulating markers of prognosis and response to treatment in patients with midgut carcinoid tumours. Gut 2006;55:1586–91.

35. Kanakis G, Kaltsas G. Biochemical markers for gastroenteropancreatic neuroendocrine tumours (GEP-NETs). Best Pract Res Clin Gastroenterol 2012;26: 791–802.

36. Metz DC, Jensen RT. Gastrointestinal neuroendocrine tumors: pancreatic endocrine tumors. Gastroenterology 2008;135:1469–92.

37. Kloppel G, Anlauf M. Epidemiology, tumour biology and histopathological classification of neuroendocrine tumours of the gastrointestinal tract. Best Pract Res Clin Gastroenterol 2005;19:507–17.

38. Oberg K, Eriksson B. Endocrine tumours of the pancreas. Best Pract Res Clin Gastroenterol 2005;19:753–81.

39. Falconi M, Plockinger U, Kwekkeboom DJ, et al. Well-differentiated pancreatic nonfunctioning tumors/carcinoma. Neuroendocrinology 2006;84:196–211.

40. Liakakos T, Roukos DH. Everolimus and sunitinib: from mouse models to treatment of pancreatic neuroendocrine tumors. Future Oncol 2011;7:1025–9.
41. Ito T, Igarashi H, Jensen RT. Pancreatic neuroendocrine tumors: clinical features, diagnosis and medical treatment: advances. Best Pract Res Clin Gastroenterol 2012;26:737–53.
42. Halfdanarson TR, Rabe KG, Rubin J, et al. Pancreatic neuroendocrine tumors (PNETs): incidence, prognosis and recent trend toward improved survival. Ann Oncol 2008;19:1727–33.
43. Falconi M, Bartsch DK, Eriksson B, et al. ENETS Consensus Guidelines for the management of patients with digestive neuroendocrine neoplasms of the digestive system: well-differentiated pancreatic non-functioning tumors. Neuroendocrinology 2012;95:120–34.
44. Plockinger U, Wiedenmann B. Diagnosis of non-functioning neuro-endocrine gastro-enteropancreatic tumours. Neuroendocrinology 2004;80(Suppl 1):35–8.
45. Jensen RT. Endocrine neoplasms of the pancreas. In: Yamada T, Alpers DH, Kalloo AN, et al, editors. Textbook of gastroenterology. 5th edition. Oxford (England): Wiley-Blackwell; 2009. p. 1875–920.
46. Roberts RE, Zhao M, Whitelaw BC, et al. GLP-1 and glucagon secretion from a pancreatic neuroendocrine tumor causing diabetes and hyperinsulinemic hypoglycemia. J Clin Endocrinol Metab 2012;97:3039–45.
47. Samyn I, Fontaine C, Van TF, et al. Paraneoplastic syndromes in cancer: Case 1. Polycythemia as a result of ectopic erythropoietin production in metastatic pancreatic carcinoid tumor. J Clin Oncol 2004;22:2240–2.
48. Ruddy MC, Atlas SA, Salerno FG. Hypertension associated with a renin-secreting adenocarcinoma of the pancreas. N Engl J Med 1982;307:993–7.
49. Chung JO, Hong SI, Cho DH, et al. Hypoglycemia associated with the production of insulin-like growth factor II in a pancreatic islet cell tumor: a case report. Endocr J 2008;55:607–12.
50. Piaditis G, Angellou A, Kontogeorgos G, et al. Ectopic bioactive luteinizing hormone secretion by a pancreatic endocrine tumor, manifested as luteinized granulosa-thecal cell tumor of the ovaries. J Clin Endocrinol Metab 2005;90:2097–103.
51. Brignardello E, Manti R, Papotti M, et al. Ectopic secretion of LH by an endocrine pancreatic tumor. J Endocrinol Invest 2004;27:361–5.
52. Fleury A, Flejou JF, Sauvanet A, et al. Calcitonin-secreting tumors of the pancreas: about six cases. Pancreas 1998;16:545–50.
53. Schneider R, Waldmann J, Swaid Z, et al. Calcitonin-secreting pancreatic endocrine tumors: systematic analysis of a rare tumor entity. Pancreas 2011;40:213–21.
54. Vinik AI, Strodel WE, Eckhauser FE, et al. Somatostatinomas, PPomas, neurotensinomas. Semin Oncol 1987;14:263–81.
55. Amrilleva V, Slater EP, Waldmann J, et al. A pancreatic polypeptide-producing pancreatic tumor causing WDHA syndrome. Case Rep Gastroenterol 2008;2:238–43.
56. Lundqvist G, Krause U, Larsson LI, et al. A pancreatic-polypeptide-producing tumour associated with the WDHA syndrome. Scand J Gastroenterol 1978;13:715–8.
57. Jensen RT, Berna MJ, Bingham DB, et al. Inherited pancreatic endocrine tumor syndromes: advances in molecular pathogenesis, diagnosis, management, and controversies. Cancer 2008;113:1807–43.
58. Grant CS. Insulinoma. Best Pract Res Clin Gastroenterol 2005;19:783–98.

59. de Herder WW, Niederle B, Scoazec JY, et al. Well-differentiated pancreatic tumor/carcinoma: insulinoma. Neuroendocrinology 2006;84:183–8.
60. Kann PH, Balakina E, Ivan D, et al. Natural course of small, asymptomatic neuroendocrine pancreatic tumours in multiple endocrine neoplasia type 1: an endoscopic ultrasound imaging study. Endocr Relat Cancer 2006;13:1195–202.
61. Won JG, Tseng HS, Yang AH, et al. Clinical features and morphological characterization of 10 patients with noninsulinoma pancreatogenous hypoglycaemia syndrome (NIPHS). Clin Endocrinol (Oxf) 2006;65:566–78.
62. Kaltsas GA, Besser GM, Grossman AB. The diagnosis and medical management of advanced neuroendocrine tumors. Endocr Rev 2004;25:458–511.
63. O'Toole D, Salazar R, Falconi M, et al. Rare functioning pancreatic endocrine tumors. Neuroendocrinology 2006;84:189–95.
64. Kindmark H, Sundin A, Granberg D, et al. Endocrine pancreatic tumors with glucagon hypersecretion: a retrospective study of 23 cases during 20 years. Med Oncol 2007;24:330–7.
65. van Beek AP, de Haas ER, van Vloten WA, et al. The glucagonoma syndrome and necrolytic migratory erythema: a clinical review. Eur J Endocrinol 2004; 151:531–7.
66. Nikou GC, Toubanakis C, Nikolaou P, et al. VIPomas: an update in diagnosis and management in a series of 11 patients. Hepatogastroenterology 2005;52:1259–65.
67. Moayedoddin B, Booya F, Wermers RA, et al. Spectrum of malignant somatostatin-producing neuroendocrine tumors. Endocr Pract 2006;12: 394–400.
68. Tanaka S, Yamasaki S, Matsushita H, et al. Duodenal somatostatinoma: a case report and review of 31 cases with special reference to the relationship between tumor size and metastasis. Pathol Int 2000;50:146–52.
69. Pacak K, Jochmanova I, Prodanov T, et al. New syndrome of paraganglioma and somatostatinoma associated with polycythemia. J Clin Oncol 2013;31: 1690–8.
70. Zhuang Z, Yang C, Lorenzo F, et al. Somatic HIF2A gain-of-function mutations in paraganglioma with polycythemia. N Engl J Med 2012;367:922–30.
71. Vu JP, Wang HS, Germano PM, et al. Ghrelin in neuroendocrine tumors. Peptides 2011;32:2340–7.
72. Chauhan A, Ramirez RA, Stevens MA, et al. Transition of a pancreatic neuroendocrine tumor from ghrelinoma to insulinoma: a case report. J Gastrointest Oncol 2015;6:E34–6.
73. Corbetta S, Peracchi M, Cappiello V, et al. Circulating ghrelin levels in patients with pancreatic and gastrointestinal neuroendocrine tumors: identification of one pancreatic ghrelinoma. J Clin Endocrinol Metab 2003;88:3117–20.
74. Tsolakis AV, Portela-Gomes GM, Stridsberg M, et al. Malignant gastric ghrelinoma with hyperghrelinemia. J Clin Endocrinol Metab 2004;89:3739–44.
75. Taupenot L, Harper KL, O'Connor DT. The chromogranin-secretogranin family. N Engl J Med 2003;348:1134–49.
76. Nobels FR, Kwekkeboom DJ, Bouillon R, et al. Its clinical value as marker of neuroendocrine tumours. Eur J Clin Invest 1998;28:431–40.
77. Panzuto F, Severi C, Cannizzaro R, et al. Utility of combined use of plasma levels of chromogranin A and pancreatic polypeptide in the diagnosis of gastrointestinal and pancreatic endocrine tumors. J Endocrinol Invest 2004;27:6–11.
78. Hart PA, Baichoo E, Bi Y, et al. Pancreatic polypeptide response to a mixed meal is blunted in pancreatic head cancer associated with diabetes mellitus. Pancreatology 2015;15(2):162–6.

79. de Herder WW. Biochemistry of neuroendocrine tumours. Best Pract Res Clin Endocrinol Metab 2007;21:33–41.
80. Carney JA, Go VL, Fairbanks VF, et al. The syndrome of gastric argyrophil carcinoid tumors and nonantral gastric atrophy. Ann Intern Med 1983;99:761–6.
81. Wynick D, Williams SJ, Bloom SR. Symptomatic secondary hormone syndromes in patients with established malignant pancreatic endocrine tumors. N Engl J Med 1988;319:605–7.
82. Jensen RT, Cadiot G, Brandi ML, et al. ENETS Consensus Guidelines for the management of patients with digestive neuroendocrine neoplasms: functional pancreatic endocrine tumor syndromes. Neuroendocrinology 2012;95:98–119.
83. Akerstrom G. Management of carcinoid tumors of the stomach, duodenum, and pancreas. World J Surg 1996;20:173–82.
84. Tomassetti P, Migliori M, Lalli S, et al. Epidemiology, clinical features and diagnosis of gastroenteropancreatic endocrine tumours. Ann Oncol 2001;12(Suppl 2):S95–9.
85. Wang GG, Yao JC, Worah S, et al. Comparison of genetic alterations in neuroendocrine tumors: frequent loss of chromosome 18 in ileal carcinoid tumors. Mod Pathol 2005;18:1079–87.
86. Kytola S, Hoog A, Nord B, et al. Comparative genomic hybridization identifies loss of 18q22-qter as an early and specific event in tumorigenesis of midgut carcinoids. Am J Pathol 2001;158:1803–8.
87. Choi IS, Estecio MR, Nagano Y, et al. Hypomethylation of LINE-1 and Alu in well-differentiated neuroendocrine tumors (pancreatic endocrine tumors and carcinoid tumors). Mod Pathol 2007;20:802–10.
88. Brandi ML, Gagel RF, Angeli A, et al. Guidelines for diagnosis and therapy of MEN type 1 and type 2. J Clin Endocrinol Metab 2001;86:5658–71.
89. Thakker RV. Multiple endocrine neoplasia type 1 (MEN1). Best Pract Res Clin Endocrinol Metab 2010;24:355–70.
90. Toumpanakis CG, Caplin ME. Molecular genetics of gastroenteropancreatic neuroendocrine tumors. Am J Gastroenterol 2008;103:729–32.
91. Capdevila J, Meeker A, Garcia-Carbonero R, et al. Molecular biology of neuroendocrine tumors: from pathways to biomarkers and targets. Cancer Metastasis Rev 2014;33:345–51.
92. Cao Y, Gao Z, Li L, et al. Whole exome sequencing of insulinoma reveals recurrent T372R mutations in YY1. Nat Commun 2013;4:2810.
93. Lewis MA, Yao JC. Molecular pathology and genetics of gastrointestinal neuroendocrine tumours. Curr Opin Endocrinol Diabetes Obes 2014;21:22–7.
94. Banck MS, Kanwar R, Kulkarni AA, et al. The genomic landscape of small intestine neuroendocrine tumors. J Clin Invest 2013;123:2502–8.
95. Jiao Y, Shi C, Edil BH, et al. DAXX/ATRX, MEN1, and mTOR pathway genes are frequently altered in pancreatic neuroendocrine tumors. Science 2011;331:1199–203.
96. Missiaglia E, Dalai I, Barbi S, et al. Pancreatic endocrine tumors: expression profiling evidences a role for AKT-mTOR pathway. J Clin Oncol 2010;28:245–55.
97. Marx SJ, Agarwal SK, Kester MB, et al. Multiple endocrine neoplasia type 1: clinical and genetic features of the hereditary endocrine neoplasias. Recent Prog Horm Res 1999;54:397–438.
98. Giri D, McKay V, Weber A, et al. Multiple endocrine neoplasia syndromes 1 and 2: manifestations and management in childhood and adolescence. Arch Dis Child 2015;100(10):994–9.

99. Piecha G, Chudek J, Wiecek A. Multiple endocrine neoplasia type 1. Eur J Intern Med 2008;19:99–103.

100. Perry R. Multiple endocrine neoplasia type 1 and MEN II. Diffuse hormonal systems and endocrine tumor syndromes. 2006.

101. Lemos MC, Thakker RV. Multiple endocrine neoplasia type 1 (MEN1): analysis of 1336 mutations reported in the first decade following identification of the gene. Hum Mutat 2008;29:22–32.

102. Thakker RV, Newey PJ, Walls GV, et al. Clinical practice guidelines for multiple endocrine neoplasia type 1 (MEN1). J Clin Endocrinol Metab 2012;97:2990–3011.

103. Gagel RF, Levy ML, Donovan DT, et al. Multiple endocrine neoplasia type 2a associated with cutaneous lichen amyloidosis. Ann Intern Med 1989;111:802–6.

104. Borst MJ, VanCamp JM, Peacock ML, et al. Mutational analysis of multiple endocrine neoplasia type 2A associated with Hirschsprung's disease. Surgery 1995;117:386–91.

105. Gertner ME, Kebebew E. Multiple endocrine neoplasia type 2. Curr Treat Options Oncol 2004;5:315–25.

106. Chen H, Sippel RS, O'Dorisio MS, et al. The North American Neuroendocrine Tumor Society consensus guideline for the diagnosis and management of neuroendocrine tumors: pheochromocytoma, paraganglioma, and medullary thyroid cancer. Pancreas 2010;39:775–83.

107. Niederle B, Sebag F, Brauckhoff M. Timing and extent of thyroid surgery for gene carriers of hereditary C cell disease–a consensus statement of the European Society of Endocrine Surgeons (ESES). Langenbecks Arch Surg 2014;399:185–97.

108. Lairmore TC, Ball DW, Baylin SB, et al. Management of pheochromocytomas in patients with multiple endocrine neoplasia type 2 syndromes. Ann Surg 1993;217:595–601.

109. Dromain C, de BT, Lumbroso J, et al. Detection of liver metastases from endocrine tumors: a prospective comparison of somatostatin receptor scintigraphy, computed tomography, and magnetic resonance imaging. J Clin Oncol 2005;23:70–8.

110. Chiti A, Fanti S, Savelli G, et al. Comparison of somatostatin receptor imaging, computed tomography and ultrasound in the clinical management of neuroendocrine gastro-entero-pancreatic tumours. Eur J Nucl Med 1998;25:1396–403.

111. Janson ET, Westlin JE, Ohrvall U, et al. Nuclear localization of 111In after intravenous injection of [111In-DTPA-D-Phe1]-octreotide in patients with neuroendocrine tumors. J Nucl Med 2000;41:1514–8.

112. Gabriel M, Decristoforo C, Kendler D, et al. 68Ga-DOTA-Tyr3-octreotide PET in neuroendocrine tumors: comparison with somatostatin receptor scintigraphy and CT. J Nucl Med 2007;48:508–18.

113. Orlefors H, Sundin A, Garske U, et al. Whole-body (11)C-5-hydroxytryptophan positron emission tomography as a universal imaging technique for neuroendocrine tumors: comparison with somatostatin receptor scintigraphy and computed tomography. J Clin Endocrinol Metab 2005;90:3392–400.

114. Geatti O, Shapiro B, Sisson JC, et al. Iodine-131 metaiodobenzylguanidine scintigraphy for the location of neuroblastoma: preliminary experience in ten cases. J Nucl Med 1985;26:736–42.

115. Doppman JL, Miller DL, Chang R, et al. Gastrinomas: localization by means of selective intraarterial injection of secretin. Radiology 1990;174:25–9.

116. Doppman JL, Chang R, Fraker DL, et al. Localization of insulinomas to regions of the pancreas by intra-arterial stimulation with calcium. Ann Intern Med 1995; 123:269–73.

117. Jackson JE. Angiography and arterial stimulation venous sampling in the localization of pancreatic neuroendocrine tumours. Best Pract Res Clin Endocrinol Metab 2005;19:229–39.

118. Strodel WE, Vinik AI, Jaffe BM, et al. Substance P in the localization of a carcinoid tumor. J Surg Oncol 1984;27:106–11.

119. Ruszniewski P, Delle FG, Cadiot G, et al. Well-differentiated gastric tumors/carcinomas. Neuroendocrinology 2006;84:158–64.

120. Rockall AG, Reznek RH. Imaging of neuroendocrine tumours (CT/MR/US). Best Pract Res Clin Endocrinol Metab 2007;21:43–68.

121. Virgolini I, Traub-Weidinger T, Decristoforo C. Nuclear medicine in the detection and management of pancreatic islet-cell tumours. Best Pract Res Clin Endocrinol Metab 2005;19:213–27.

122. Gibril F, Jensen RT. Diagnostic uses of radiolabelled somatostatin receptor analogues in gastroenteropancreatic endocrine tumours. Dig Liver Dis 2004; 36(Suppl 1):S106–20.

123. Sundin A, Garske U, Orlefors H. Nuclear imaging of neuroendocrine tumours. Best Pract Res Clin Endocrinol Metab 2007;21:69–85.

124. Pavel M, Baudin E, Couvelard A, et al. ENETS Consensus Guidelines for the management of patients with liver and other distant metastases from neuroendocrine neoplasms of foregut, midgut, hindgut, and unknown primary. Neuroendocrinology 2012;95:157–76.

125. Bhattacharyya S, Toumpanakis C, Caplin ME, et al. Usefulness of N-terminal pro-brain natriuretic peptide as a biomarker of the presence of carcinoid heart disease. Am J Cardiol 2008;102:938–42.

126. Lipton A, Costa L, Ali S, et al. Use of markers of bone turnover for monitoring bone metastases and the response to therapy. Semin Oncol 2001;28:54–9.

127. Brown JE, Cook RJ, Major P, et al. Bone turnover markers as predictors of skeletal complications in prostate cancer, lung cancer, and other solid tumors. J Natl Cancer Inst 2005;97:59–69.

Surgical Treatment of Small Bowel Neuroendocrine Tumors

Heather A. Farley, MD[a], Rodney F. Pommier, MD[b],*

KEYWORDS

- Neuroendocrine • Primary tumor • Mesenteric nodal mass • Liver • Metastasis
- Resection • Ablation

KEY POINTS

- Primary tumors tend to remain small and have metastasis, which is different than the typical cancer paradigm.
- Resection of the primary tumor may be associated with improved survival rates, even in the setting of unresectable metastases.
- Tumors tend to metastasize to nodes at the root of the mesentery, resulting in bowel obstruction and ischemia to vital organs. Aggressive resection should be considered.
- Patients with neuroendocrine liver metastases may benefit from an aggressive surgical approach even if they do not receive a complete resection and have extrahepatic disease.
- Radiofrequency ablation is an important adjunct to resection and can be used to help preserve hepatic parenchyma or in patients who are not surgical candidates.

INTRODUCTION: NATURE OF THE PROBLEM

Neuroendocrine tumors of the small bowel (carcinoids) are rare and slow-growing tumors that arise from neuroendocrine cells in the gastrointestinal tract. They have a high propensity to metastasize to nodes at the root of the mesentery and to the liver. They are also capable of producing hormones that, when released from the liver, cause carcinoid syndrome of flushing, diarrhea, and congestive heart failure. Approximately 80% of patients who die of disease die of liver failure, with 16% dying of bowel obstruction. Surgical treatment can have a significant impact on these outcomes as well as relieving symptoms and improving quality of life.

[a] Department of Surgery, Oregon Health & Science University, 3181 Southwest Sam Jackson Park Road, Mail Code L 619, Portland, OR 97329, USA; [b] Division of Surgical Oncology, Oregon Health & Science University, 3181 Southwest Sam Jackson Park Road, Mail Code L 619, Portland, OR 97329, USA
* Corresponding author.
E-mail address: pommierr@ohsu.edu

Hematol Oncol Clin N Am 30 (2016) 49–61
http://dx.doi.org/10.1016/j.hoc.2015.09.001
0889-8588/16/$ – see front matter © 2016 Elsevier Inc. All rights reserved.

THE ALTERNATE TUMOR PARADIGM OF NEUROENDOCRINE TUMORS

Most physicians are trained in the standard cancer paradigm. This paradigm can be represented as a pyramid structure (**Fig. 1**). The cancer originates in the primary tumor, represented by the bottom layer of the pyramid. The primary tumor has to grow to a substantial size before it spreads to the next level, which is lymph node metastases. The volume of the lymph node metastases is expected to remain smaller than that of the primary tumor. There has to be a large primary tumor and a high number of positive lymph nodes before we expect the disease go to the next level, which is distant metastases, represented by the capstone of the pyramid. This is the entire basis of the tumor–nodes–metastases (TNM) staging system. Thus, when patients present with metastatic disease, we expect the primary tumor to be large and easily detectable on physical examination, imaging, or endoscopy. In the unusual cases when it is not, the primary tumor is considered occult and unlikely to ever be found.

Small bowel neuroendocrine tumors follow a different paradigm, represented by an upside-down pyramid (**Fig. 2**). The majority of patients present with numerous liver metastases (**Fig. 3**). Imaging searches for the primary tumor find at most a very large nodal mass at the root of the mesentery with surrounding desmoplastic reaction (**Figs. 4 and 5**), represented by the middle layer of the pyramid. Ironically, the primary tumor that produced such voluminous metastatic liver and nodal disease is still so small (**Fig. 6**), represented by the tip of the upside-down pyramid, that it eludes detection on virtually all localizing tests and examinations. When the search fails to find a primary tumor, physicians subscribing to the standard cancer paradigm conclude that the primary tumor is in fact occult and can never be found. However, with the neuroendocrine tumor paradigm, the primary tumor is actually expected to be small. Importantly, this does not imply that it is truly occult and unable to ever be found.

SUCCESSFULLY LOCATING "OCCULT" PRIMARY NEUROENDOCRINE TUMORS

Our institution published a series of 63 patients presenting with metastatic neuroendocrine tumors.[1] These 63 patients were evaluated with a total of 177 computed tomography scans, MRI scans, gastrointestinal contrast studies, scintigraphy with radiolabeled octreotide (OctreoScans, Mallinckrodt Inc, St. Louis, MO), endoscopies,

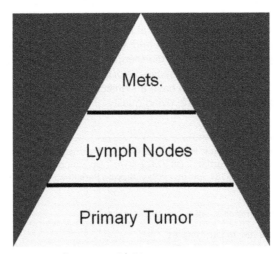

Fig. 1. Standard cancer paradigm pyramid. Mets, metastases.

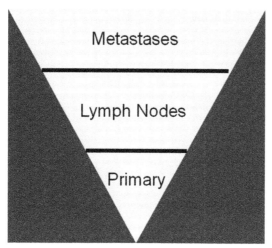

Fig. 2. Neuroendocrine tumor paradigm pyramid.

and capsule videography to search for their primary tumors. Only 6.2% of these tests correctly located a primary tumor. Unfortunately, this true-positive rate was confounded by a false-positive rate nearly as high at 4.7%. However, surgical exploration found the primary tumor in 80% of cases. Eighty percent of the successfully located tumors were found laparoscopically. If tumors were not visualized laparoscopically, the periumbilical incision for the laparoscope was enlarged slightly and the small bowel was eviscerated a few centimeters at a time through that incision, palpated, and replaced. This resulted in finding additional primary tumors not visible by laparoscopy. All tumors would have been found without preoperative knowledge of their location.

PRIMARY TUMOR RESECTION

With most other types of cancer, resecting a primary tumor in the presence of distant metastases does not affect survival, but this may not be the case with small bowel neuroendocrine tumors. One of the first reports of improved outcomes in patients

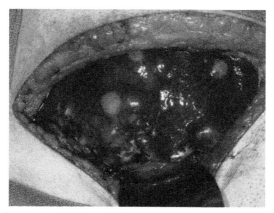

Fig. 3. Numerous liver metastases in a patient with a small bowel neuroendocrine tumor.

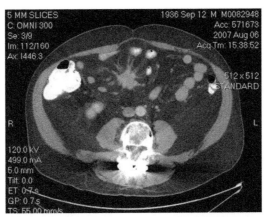

Fig. 4. Computed tomography scan showing classic findings of a large mesenteric nodal mass with desmoplastic reaction at the root of the mesentery.

with metastatic disease came from Hellman and colleagues.[2] They reported 314 patients with small bowel neuroendocrine tumors with mesenteric nodal or liver metastases. Patients whose primary tumors were resected had significantly longer median survival of 7.4 years compared with 4.0 years for those whose primary tumors were not resected. However, there were 65 patients in the series with no liver metastases who were likely in the primary tumor resected group, whereas most of the patients who did not have their primary tumor resected likely had liver metastases. Therefore, it is possible that some of the difference in survival may be owing to a difference in distribution of patients with liver metastases between the 2 comparison groups.

In 2006, our institution reported a group of 84 patients with small bowel neuroendocrine tumors, all of whom had inoperable liver metastases.[3] Sixty patients had their primary tumors resected and 24 did not. The 2 groups were comparable with respect to all other clinical factors examined. Median time to liver progression was 56 months for patients whose primary tumors were resected compared with 25 months for those whose primary tumors were not resected. Furthermore, the median survival of patients whose primary tumors were resected was 159 months compared with 47 months for those whose primary tumors were not resected. Because, unlike in the series reported

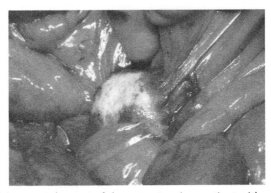

Fig. 5. Large nodal mass at the root of the mesentery in a patient with small bowel neuroendocrine tumor.

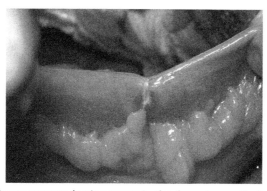

Fig. 6. A small primary neuroendocrine tumor in the ileum in a patient with large mesenteric nodal and extensive liver metastases.

by Hellman and associates, all the patients in this series had inoperable liver metastases, the difference in survival cannot be attributed to lack of liver metastases in some of the patients who underwent primary tumor resection.

In 2009, Ahmed and colleagues[4] published a review of 360 patients from the United Kingdom and Ireland with liver metastases from small bowel neuroendocrine tumors. Primary tumor resection was one of several factors associated with improved survival on univariate analysis. More important, primary tumor resection remained a significant predictor of improved survival on multivariate analysis. The authors concluded that primary tumor resection is an independent factor associated with improved survival in patients with liver metastases.

These data are retrospective and may have been influenced by selection bias and/or referral bias, and it is highly unlikely that randomized prospective data will be forthcoming in the foreseeable future. However, based on the findings of these 3 independent series, we recommend operative exploration to locate and resect primary small bowel neuroendocrine tumors, even among patients with unresectable liver metastases, with the minimal goals of relieving symptoms and preventing future complications and bowel obstruction, even though the data on survival benefit are not definitive. Understandably, there may be hesitance to submit patients with unresectable liver metastases to a major abdominal operation to locate their primary tumor when no target has been identified preoperatively and therefore considered unlikely to be successful. However, as demonstrated in the series from our institution,[1] primary tumors can be located successfully surgically in the vast majority of patients despite extensive negative preoperative testing. Furthermore, it can usually be accomplished laparoscopically or through a very small extension of the periumbilical incision used to insert the laparoscope. These techniques quickly identify patients in whom the primary tumor can actually be located before proceeding with a larger operation. Furthermore, the few patients in whom the primary tumor could not be located all went home the same day with only a small periumbilical incision.[1]

MESENTERIC NODAL MASSES

Despite their small size, small bowel neuroendocrine tumors have a high propensity to metastasize to nodes at the root of the mesentery (see **Figs. 4** and **5**). This region is replete with vital structures, such as the superior mesenteric vein, the superior mesenteric artery, the cysterna chyli, pancreas, and the transverse duodenum.

The volume of tumor in the mesenteric nodes is magnitudes greater than the volume of the primary tumor and produces a correspondingly large volume of hormones that induce an intense desmoplastic reaction and peritoneal fibrosis in the region. The desmoplastic reaction causes shortening, folding, and accordion pleating of the mesentery, creating multiple hairpin turns in the small bowel (**Fig. 7**). Nodal disease can impinge on or encase the superior mesenteric vessels and disrupt the cysterna chyli. It can also impinge on the duodenum and pancreas.

Thus, mesenteric nodal masses can produce a number of clinically challenging problems. Accordion pleating can result in severe abdominal pain after eating and eventually cause small bowel obstruction. Compression of the duodenum can result in duodenal obstruction. Obstruction of the superior mesenteric vein results in the formation of large venous collaterals that predispose patients to gastrointestinal hemorrhage. Encasement of the superior mesenteric vessels can preclude the normal vasodilation that occurs after eating, resulting in intestinal angina. Vascular occlusion can also produce loops of ischemic or infarcted bowel (**Fig. 8**). Accordion pleating, intestinal angina, bowel ischemia, or any combination thereof, can result in "food fear," with patients avoiding food to avoid pain. This avoidance results in weight loss, malnourishment, and nutritional bankruptcy. Disruption of the cysterna chyli can cause chylous ascites.

Accordingly, it is recommended to resect mesenteric nodal masses whenever possible to prevent or relieve these complications. The root of the mesentery is commonly referred to by surgeons as "tiger territory," implying that operating in this region often results in surgical misadventure. Accordingly, many surgeons declare mesenteric nodal masses at the root of the mesentery to be unresectable.

However, mesenteric nodal masses can often be resected while avoiding injury to superior mesenteric vessels, the duodenum, and the pancreas, and limiting bowel resection. Extensive mobilization of the bowel and mesentery is a key to successful resection. Mobilization is begun from the right colic gutter, successively elevating the right colon, cecum, and terminal ileum, permitting elevation of the mesenteric mass off the retroperitoneum. The main trunks of the superior mesenteric artery and vein can be identified crossing the transverse duodenum. The ability to approach the mass from a posterior as well as an anterior aspect allows it to be separated safely from the duodenum and pancreas.

Dividing the mesentery on the proximal and distal sides of the primary tumor (and any ischemic bowel) also releases peritoneal fibrosis and further mobilizes the

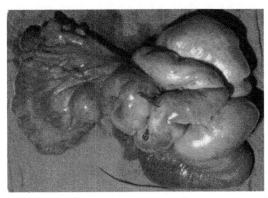

Fig. 7. Hairpin turns in the small bowel from desmoplastic reaction of the mesentery to nodal metastasis.

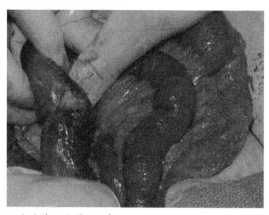

Fig. 8. Primary tumor in ischemic ileum from vascular occlusion caused by mesenteric nodal mass.

mesenteric mass. Using blunt and sharp techniques, the mass can be often be dissected carefully off the vessels.

Outcomes of mesenteric nodal mass resection are very good.[2,5–7] Boudreaux and colleagues[7] reported that, with an aggressive surgical approach, 93% of patients had relief of obstruction and 83% had relief of mesenteric vascular encasement and bowel ischemia. Mean Karnofsky performance status improved from a score of 65 preoperatively to 85 postoperatively, with 5 "terminal" patients rescued. Hellman and colleagues[2] also reported significantly longer survival in patients whose mesenteric nodal masses were resected. Patients may need nutritional rescue before operation, and this may require months of total parenteral nutrition in some cases. Not all patients may benefit from aggressive surgical resection. These results come from major centers with extensive experience at resecting mesenteric nodal masses, exercising careful selection of patients from a population exhibiting a wide spectrum of disease burdens. For example, asymptomatic patients with extensive hepatic metastases may not benefit from an aggressive resection of their mesenteric mass and patients who already have diarrhea from carcinoid syndrome will have a decreased quality of life and performance status if aggressive resection results in substantial loss of bowel, compounding their diarrhea with the addition of short bowel syndrome. Referral to major centers that frequently perform mesenteric mass resections may be advisable for complicated cases.

LIVER METASTASES

With other cancers, the eligibility criteria for liver resection generally are strict. If a complete resection cannot be accomplished, then surgery is not undertaken. This decision is based on outcomes data showing that incomplete resection and positive margins lead to rapid recurrence and poor outcomes. Resection for most cancers should be limited to 1 portion of the liver, leave an adequate hepatic remnant, and have negative margins. Negative margins of resection are required because primary liver tumors and colorectal metastases are infiltrative, with microscopic extensions continuing a considerable distance beyond the grossly visible tumor.

As demonstrated in this review of the literature, these strict criteria do not apply to liver resection for neuroendocrine metastases. Neuroendocrine liver metastases are not infiltrative, but instead expansive, pushing aside the liver parenchyma. This makes it possible to separate tumor masses from the surrounding liver tissue and essentially enucleate them with very little blood loss and sparing liver parenchyma (**Fig. 9**). In

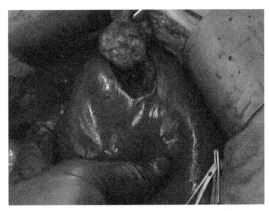

Fig. 9. Enucleation of a small bowel neuroendocrine metastasis from the liver.

reviewing the literature, there is usually no difference in survival outcomes between R0 and R1 resections and major debulking yields equivalent benefit to a complete resection. In addition, the presence of extrahepatic disease is not a contraindication to resection. Most patients die from liver failure and several series demonstrate no difference in survival between patients with or without extrahepatic disease. In addition, patients with functional neuroendocrine liver metastases may experience an improvement in hormonal symptoms after liver resection that is not possible for patients with other types of liver tumors.

Prospective randomized data on the outcomes of surgical treatment of neuroendocrine liver metastases are lacking. Recommendations were based initially on small single institution experiences compared with historical controls. Published series between 1990 and 2001 had small numbers of patients (range, 4–34; mean, 19), and patients usually had complete resections of all liver disease.[8–10] Reported rates of symptomatic relief, were high (88%–100%) and survival rates at 3 to 5 years were encouraging.

McEntee and colleagues[11] were among the first, in 1990, to advocate surgical debulking when at least 90% of the grossly visible metastases could be resected. The chief justification for incomplete resection was relief of hormonal symptoms. Therefore, it would be difficult to justify incomplete resection in patients with nonfunctional tumors.

In 2003, Sarmiento and colleagues[12] published a landmark retrospective series of 170 patients who underwent surgical resection with a debulking threshold of 90% of the grossly visible disease endeavoring to determine if a survival advantage could also be demonstrated. They further endeavored to determine if the operations could be done with acceptable morbidity and mortality.

Their series included patients with liver metastases from carcinoid, pancreatic, and unknown primary tumors. They had functional and nonfunctional tumors and included patients with extrahepatic disease. They found that the major and minor complication rates were 17% and 4%, respectively, and the mortality rate was 1.2%. Ninety-six percent of patients with functional tumors had symptom relief, with a median time to recurrence of 45.5 months. Symptom recurrence rates were lower with complete resection. Tumor progression and recurrence rates, based on imaging or recurrence of symptoms, were high at 84% at 5 years and 95% at 10 years. There were no differences in recurrence rates between small bowel and pancreatic neuroendocrine tumor patients.

The 5- and 10-year overall survival rates were 61% and 35%, respectively, and the median survival was 81 months. No differences in survival rates were noted between patients with pancreatic neuroendocrine tumors and carcinoid tumors or between patients who had functional and nonfunctional tumors. The authors compared their results with historical data from patients with untreated neuroendocrine liver metastases showing 5-year survival rates of 30% to 40% and median survival times of 24 to 48 months. The final conclusion by these authors was that surgical debulking doubled the survival with acceptable morbidity and mortality rates and was justified in these patients.

A similar series was published by Glazer and colleagues[13] in 2010, which demonstrated a complication rate of 24% and no perioperative deaths. The series included 182 patients with carcinoid and pancreatic neuroendocrine liver metastases, 140 of whom underwent some type of hepatic resection. Some patients had radiofrequency ablation (RFA) of some lesions. Forty-nine percent had bilobar disease. No patients had extrahepatic disease. Forty-seven percent had recurrence of their disease. The 5- and 10-year survival rates were 77% and 50%, respectively, and the median survival was 9.6 years. The authors noted that positive margins (R1 or R2) were not associated with significantly worse recurrence-free or overall survival. Thus, the authors concluded that patients with neuroendocrine liver metastases benefit from an aggressive surgical approach, even if they do not undergo complete resection.

Also in 2010, Mayo and colleagues[14] published a review of surgical treatment of neuroendocrine liver metastases by compiling the databases of 8 international major hepatobiliary centers. This large cohort included 339 patients, of whom 40% had pancreatic primaries and 25% had small bowel primaries. Seventy-eight percent of patients had hepatic resection, 3% had ablation, and 19% had hepatic resection combined with ablation. Forty-five percent of hepatic resections were major resections. Sixty percent of patients had bilobar disease. The debulking threshold was not defined, but patients were divided into groups based on whether they had R0, R1, or R2 resections; 19% had R2 resections.

Ninety-four percent of patients had recurrence at 5 years. The 5- and 10-year overall survival rates were 74% and 51%, respectively, and the median survival was 125 months. This median survival time was therefore more than 3 times that of the historical median survival times in patients with untreated neuroendocrine liver metastases with which Sarmiento and colleagues[12] compared their results. Patients with functional tumors and R0 or R1 resections derived the most benefit from surgery. On multivariate analysis, synchronous liver metastases, nonfunctional tumors, and extrahepatic disease were significantly associated with decreased survival. However, survival rates for those groups were still very good. Median survival time for patients with extrahepatic disease was 85 months. The median survival time for patients with nonfunctional tumors and R2 resections, a combination of 2 adverse factors, was in excess of 84 months.

In an effort to expand the pool of patients with neuroendocrine liver metastases eligible for liver debulking, our institution published a series of 52 carcinoid patients in whom the eligibility criteria were expanded to include a debulking threshold of 70%, allowing positive margins, and allowing extrahepatic disease.[15] Ninety percent of patients had bilobar disease. Sixty-five percent had extrahepatic disease, and 35% still had extrahepatic disease after operation. The mean number of tumors resected per patient was 22 (range, 1–131) **(Fig. 10)**. Many patients also had their primary tumor located and resected and their mesenteric nodal mass resected at the same operation. More than 200 resected metastases were graded histologically and 33% of patients had at least 1 intermediate grade metastasis despite all reviewed primary tumors being low grade.

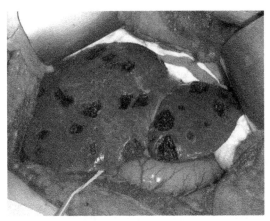

Fig. 10. A liver with 42 metastases removed without major hepatic resection.

The median time to liver progression was 71.6 months. Progression did not correlate with the number or size of tumors resected, grade of metastases, type of hepatic resection, percentage of disease debulked, or the presence of extrahepatic disease. The only factor that correlated with time to liver progression was age. Patients younger than 50 years of age had a median time to liver progression of 39 months, whereas the median time to liver progression in patients age 50 and older had not been reached.

The 5-year disease-specific survival rate was 90%. All disease-specific deaths were owing to liver failure; no patient died of extrahepatic disease. Again, none of the clinical or pathologic factors correlated with survival, except age. Patients younger than 50 years of age had a 5-year survival rate of 73%, similar to the overall 5-year survival rates reported in many of series reported. However, the 5-year survival rate for patients age 50 and older was a remarkable 97%.

The complication rates for hepatic resection have generally been reported to be 16% to 24%. The most commonly reported complications are hemorrhage, bile leak, intraabdominal abscess, pleural effusion, cardiac arrhythmia, and urinary tract infection.[12–14]

Again, these data are retrospective and definitive randomized prospective data are unlikely to be forthcoming in the foreseeable future. The importance of clinical judgment and appropriate patient selection in these series is emphasized.

RADIOFREQUENCY ABLATION

RFA is another technique used to treat neuroendocrine metastases to the liver, but it has limitations. One can ablate a limited number of lesions (generally ≤5) of limited size (generally <5 cm in diameter), provided they are not in close proximity to major hepatic veins and portal radicals. Usually, lesions that fit those criteria can be surgically resected, so it is not preferred over surgery unless the patient is not a good candidate for surgery. In such cases, the procedure can be performed by an interventional radiologist. Its greatest utility is in patients as an adjunct to when there is a significant metastasis in the hepatic remnant that would also require major resection. RFA can be used to still meet the debulking threshold without further resection. It is also useful in patients with inadequate hepatic reserves for resection, where it can be done open or laparoscopically.[16,17]

Data on treating neuroendocrine liver metastases by RFA alone indicate it is well tolerated with a 4% to 5% morbidity rate. Complications include bleeding, wound infections, pneumonias, urinary tract infections, and liver abscess. Mean hospital stay for RFA is 1.1 days.[17] Some degree of subjective relief of symptoms is reported in up to 95% of patients,[9] with significant symptom relief occurring in 70% to 80% of patients.[9,10] Sixty-five percent to 75% of patients show reduction in their tumor markers, such as 24-hour urinary 5-hydroxyindoleacetic acid or serum chromogranin A levels.[18] Survival data for patients with neuroendocrine tumors treated primarily by RFA are scant, but the Cleveland Clinic group reports a median survival time of 3.9 years from the time of first ablation among 63 patients undergoing 80 ablation procedures.[17]

The real usefulness of RFA in the treatment of neuroendocrine liver metastases for surgeons is as an adjunct to surgical resection. As seen in the surgical series reviewed herein, it is sometimes combined with surgical resection. The greatest usefulness of the technique comes in cases in which substantial liver debulking requires a major hepatic resection, yet there is a lesion or lesions deep in the future hepatic remnant that would also require a major hepatic resection. RFA offers a reasonable way to still achieve the debulking goal and not compromise the hepatic remnant.

PROPHYLACTIC CHOLECYSTECTOMY

Prophylactic cholecystectomy is recommended during any abdominal operation in patients with liver metastases.[19] Somatostatin analogs, which cause cholestasis and the formation of gallstones, are given to most patients with liver metastases and cholecystectomy avoids potential complications.

SUMMARY

Typically, the paradigm for cancer and the presence or absence of metastasis relates to the primary tumor size; larger primaries have a greater risk of metastases. Small bowel neuroendocrine primaries do not follow this paradigm and tend to remain small while there is metastatic disease. The treatment parameters differ as well. There is evidence that primary tumor resection is associated with improved survival rates, even in the setting of unresectable metastases. Metastasis tends to be to nodes at the root of the mesentery and the liver. The mesentery reacts to the local hormonal effects, creating a large amount of fibrosis. This results in bowel obstruction and vascular impingement to vital structures. Resection can be challenging, but an aggressive surgical approach is recommended. Criteria for liver resection also differ from standard criteria. Incomplete resection can improve symptoms and survival. Enucleation of liver lesions can spare liver parenchyma and decrease blood loss compared with major hepatic resections with wide margins required for other tumors. RFA is a useful adjunct to operative resection to achieve the debulking threshold without compromising the hepatic remnant. Unfortunately, many patients liver metastasis and extrahepatic disease are deemed unresectable inappropriately. Failure to consult a surgeon familiar with these principles could result in denial of appropriate treatment.[20] Application of these principles could greatly expand the pool of eligible patients for liver debulking surgery.

A better understanding of the principles outlined in this article will hopefully lead to appropriate treatment of patients with small bowel neuroendocrine tumors, which will result in improved quality of life and increased survival.

REFERENCES

1. Massimino KP, Han E, Pommier SJ, et al. Laparoscopic surgical exploration is an effective strategy for location occult primary neuroendocrine tumors. Am J Surg 2012;203(5):628–31.
2. Hellman P, Lundstrom T, Ohrvall U, et al. Effect of surgery on outcome of midgut carcinoid disease with lymph node and liver metastases. World J Surg 2002;26: 991–7.
3. Givi B, Pommier SJ, Thompson AK, et al. Operative resection of primary carcinoid neoplasms in patients with liver metastases yields significantly better survival. Surgery 2006;140:891–8.
4. Ahmed A, Turner G, King B, et al. Midgut neuroendocrine tumours with liver metastases: results of the UKINETS study. Endocr Relat Cancer 2009;16: 885–94.
5. Akerstrom G, Hellman P, Hessman O, et al. Management of midgut carcinoids. J Surg Oncol 2005;89:161–9.
6. Chamber AJ, Pasieka JL, Dixon E, et al. The palliative benefit of aggressive surgical intervention for both hepatic and mesenteric metastases from neuroendocrine tumors. Surgery 2008;144:645–54.
7. Boudreaux JP, Putty B, Frey DJ, et al. Surgical treatment of advanced stage carcinoid tumor: lessons learned. Am J Surg 2005;241:839–45.
8. Chen H, Hardacre JM, Uzar A, et al. Isolated liver metastases from neuroendocrine tumors: does resection prolong survival? J Am Coll Surg 1998;187: 88–93.
9. Chamberlain RS, Canes D, Brown KT, et al. Hepatic neuroendocrine metastases: does intervention alter outcomes? J Am Coll Surg 2000;190:432–45.
10. Yao KA, Talamonti MS, Nemcek A, et al. Indications and results of liver resection and hepatic chemoembolization for metastatic gastrointestinal neuroendocrine tumors. Surgery 2001;130:677–85.
11. McEntee GP, Nagorney DM, Brown KT, et al. Cytoreductive hepatic surgery for neuroendocrine tumors. Surgery 1990;108:1091–6.
12. Sarmiento JM, Heywood G, Rubin J, et al. Surgical treatment of neuroendocrine metastases to the liver; a plea for resection to increase survival. J Am Coll Surg 2003;197:29–37.
13. Glazer ES, Tseng JF, Al-Refaie W, et al. Long-term survival after surgical management of neuroendocrine hepatic metastases. HPB (Oxford) 2010;12: 427–33.
14. Mayo SC, de Jong MC, Pulitano C, et al. Surgical management of hepatic neuroendocrine tumor metastasis: results from an international multi-institutional analysis. Ann Surg Oncol 2010;17:3129–36.
15. Graff-Baker AN, Sauer DA, Pommier SJ, et al. Expanded criteria for carcinoid liver debulking: maintaining survival and increasing the number of eligible patients. Surgery 2014;156:1369–77.
16. Berber E, Flesher N, Siperstein AE. Laparoscopic radiofrequency ablation of neuroendocrine liver metastases. World J Surg 2002;26(8):985–90.
17. Mazzaglina PJ, Berber E, Milas M, et al. Laparoscopic radiofrequency ablation of neuroendocrine liver metastases: a 10-year experience evaluation predictors of survival. Surgery 2007;142(1):10–9.
18. Eriksson J, Stålberg P, Nilsson A, et al. Surgery and radiofrequency ablation for treatment of liver metastases from midgut and foregut carcinoids and endocrine pancreatic tumors. World J Surg 2008;32(5):930–8.

19. Boudreaux JP, Klimstra DS, Hassan MM, et al. The NANETS consensus guideline for the diagnosis and management of neuroendocrine tumors: well-differentiated neuroendocrine tumors of the jejunum, ileum, appendix, and cecum. Pancreas 2010;39:753–66.
20. Kelz RR, Fraker DL. Metastatic carcinoid: don't forget the surgical consultation. Surgery 2014;156:1367–8.

Systemic Therapies for Advanced Gastrointestinal Carcinoid Tumors

Claire K. Mulvey, MD[a], Emily K. Bergsland, MD[b],*

KEYWORDS

- Gastrointestinal neuroendocrine tumors • Somatostatin analogues
- Carcinoid syndrome • Carcinoid tumor
- Mammalian target of rapamycin (mTOR) pathway

KEY POINTS

- Low- and intermediate-grade neuroendocrine tumors are an indolent group of malignancies that can cause symptoms from hormone hypersecretion and/or tumor mass.
- Somatostatin analogues are the mainstay of therapy for the control of symptoms associated with carcinoid syndrome.
- Systemic treatment of advanced disease remains a challenge; only somatostatin analogues have proven antitumor activity in advanced gastrointestinal neuroendocrine tumors.
- Gastrointestinal neuroendocrine tumors represent an active area of research. Clinical trials with peptide receptor radionuclide therapy, inhibitors of the mammalian target of rapamycin and vascular endothelial growth factor signaling pathways, immunotherapy, and other therapeutic approaches are ongoing.
- Improved understanding of the underlying molecular biology may lead to additional treatment advances.

INTRODUCTION

Neuroendocrine tumors (NETs) are a relatively rare, heterogeneous group of neoplasms arising nearly anywhere in the body with an annual incidence of 5 cases per 100,000 people in the United States.[1] The updated World Health Organization

Disclosures: C.K. Mulvey has no conflict of interests to disclose. E.K. Bergsland has received support for clinical trials from Novartis Oncology, Genentech BioOncology/Roche, and Lexicon Pharmaceuticals, Inc. She has served as an advisor (uncompensated) for Ipsen Biopharmaceuticals, Inc and Genentech BioOncology.
[a] Department of Medicine, University of California, San Francisco, 505 Parnassus Avenue, Box 0119, San Francisco, CA 94143, USA; [b] Division of Hematology/Oncology, Department of Medicine, University of California, San Francisco, 1600 Divisadero Street, A727, San Francisco, CA 94115, USA
* Corresponding author.
E-mail address: emily.bergsland@ucsf.edu

Hematol Oncol Clin N Am 30 (2016) 63–82
http://dx.doi.org/10.1016/j.hoc.2015.09.002
0889-8588/16/$ – see front matter © 2016 Elsevier Inc. All rights reserved.

classification system of gastroenteropancreatic NETs emphasizes the tumor site of origin, clinical syndrome, and degree of differentiation when categorizing these malignancies. Well-differentiated NETs (formerly known as carcinoid tumors) arising from the tubular gastrointestinal tract tend to be indolent and slow growing, in contrast to poorly differentiated neuroendocrine carcinomas (NECs), which are more aggressive and associated with a poor prognosis. The treatment of well-differentiated NETs depends on the presence of symptoms and the tumor site of origin. Pancreatic NETs are distinguished from nonpancreatic gastrointestinal NETs (GINETs) given evidence suggesting a differential response to therapy and differences in the molecular underpinnings of each disease.

Somatostatin analogues (SSAs) continue to play a key role in controlling hormone-mediated symptoms. In addition, clinical trials completed in the last decade have definitively demonstrated the antitumor properties of these agents in patients with advanced disease. Based on an improved understanding of the mechanisms underlying NET tumor progression, several novel therapeutic targets have been identified, including the vascular endothelial growth factor (VEGF) and mammalian target of rapamycin (mTOR) signaling pathways. Therapeutic clinical trials of novel agents are ongoing, but none has been definitively validated in GINETs. As a result, the systemic treatment of unresectable disease remains a challenge, and there is a significant unmet medical need for additional systemic treatments.

SYSTEMIC THERAPY FOR THE CONTROL OF SYMPTOMS FROM HORMONE HYPERSECRETION
Somatostatin Analogues

GINETs can be classified as functional or nonfunctional. Nonfunctional tumors do not secrete hormones and present with symptoms from tumor mass and growth, such as obstruction, abdominal pain, and bleeding. Functional tumors can secrete several biologically active hormones and peptides, including serotonin, histamine, amines, and prostaglandins. Carcinoid syndrome is an uncommon, but potentially dramatic manifestation of functional GINETs, affecting approximately 20% of patients with advanced well-differentiated tumors of the jejunum or ileum.[2] The symptoms are intermittent, attributable to hormonal hypersecretion, and may include flushing, diarrhea, rhinorrhea, wheezing, and ultimately can result in right-sided valvular heart disease. Most GINETs are associated with carcinoid syndrome only after they have metastasized to the liver, as hormones produced by tumor cells (most commonly serotonin) can be released directly into the systemic circulation, thus bypassing hepatic metabolism.[3]

For patients with hormone-mediated symptoms from a GINET, therapy with a somatostatin analogue (SSA) is appropriate. Somatostatin is a small, 14-amino acid peptide that inhibits the secretion and synthesis of many gastrointestinal (GI) hormones. Effects of native somatostatin include inhibition of endocrine and exocrine secretion, gastric and intestinal motility, gallbladder contraction, angiogenesis, and cell proliferation. Somatostatin's effects are mediated through 5 high-affinity G-protein coupled receptors. Most GINETs express a receptor for somatostatin, and somatostatin analogues have been shown to be highly effective at controlling the debilitating symptoms of NETs.[4] The 2 synthetic SSAs that are used clinically, octreotide and lanreotide, have significantly longer half-lives than native somatastatin, which has a half-life of approximately 1 to 2 minutes. These analogues have high affinity for somatostatin receptor 2 and 5, in particular. The antisecretory effect of somatostatin has made SSA essential for managing GINETs.

Approximately 50% to 90% of patients experience improvement in hormone-mediated symptoms (carcinoid syndrome) as a result of SSA therapy.[5–10] Octreotide has been approved by the US Food and Drug Administration (FDA) for this indication.[11] Lanreotide autogel is also a long-acting SSA. Its receptor binding profile is similar to that of octreotide, but it is administered as a depot deep subcutaneous injection (every 4 weeks).[12] Both octreotide LAR (long-acting release) and lanreotide afford an approximately 70% symptomatic response rate overall.[13] Although there is no standard protocol preoperative administration of octreotide can reduce the incidence of carcinoid crisis and is recommended for patients with a history of carcinoid syndrome who undergo surgical procedures or related interventions.[14,15] It remains unclear whether the use of SSA therapy per se can inhibit or reverse the progression of carcinoid heart disease.[16]

Additional SSAs with broader receptor binding profiles are currently in development. Pasireotide has increased affinity for receptor subtypes 1, 3, and 5 compared with other somatostatin analogues, which preferentially target receptor subtype 2. In 1 study, pasireotide 600 to 900 μg subcutaneously twice daily controlled the symptoms of diarrhea and flushing in 27% of patients who had refractory symptoms despite octreotide LAR.[17] However, a phase III study that compared pasireotide with octreotide LAR in patients with inadequate symptom control despite maximum doses of somatostatin analogues was terminated early because of futility with regard to incremental impact on symptom control.[18] However, as discussed later, there is still interest in the potential antitumor activity of pasireotide.

Tryptophan Hydroxylase Inhibitors

Some patients with carcinoid syndrome have residual symptoms despite the use of somatostatin analogues, so there has been interest in developing alternative strategies for reducing serotonin-mediated resulting from functional tumors. Telotristat is an oral small-molecule inhibitor of the enzyme tryptophan hydroxylase, which catalyzes the conversion of tryptophan to 5-hydroxytryptophan, the rate-limiting step in the synthesis of serotonin. Telotristat is designed to inhibit peripheral serotonin synthesis without altering brain serotonin levels. The TELESTAR randomized phase III trial enrolled patients with refractory diarrhea despite being on a stable dose of SSA. Recently released results suggest that telotristat reduces the average number of bowel movements in patients with NET compared with placebo.[19] Several other clinical trials are ongoing to assess the usefulness of telotristat and other novel formulations of somatostatin analogues (**Table 1**) to treat patients with refractory symptoms.

Interferon

Before SSAs were widely available, interferon was shown to reduce the symptoms of carcinoid syndrome in roughly 30% to 70% of patients (with some studies suggesting a superior effect on flushing compared with diarrhea).[20–22] However, routine use of interferon for symptom control is limited by its relatively unfavorable side-effect profile (including fatigue, depression, myelosuppression, weight loss, flulike syndrome, and thyroid abnormalities). Instead, interferon alpha is typically reserved for patients with advanced GINETs with inadequate symptom control on SSAs or patients who are intolerant of SSAs.[23]

SYSTEMIC THERAPY FOR THE CONTROL OF TUMOR GROWTH
Somatostatin Analogues

In addition to controlling symptoms, SSAs have also been shown to inhibit the growth of well-differentiated GI and pancreatic NETs. Somatostatin inhibits the production of

Table 1
Ongoing clinical trials for supportive care for patients with well-differentiated neuroendocrine tumors

Study ID	Phase	Study Arms	Outcome	Condition	Sponsor
Telotristat Etiprate for Carcinoid Syndrome Therapy (TELECAST)[a]	III randomized	Telotristat vs placebo[b]	Incidence of treatment-emergent adverse events and urine 5-HIAA levels	Well-differentiated NETs with a history of carcinoid syndrome refractory to stable somatostatin analogue therapy	Lexicon Pharmaceuticals
TELESTAR (Telotristat Etiprate for Somatostatin Analogue Not Adequately Controlled Carcinoid Syndrome)[a]	III randomized	Telotristat vs placebo; both in addition to somatostatin analogue[b]	Incidence of adverse events and number of bowel movements	Well-differentiated NETs with a history of carcinoid syndrome refractory to stable somatostatin analogue therapy	Lexicon Pharmaceuticals
An Efficacy and Safety Study of Somatuline Depot (Lanreotide) Injection to Treat Carcinoid Syndrome (ELECT)[a]	III randomized	Lanreotide depot vs placebo[b]	Use of rescue octreotide to control symptoms	Carcinoid (including unknown primary) with carcinoid syndrome (flushing ± diarrhea); treatment naive or responsive to octreotide	Beaufour Ipsen International SNC
Telotristat Etiprate - Expanded Treatment for Patients With Carcinoid Syndrome Symptoms (TELEPATH)	III	Telotristat	Long-term extension study of adverse events	Patients with well-differentiated NETs with a history of carcinoid syndrome who are participating in other trials of telotristat	Lexicon Pharmaceuticals
Phase II Study of Subcutaneous Injection Depot of Octreotide in Patients With Acromegaly and Neuroendocrine Tumors	II	Two doses of CAM2029 (octreotide FluidCrystal injection depot)	Pharmacokinetic study with secondary outcomes of adverse events and symptom relief	Acromegaly or a functional, well-differentiated NET, with carcinoid symptoms despite octreotide LAR	Camurus AB

[a] Enrollment completed, results not yet published.
[b] Randomized, placebo-controlled trial.
Data from http://www.clinicaltrials.gov. Accessed June, 2015.

growth factors and hormones that promote tumor growth through paracrine and autocrine pathways, blocking tumor cell proliferation, invasion, and tumor angiogenesis, along with induction of apoptosis.[24] Somatostatin seems to directly inhibit tumor growth and metastatic spread through the 5 somatostatin receptor subtypes, which are expressed by both tumor cells and endothelial cells in the tumor microenvironment.

The results of the PROMID (Placebo controlled, double blind, prospective, Randomized study on the effect of octreotide LAR in the control of tumor growth in patients with metastatic neuroendocrine MIDgut tumors) trial demonstrated that octreotide slows progression of midgut NETs compared with placebo in treatment-naive patients. Use of octreotide LAR 30 mg monthly improved median time to tumor progression from 6 months in the placebo group to 14.3 months in the treatment group.[25] Both functional and nonfunctional tumors seemed to benefit. In 2014, results from the Controlled Study of Lanreotide Antiproliferative Response in Neuroendocrine Tumors (CLARINET) study were published. Treatment with extended-release lanreotide treatment resulted in prolonged progression-free survival (PFS) compared with placebo (median PFS, 18 months v NR [versus not reached]) in metastatic, nonfunctional, well-differentiated, and moderately differentiated GI and pancreatic NETs.[26] As a result, lanreotide was approved by the FDA for tumor control in GINETs and pancreatic NETs. The most common side effect was mild diarrhea in 26% of patients, followed by abdominal pain and gallstones. Serious side effects were rare.

An exploratory post hoc data analysis of the negative phase III study originally designed to evaluate the effect of pasireotide on carcinoid symptoms demonstrated that pasireotide LAR increased PFS by 5 months, suggesting potential antitumor activity.[18] A follow-up phase II clinical trial in treatment-naive patients with metastatic grade 1 or 2 NETs demonstrated a median PFS of 11 months with pasireotide LAR.[27] There was a high incidence of hyperglycemia (14% grade 3 hyperglycemia), raising concerns about the suitability of pasireotide as a first-line agent. Another prospective open-label phase II clinical trial (COOPERATE-2) examined the effects of pasireotide in combination with everolimus compared with everolimus alone in advanced, progressive pancreatic NETs. The addition of pasireotide did not seem to improve tumor control.[28] See **Table 2** for a list of ongoing clinical trials with pasireotide and other somatostatin analogues.

Interferon

Interferon receptors are expressed by GINETs.[29] After binding to its receptor, interferon initiates a signal transduction cascade and exerts antitumor effects through a variety of mechanisms, including stimulation of T cells, induction of cell cycle arrest, and/or inhibition of angiogenesis.[30,31] Several studies have been conducted comparing SSAs with or without interferon alpha. The results of 1 small study suggested prolonged 5-year survival in the combination group, but this difference was not statistically significant.[32] Another 3-arm trial compared lanreotide alone, interferon alone, or combination therapy; tumor progression rates were essentially identical in all arms.[33] A third randomized trial of 109 patients compared octreotide alone or in combination with interferon and demonstrated a nonsignificant increase in survival with the combination.[34] Response rates across all arms were generally low. Taken together, the data preclude making definitive conclusions about the antitumor effects of interferon. Thus, the role for interferon remains controversial in GINETs and its use is typically reserved for SSA-refractory disease.

Table 2
Selected ongoing clinical trials of somatostatin analogues in well-differentiated neuroendocrine tumors

Study ID	Phase	Outcome	Population	Sponsors
Study to Allow Access to Pasireotide for Patients Benefiting From Pasireotide Treatment in a Novartis-sponsored Study	IV	Number of patients receiving pasireotide; adverse events	Patients who completed a previous Novartis-sponsored Pasireotide study	Novartis Pharmaceuticals Corporation
A Study Evaluating Lanreotide as Maintenance Therapy in Patients With Non-Resectable Duodeno-Pancreatic Neuroendocrine Tumors (REMINET)[a]	II/III randomized	PFS at 6 mo	Advanced well-differentiated duodenopancreatic NETs; patients who progressed after first-line treatment with either chemotherapy or biotherapy	Federation Francophone de Cancerologie Digestive
Study of Pasireotide Long Acting Release (LAR) in Patients With Metastatic Neuroendocrine Tumors (NETs)[b]	II	PFS	Locally unresectable or metastatic carcinoid or pancreatic NETs	H. Lee Moffitt Cancer Center and Research Institute at University of South Florida; Novartis Pharmaceuticals Corporation
Study of Pasireotide in Patients With Rare Tumors of Neuroendocrine Origin[b]	II	Change in primary tumor biomarkers	Rare tumors of neuroendocrine origin (including pancreatic neuroendocrine)	Novartis Pharmaceuticals Corporation
Combination of Lanreotide Autogel 120 mg and Temozolomide in Progressive GEP-NET (SONNET)	II	Disease control rate at 6 mo	Low- or intermediate- grade gastroenteropancreatic NET	Ipsen
Safety and Tolerability of Pasireotide LAR in Combination With Everolimus in Advanced Metastatic NETs (COOPERATE-1)[c]	I	Safety and tolerability	Grade 1 or 2 advanced pulmonary or gastroenteropancreatic NETs	Novartis Pharmaceuticals Corporation
Dose Escalation Study of Pasireotide (SOM230) in Patients With Advanced Neuroendocrine Tumors (NETs)[b]	I	Pharmacokinetic/safety study	Well-differentiated or moderately differentiated NETs	Novartis Pharmaceuticals Corporation

[a] Randomized, placebo-controlled trial.
[b] Enrollment completed, trial ongoing.
[c] Study completed, results not published.
Data from http://www.clinicaltrials.gov. Accessed June, 2015.

Everolimus

Small-molecule tyrosine inhibitors are a class of targeted therapies that hold promise for the treatment of GINETs. mTOR is a serine-threonine kinase that regulates cell growth, proliferation, and survival signaling in response to metabolic factors.[35] mTOR mediates downstream signaling in several growth factor pathways active in NETs, including the VEGF and insulinlike growth factor signaling pathways.[36] In addition, mTOR regulates angiogenesis by controlling the production of hypoxia inducible factor. Overactivation of the mTOR pathway by hyperphosphorylation has been demonstrated in some well-differentiated NETs,[37–39] and inhibition of the mTOR pathway has antiproliferative effects in NET cell lines in vitro.[38,40] As a result, there has been interest in developing inhibitors of mTOR as a novel treatment mechanism for advanced GINETs.

Everolimus (also known as RAD001) is an oral mTOR inhibitor that is already FDA-approved for the treatment of panNETs based on improvements in PFS.[41] Treatment with everolimus showed a trend toward improved PFS in the randomized phase III RADIANT-2 study of 429 patients with advanced nonpancreatic NETs, a history of carcinoid syndrome, and radiologic disease procession.[42] An investigator-initiated exploratory analysis that corrected for randomization imbalances found that everolimus plus octreotide reduced the risk of progression by 38% compared with octreotide alone, but the drug has not yet been approved by the FDA for this indication.[43] There were also discordances between the central and investigator (local) radiologic review, highlighting the challenges associated with interpreting cross-sectional imaging of highly vascular GINETs and resulting in significant censoring for the final analysis, thus reducing the total number of events and the statistical power for the primary end point. There was no significant difference in overall survival between the 2 groups. However, patients who were randomized to placebo were permitted to cross over into the active treatment group, confounding interpretation of the survival data.

A follow-up phase III study in 279 patients with advanced, progressive low-grade or intermediate-grade, nonfunctional NETs of GI or lung origin has been completed (RADIANT-4). Patients were randomized to either everolimus 10 mg daily or placebo. Recently reported results suggest that everolimus extends PFS in these patients, but the drug is not yet approved for this indication.[44] Several other clinical trials are ongoing in patients with low-grade or intermediate-grade GINETs (**Table 3**).

Vascular Endothelial Growth Factor Inhibitors

NETs are among the most highly vascular solid tumors. Frequently, NETs express VEGF, a potent regulator of tumor angiogenesis and its receptors; expression has been linked to metastases and decreased PFS.[45] Disruption of the VEGF signaling pathway is a promising treatment strategy for GINETs. In preclinical models, inhibition of the VEGF pathway inhibits NET cell growth and metastasis.[46] However, emerging data from clinical trials with VEGF pathway inhibitors in GINETS suggest that these agents are cytostatic—generally leading to disease stabilization, not shrinkage (and associated with a low radiographic response rate). This suggests that PFS may be a better outcome measure than radiographic response when evaluating VEGF inhibitors in GINETs. The use of adequate controls is also critically important given the potential for well-differentiated NETs to progress slowly even in untreated patients. Several tyrosine kinase inhibitors and antibody-based strategies have been or are under evaluation in clinical trials (see **Table 3**).

Bevacizumab was evaluated in a phase II trial of 44 patients with advanced GINETs randomized to bevacizumab or pegylated interferon alpha-2b for 18 weeks, after which they received both agents in combination.[47] Rates of PFS after 18 weeks of

Table 3
Targeted therapies for well-differentiated neuroendocrine tumors: selected ongoing trials of VEGF inhibitors, mTOR inhibitors, and novel therapeutic targets

Study ID	Phase	Study Arms	Population	Sponsors
mTOR inhibitors				
Everolimus Roll-over Protocol for Patients Who Have Completed a Previous Novartis-sponsored Everolimus Study	IV	Everolimus	Patients receiving everolimus in a Novartis-sponsored, Oncology Clinical Development & Medical Affairs study	Novartis Pharmaceuticals Corporation
Everolimus Plus Best Supportive Care vs Placebo Plus Best Supportive Care in the Treatment of Patients With Advanced Neuroendocrine Tumors (GI or Lung Origin) (RADIANT-4)[c]	III randomized	Everolimus vs placebo[b]	Advanced, well-differentiated gastrointestinal or lung NETs	Novartis Pharmaceuticals Corporation
Phase II Study of Everolimus Combined With Octreotide LAR to Treat Advanced GI NET (EVERLAR)[a]	II	Everolimus and octreotide LAR combination	Advanced, nonfunctioning, well-differentiated GINETs	Grupo Espanol de Tumores Neuroendocrinos
Study of Everolimus Treatment in Newly-diagnosed Patients With Advanced Gastrointestinal Neuroendocrine Tumors	II	Everolimus	Well-differentiated or moderately differentiated advanced (metastatic or unresectable) gastrointestinal or pancreatic NETs	Hellenic Cooperative Oncology Group
RAMSETE: RAD001 in Advanced and Metastatic Silent Neuro-endocrine Tumors in Europe (RAMSETE/CDE16)[a]	II	Everolimus	Progressive, low- or intermediate-grade, nonfunctional, nonpancreatic NET	Novartis Pharmaceuticals Corporation
Safety and Tolerability of Pasireotide LAR in Combination With Everolimus in Advanced Metastatic NETs (COOPERATE-1)[c]	I	Pasireotide in combination with everolimus	Grade 1 or 2 advanced pulmonary or gastroenteropancreatic NET	Novartis Pharmaceuticals Corporation
Pasireotide in Combination With RAD001 in Patients With Advanced Neuroendocrine Tumors[a]	I	Pasireotide in combination with Everolimus	Low-grade or intermediate-grade locally unresectable or metastatic NETs	Dana-Farber Cancer Institute; Beth Israel Deaconess Medical Center; Brigham and Women's Hospital; Massachusetts General Hospital; Novartis
Cixutumumab, Everolimus, and Depot Octreotide Acetate in Patients With Advanced Low- to Intermediate-Grade Neuroendocrine Carcinoma[a]	I	Combination of cixutumumab, everolimus, and octreotide	Low- or intermediate-grade neuroendocrine carcinoma	M.D. Anderson Cancer Center at University of Texas; National Cancer Institute

VEGF inhibitors

Title	Phase	Treatment	Description	Sponsor
Pazopanib Hydrochloride in Treating Patients With Progressive Carcinoid Tumors (A021202)	II randomized	Pazopanib vs placebo[b]	Progressive low- or intermediate-grade neuroendocrine carcinoma (foregut, midgut, hindgut origin; nonpancreatic)	National Cancer Institute; Alliance for Clinical Trials
A Study of Sunitinib vs Placebo in Combination With Lanreotide in Patients With Progressive Advanced/ Metastatic Midgut Carcinoid Tumors (SUNLAND)	II randomized	Lanreotide plus either sunitinib or placebo[b]	Midgut low- or intermediate-grade NETs	Groupe Cooperateur Multidisciplinaire en Oncologie (GERCOR) Pfizer Ipsen
Pazopanib as Single Agent in Advanced NETs[a]	II	Pazopanib	Pancreatic islet cell tumors, well-differentiated GINETs, pulmonary carcinoids, and well-differentiated thymic carcinoids	Grupo Espanol de Tumores Neuroendocrinos
A Study of Axitinib in Advanced Carcinoid Tumors[a]	II	Axitinib	Well-differentiated and moderately differentiated NETs of the aerodigestive tract, as well as rare primary sites (renal, ovarian, thymic, hepatic)	H. Lee Moffitt Cancer Center; National Comprehensive Cancer Network Pfizer
Ziv-Aflibercept for Advanced Progressive Carcinoid Tumors[a]	II	Ziv-aflibercept plus octreotide	Well-differentiated or moderately differentiated neuroendocrine tumors	Dana-Farber Cancer Institute
Nintedanib in Treating Patients With Locally Advanced or Metastatic Neuroendocrine Tumors	II	Nintedanib	Low- or intermediate-grade NETs of nonpancreatic origin; patients on stable dose of octreotide	Roswell Park Cancer Institute; National Cancer Institute
A Study of Famitinib in Patients With Advanced or Metastatic Gastroenteropancreatic Neuroendocrine Tumor	II	Famitinib	Metastatic low- or intermediate-grade gastroenteropancreatic NET	Jiangsu HengRui Medicine Co., Ltd; Cancer Institute and Hospital, Chinese Academy of Medical Sciences
Cabozantinib in Advanced Pancreatic Neuroendocrine and Carcinoid Tumors	II	Cabozantinib (XL184)	Carcinoid or pancreatic NET; patients with pancreatic NET must have had previous VEGF inhibitor treatment	Massachusetts General Hospital
Regorafenib in Treating Patients With Advanced or Metastatic Neuroendocrine Tumors[d]	II	Regorafenib	Advanced metastatic, progressing carcinoid, or pancreatic islet cell cancers	University of Southern California; National Cancer Institute (NCI)

(continued on next page)

Table 3
(continued)

Study ID	Phase	Study Arms	Population	Sponsors
Other				
YF476 in Patients With Type II Gastric Carcinoids Associated With Zollinger-Ellison Syndrome	II	YF476 (gastrin antagonist)	Patients with Zollinger-Ellison syndrome and type II gastric carcinoids or their precancerous cells	National Institute of Diabetes and Digestive and Kidney Diseases
A Phase 2 Study of Fosbretabulin in Subjects With Gastrointestinal Neuroendocrine Tumors With Elevated Biomarkers	II	Fosbretabulin tromethamine	Well-differentiated, low- to intermediate-grade GINETs with increased levels of biomarkers and progressive disease	OXiGENE
Carfilzomib for the Treatment of Patients With Advanced Neuroendocrine Cancers	II	Carfilzomib (proteasome inhibitor)	Advanced (unresectable or metastatic) well-differentiated or moderately differentiated NETs including typical carcinoid and pNETs	SCRI Development Innovations, LLC; Onyx Pharmaceuticals
A Pilot Study of Metformin Treatment in Patients With Well-differentiated Neuroendocrine Tumors (MetNet)	II	Metformin	Metastatic well-differentiated NET grade 1 or 2	Instituto do Cancer do Estado de São Paulo
Recombinant Anti-tumor and Anti-virus Protein for Injection to Treat Advanced Neuroendocrine Tumors[d]	II	Novaferon	Low- or intermediate-grade advanced (unresectable or metastatic) NETs	The Affiliated Hospital of the Chinese Academy of Military Medical Sciences

Study	Phase	Agent	Tumor Type	Sponsor
LEE011 in Neuroendocrine Tumors of Foregut Origin[d]	II	LEE011 (CDK4/6 inhibitor)	Well-differentiated foregut NETs	M.D. Anderson Cancer Center; Novartis Pharmaceuticals Corporation
A Study to Determine Safety, Pharmacokinetics and Pharmacodynamics of Intravenous TKM 080301 in Neuroendocrine Tumors (NET) and Adrenocortical Carcinoma (ACC) Patients[a]	I/II	TKM-080301 (small interfering RNA directed against poliolike kinase 1)	Refractory NETs or adrenocortical carcinomas	Tekmira Pharmaceuticals Corporation
Biological Study of Resveratrol's Effects on Notch-1 Signaling in Subjects With Low Grade Gastrointestinal Tumors[a]	I	Resveratrol	Low-grade GINETs	University of Wisconsin Paul P. Carbone Comprehensive Cancer Center

[a] Enrollment completed, study ongoing.
[b] Randomized, placebo-controlled clinical trial.
[c] Trial completed, no results published yet.
[d] Active, not yet recruiting.
Data from http://www.clinicaltrials.gov. Accessed June, 2015.

monotherapy were 95% in the bevacizumab group compared with 68% in the interferon arm. Based on these results, 402 eligible patients were enrolled in a phase III trial (SWOG 0518) comparing octreotide LAR plus interferon with octreotide LAR plus bevacizumab in patients with advanced NET with a poor prognosis.[48] The median PFS by central review was 16.6 months (95% confidence interval [CI], 12.9–19.6) in bevacizumab-treated patients and 15.4 months (95% CI, 9.6–18.6) for interferon-treated patients (hazard ratio [HR], 0.93; 95% CI, 0.73–1.18; P = .55). Time to treatment failure (TTF) was significantly longer with bevacizumab compared with interferon (HR, 0.72; 95% CI, 0.58–0.89; P = .003). Median TTF was 9.9 months (95% CI, 7.3–11.1) in the bevacizumab arm and 5.6 (95% CI, 4.3–6.4) months in the interferon arm. Confirmed radiologic response rates were 12% (95% CI, 8%–18%) in the bevacizumab arm and 4% (95% CI, 2%–8%) in the interferon arm. Overall, bevacizumab and interferon seemed to have similar activity in this population (ie, the potential benefit of bevacizumab might have been masked by an active control arm).

Bevacizumab has also been assessed in combination with cytotoxic chemotherapy in an effort to achieve a synergistic effect.[49,50] Bevacizumab plus octreotide and metronomic capecitabine was evaluated in 45 patients with metastatic well-differentiated and moderately differentiated NETs arising from various primary sites.[51] Partial response was obtained in 8 patients (17.8%), with response being more frequent in pancreatic malignancies compared with nonpancreatic malignancies. Median PFS was 14.9 months in this trial.

Oral small-molecule receptor tyrosine kinase inhibitors with activity against the VEGF receptor (eg, sunitinib, sorafenib, and pazopanib) are also of interest in NETs. Sunitinib is already approved for use in pancreatic NETs based on its ability to delay tumor progression compared with placebo (median PFS, 11.4 months vs 5.5 months).[52] In a non-randomized trial of patients with advanced pancreatic and GINETs treated with sunitinib, an objective response rate of 16.7% was noted for pancreatic NETs but only 2.4% for nonpancreatic GINETs, suggesting a differential response to therapy based on the site of origin.[53] A randomized phase II trial in tumors of midgut origin is ongoing (SUNLAND trial; lanreotide plus placebo or sunitinib) (see **Table 3**).

Pazopanib is also under study in NETs. Ahn and colleagues[54] reported on a non-randomized, open-label phase II study of patients with unresectable low- to intermediate-grade pancreatic GINETs. The objective response rate was 18.9% and the disease control rate was 75.7% (pooled NETs). Another phase II cohort study was completed for patients with metastatic low- or intermediate-grade pancreatic NETs or GINETs.[55] Patients received pazopanib 800 mg orally once a day and octreotide. Treatment with pazopanib was associated with a tumor response in 7 of 32 patients (21.9%) with pancreatic NETs. There were no radiographic responses in the 20 patients accrued in the first stage of the carcinoid tumor cohort, however, the waterfall plots were suggestive of cytostatic activity. A randomized, phase II clinical trial (A021202) in patients with progressive advanced GINETs (both functional and nonfunctional) is ongoing (see **Table 3**). Other VEGF receptor tyrosine kinase inhibitors are also under study.[56]

CHEMOTHERAPY

The precise role of cytotoxic chemotherapy for advanced GINETs is debated; thus, there is no standard treatment approach and chemotherapy is typically reserved for patients without additional therapeutic options. There seems to be site-specific sensitivity to chemotherapy, with GINETs appearing less sensitive than panNETs on average. The potential benefits must be carefully weighed against the risk of significant side effects in a disease that often progresses slowly even without treatment.

Single-agent capecitabine showed some promise in a recent phase II clinical trial of patients with metastatic predominantly GINETs, with 13 of 19 patients experiencing radiographically stable disease.[57] Other chemotherapy agents such as the taxanes,[58] topotecan,[59] and gemcitabine[60] have shown little activity as single agents. Streptozotocin-based combinations are perhaps the best studied, with response rates range from 16% to 33%.[61–63] In a phase III trial, streptozotocin/5-fluorouracil (FU) was compared with doxorubicin/5-FU, with a response rate of 16% in both arms but a statistically significant improvement in overall survival in the streptozotocin-containing arm (24.3 vs 15.7 months).[62] However, more than one-third of patients in the streptozotocin arm also developed mild to moderate renal toxicity.

In a study of 56 patients with metastatic GINETs receiving single-agent dacarbazine, the overall response rate was 16%. There was significant toxicity, with 88% of patients reporting nausea and vomiting.[64] Temozolomide, an oral analogue of dacarbazine, seems to be better tolerated, but has limited activity in GINETs. In 1 study, only 1 of 44 patients (2%) with GINET experienced an objective tumor response, compared with 18 of 53 patients (34%) with pancreatic NETs treated with temozolomide.[65] The combination of temozolomide and bevacizumab was associated with a 33% response rate (5 of 15) in patients with pancreatic NETs compared with 0 of 19 patients with traditional carcinoid tumors.[66] The combination of capecitabine and temozolomide (CAPTEM) has also been studied.[67] Interim results from a phase II trial in patients with metastatic, well-differentiated or moderately differentiated NETs with progression despite octreotide were promising, however, the final analysis has not been reported.[68] Larger prospective trials will be needed to elucidate the potential activity of the CAPTEM regimen in advanced GINETs.

NOVEL SYSTEMIC THERAPIES
Peptide Receptor Radionuclide Therapy

Peptide receptor radionuclide therapy (PRRT) targets radiation directly to advanced NETs by taking advantage of somatostatin receptor expression by these tumors. Clinical trials with radionuclide therapy for NETs have primarily focused on 2 radionuclides, yttrium-90 and lutetium-177, used to label somatostatin analogues. These agents have been evaluated in phase II trials of combined pancreatic and GINETs. Objective tumor response rates as high as 30% have been reported, with improvement in symptoms in one-third of patients.[69,70] Long-term side effects include cytopenias and loss of renal function. Although encouraging, these data should be interpreted with caution as randomized studies are needed to definitively establish the efficacy and safety of PRRT (**Table 4** for ongoing trials). Thus, use of radiolabeled somatostatin analogues remains investigational in the United States. Furthermore, its use is limited to selected centers with the expertise to generate and administer the radiolabeled somatostatin analogue.[71–73] The NETTER-1 study is of particular interest as it is an international randomized trial evaluating ^{177}Lu-DOTA0-Tyr3-octreotate compared with high-dose octreotide LAR (60 mg monthly) in patients with inoperable, somatostatin receptor-positive metastatic midgut NETs with progressive disease on standard doses of octreotide LAR. Recently release results from the NETTER-1 study suggest that PRRT significantly improves progression- free survival in patients with mid gut neuroendocrine tumours.[74]

Immunotherapy

Although their relatively low mutation rate suggests that well-differentiated NETs may not be immune-sensitive tumors, immunotherapy for the treatment of NETs remains

Table 4
Peptide receptor radionuclide therapy for well-differentiated neuroendocrine tumors: selected ongoing trials

Study ID	Phase	Population	Sponsor
A Study Comparing Treatment With 177Lu-DOTA0-Tyr3-Octreotate to Octreotide LAR in Patients With Inoperable, Progressive, Somatostatin Receptor Positive Midgut Carcinoid Tumors (NETTER-1)	III randomized[a]	Progressive mi-gut carcinoid	Advanced Accelerator Applications; Pierrel Research Europe GmbH
Randomized Phase III of PRRT vs Interferon (CASTOR)[b]	III randomized[a]	Unresectable nonpancreatic GINETs resistant to therapy with somatostatin analogues	Jules Bordet Institute
Safety and Efficacy Study of In-111 Pentetreotide to Treat Neuroendocrine Tumors[c]	II/III	NETs with previous chemotherapy and/or radiation	Radio Isotope Therapy of America; Excel Diagnostic Imaging Clinics; RadioMedix; CHI St. Luke's Health
90Y DOTA/Retinoic Acid for Neuroblastoma and Neuroendocrine Tumor (NET)[c]	II randomized[a]	Children and young adults with recurrent, somatostatin receptor-positive tumors	University of Iowa; Molecular Insight Pharmaceuticals, Inc
177Lutetium-DOTA-Octreotate Therapy in Somatostatin Receptor-Expressing Neuroendocrine Neoplasms	II	Somatostatin receptor-expressing neuroendocrine neoplasms	Radio Isotope Therapy of America; Excel Diagnostics and Nuclear Oncology Center
A Trial to Assess the Safety and Effectiveness of Lutetium-177 Octreotate Therapy in Neuroendocrine Tumors	II	Somatostatin receptor-expressing neuroendocrine neoplasms	AHS Cancer Control Alberta

[a] Randomized clinical trial.
[b] Approved, not yet recruiting.
[c] Enrollment completed, study ongoing.
Data from http://www.clinicaltrials.gov. Accessed June, 2015.

an area of active research, stemming in part from the data suggesting that interferon alpha has activity in the disease. The adverse side effects of interferon limit its usefulness, but more targeted immunomodulatory therapies hold promise. Recent efforts have focused on blocking the inhibitory immune receptors cytotoxic T-lymphocyte-associated protein 4 (CTLA4) and programmed death-ligand 1 (PD-L1).[75] Clinical testing with these and other immunomodulatory agents in NETs (including modified chimeric antigen receptor T cells that target the somatostatin receptor type 2) are planned or ongoing, as is further characterization of the immune microenvironment in GINETs.

Additional Targets

Numerous other new therapeutic targets have been identified for well-differentiated NETs. Several agents that target other components of growth factor signaling are under investigation, including agents that target insulinlike growth factor 1 receptor, protein kinase B, and TORC1/2.[76,77] See **Table 3** for a list of ongoing clinical trials that may lead to novel single-agent or combination regimens with somatostatin analogues, VEGF inhibitors, and/or mTOR inhibitors.

SUMMARY

After the largely disappointing results of clinical trials with systemic chemotherapy in GINETs, the PROMID and CLARINET phase III studies definitively demonstrated the antitumor activity of somatostatin analogues in this patient population. SSAs remain the mainstay of therapy in GINETs for palliation of symptoms as well as control of tumor growth in patients with advanced disease. Given the cost and relative inconvenience of monthly injections, many defer use of SSAs until there is evidence of disease progression in asymptomatic patients. However, the optimal timing of SSA initiation and whether or not an SSA should be continued beyond progression remains unclear. Cytotoxic chemotherapy and interferon are typically reserved for select patients with progressive tumors given their unfavorable side-effect profiles and limited efficacy. Several novel treatment strategies are under study, such as VEGF signaling pathway inhibition, immunotherapy, and additional targeted agents. Randomized trials incorporating PRRT are also underway. Everolimus holds particular promise in patients with nonfunctional tumors, and telotristat provides symptom control in patients with refractory diarrhea.

Despite being an active area of investigation, there remains a serious unmet need for approved systemic treatments in advanced GINETs. The rarity of these tumors makes it difficult to study large numbers of potential therapies either alone or in combinations. This challenge is augmented by the inherent biologic heterogeneity of GINETs, which can vary by the presence or absence of carcinoid syndrome, primary site, proliferative index, and grade. Furthermore, with a natural disease course measured in years, or even decades, the optimal timing of interventions including first-line therapy remains unclear, as is the role of systemic therapy compared with liver-directed treatments. Moving forward, optimizing patient selection based on particular clinical features or novel biomarkers holds promise for identifying those individuals most likely to benefit from therapy. Advances in molecular classification of NETs may also enhance our ability to tailor therapy for a particular patient in the future.

REFERENCES

1. Yao JC, Hassan M, Phan A, et al. One hundred years after "carcinoid": epidemiology of and prognostic factors for neuroendocrine tumors in 35,825 cases in the United States. J Clin Oncol 2008;26:3063–72.
2. Ramage JK, Ahmed A, Ardill J, et al. Guidelines for the management of gastroenteropancreatic neuroendocrine (including carcinoid) tumours (NETs). Gut 2012;61:6–32.
3. Modlin IM, Kidd M, Latich I, et al. Current status of gastrointestinal carcinoids. Gastroenterology 2005;128:1717–51.
4. Reubi JC, Kvols LK, Waser B, et al. Detection of somatostatin receptors in surgical and percutaneous needle biopsy samples of carcinoids and islet cell carcinomas. Cancer Res 1990;50:5969–77.

5. Kvols LK, Moertel CG, O'Connell MJ, et al. Treatment of the malignant carcinoid syndrome. Evaluation of a long-acting somatostatin analogue. N Engl J Med 1986;315:663–6.
6. Toumpanakis C, Garland J, Marelli L, et al. Long-term results of patients with malignant carcinoid syndrome receiving octreotide LAR. Aliment Pharmacol Ther 2009;30:733–40.
7. Anthony L, Vinik AI. Evaluating the characteristics and the management of patients with neuroendocrine tumors receiving octreotide LAR during a 6-year period. Pancreas 2011;40:987–94.
8. Janson ET, Oberg K. Long-term management of the carcinoid syndrome. Treatment with octreotide alone and in combination with alpha-interferon. Acta Oncol 1993;32:225–9.
9. Oberg K, Norheim I, Theodorsson E. Treatment of malignant midgut carcinoid tumours with a long-acting somatostatin analogue octreotide. Acta Oncol 1991;30:503–7.
10. di Bartolomeo M, Bajetta E, Buzzoni R, et al. Clinical efficacy of octreotide in the treatment of metastatic neuroendocrine tumors. A study by the Italian Trials in Medical Oncology Group. Cancer 1996;77:402–8.
11. Rubin J, Ajani J, Schirmer W, et al. Octreotide acetate long-acting formulation versus open-label subcutaneous octreotide acetate in malignant carcinoid syndrome. J Clin Oncol 1999;17:600–6.
12. Ruszniewski P, Ducreux M, Chayvialle JA, et al. Treatment of the carcinoid syndrome with the longacting somatostatin analogue lanreotide: a prospective study in 39 patients. Gut 1996;39:279–83.
13. Modlin IM, Pavel M, Kidd M, et al. Review article: somatostatin analogues in the treatment of gastroenteropancreatic neuroendocrine (carcinoid) tumours. Aliment Pharmacol Ther 2010;31:169–88.
14. Castillo JG, Filsoufi F, Adams DH, et al. Management of patients undergoing multivalvular surgery for carcinoid heart disease: the role of the anaesthetist. Br J Anaesth 2008;101:618–26.
15. Vaughan DJ, Brunner MD. Anesthesia for patients with carcinoid syndrome. Int Anesthesiol Clin 1997;35:129–42.
16. Palaniswamy C, Frishman WH, Aronow WS. Carcinoid heart disease. Cardiol Rev 2012;20:167–76.
17. Kvols LK, Oberg KE, O'Dorisio TM, et al. Pasireotide (SOM230) shows efficacy and tolerability in the treatment of patients with advanced neuroendocrine tumors refractory or resistant to octreotide LAR: results from a phase II study. Endocr Relat Cancer 2012;19:657–66.
18. Wolin EM, Jarzab B, Eriksson B, et al. Phase III study of pasireotide long-acting release in patients with metastatic neuroendocrine tumors and carcinoid symptoms refractory to available somatostatin analogues. Drug Des Devel Ther 2015;3(9):5075–86.
19. Kulke MH, Hörsch D, Caplin M, et al. Telotristat etiprate is effective in treating patients with carcinoid syndrome that is inadequately controlled by somatostatin analog therapy (the phase 3 TELESTAR clinical trial). Presented at: 2015 European Cancer Congress; September 25–29; Vienna, Austria. Abstract 37LBA.
20. Oberg K, Funa K, Alm G. Effects of leukocyte interferon on clinical symptoms and hormone levels in patients with mid-gut carcinoid tumors and carcinoid syndrome. N Engl J Med 1983;309:129–33.
21. Eriksson B, Oberg K, Alm G, et al. Treatment of malignant endocrine pancreatic tumours with human leucocyte interferon. Lancet 1986;2:1307–9.

22. Boudreaux JP, Klimstra DS, Hassan MM, et al. The NANETS consensus guideline for the diagnosis and management of neuroendocrine tumors: well-differentiated neuroendocrine tumors of the jejunum, ileum, appendix, and cecum. Pancreas 2010;39:753–66.

23. Strosberg JR, Cheema A, Kvols LK. A review of systemic and liver-directed therapies for metastatic neuroendocrine tumors of the gastroenteropancreatic tract. Cancer Control 2011;18:127–37.

24. Bousquet C, Lasfargues C, Chalabi M, et al. Clinical review: Current scientific rationale for the use of somatostatin analogs and mTOR inhibitors in neuroendocrine tumor therapy. J Clin Endocrinol Metab 2012;97:727–37.

25. Rinke A, Muller HH, Schade-Brittinger C, et al. Placebo-controlled, double-blind, prospective, randomized study on the effect of octreotide LAR in the control of tumor growth in patients with metastatic neuroendocrine midgut tumors: a report from the PROMID Study Group. J Clin Oncol 2009;27:4656–63.

26. Caplin ME, Pavel M, Cwikla JB, et al. Lanreotide in metastatic enteropancreatic neuroendocrine tumors. N Engl J Med 2014;371:224–33.

27. Cives M, Kunz PL, Morse B, et al. Phase II clinical trial of pasireotide long-acting repeatable in patients with metastatic neuroendocrine tumors. Endocr Relat Cancer 2015;22:1–9.

28. Kulke MH. A randomized open-label phase II study of everolimus alone or in combination with pasireotide LAR in advanced, progressive pancreatic neuroendocrine tumors (pNET): COOPERATE-2 trial. Eur Neuroendocrine Tumor Soc 2015. Available at: http://www.enets.org/barcelona2015.html.

29. Oberg K. The action of interferon alpha on human carcinoid tumours. Semin Cancer Biol 1992;3:35–41.

30. Detjen KM, Welzel M, Farwig K, et al. Molecular mechanism of interferon alfa-mediated growth inhibition in human neuroendocrine tumor cells. Gastroenterology 2000;118:735–48.

31. Rosewicz S, Detjen K, Scholz A, et al. Interferon-alpha: regulatory effects on cell cycle and angiogenesis. Neuroendocrinology 2004;80(Suppl 1):85–93.

32. Kolby L, Persson G, Franzen S, et al. Randomized clinical trial of the effect of interferon alpha on survival in patients with disseminated midgut carcinoid tumours. Br J Surg 2003;90:687–93.

33. Faiss S, Scherubl H, Riecken EO, et al. Interferon-alpha versus somatostatin or the combination of both in metastatic neuroendocrine gut and pancreatic tumours. Digestion 1996;57(Suppl 1):84–5.

34. Arnold R, Rinke A, Klose KJ, et al. Octreotide versus octreotide plus interferon-alpha in endocrine gastroenteropancreatic tumors: a randomized trial. Clin Gastroenterol Hepatol 2005;3:761–71.

35. Vignot S, Faivre S, Aguirre D, et al. mTOR-targeted therapy of cancer with rapamycin derivatives. Ann Oncol 2005;16:525–37.

36. Zoncu R, Efeyan A, Sabatini DM. mTOR: from growth signal integration to cancer, diabetes and ageing. Nat Rev Mol Cell Biol 2011;12:21–35.

37. von Wichert G, Jehle PM, Hoeflich A, et al. Insulin-like growth factor-I is an autocrine regulator of chromogranin A secretion and growth in human neuroendocrine tumor cells. Cancer Res 2000;60:4573–81.

38. Missiaglia E, Dalai I, Barbi S, et al. Pancreatic endocrine tumors: expression profiling evidences a role for AKT-mTOR pathway. J Clin Oncol 2010;28:245–55.

39. Righi L, Volante M, Rapa I, et al. Mammalian target of rapamycin signaling activation patterns in neuroendocrine tumors of the lung. Endocr Relat Cancer 2010;17:977–87.

40. Moreno A, Akcakanat A, Munsell MF, et al. Antitumor activity of rapamycin and octreotide as single agents or in combination in neuroendocrine tumors. Endocr Relat Cancer 2008;15:257–66.
41. Yao JC, Shah MH, Ito T, et al. Everolimus for advanced pancreatic neuroendocrine tumors. N Engl J Med 2011;364:514–23.
42. Pavel ME, Hainsworth JD, Baudin E, et al. Everolimus plus octreotide long-acting repeatable for the treatment of advanced neuroendocrine tumours associated with carcinoid syndrome (RADIANT-2): a randomised, placebo-controlled, phase 3 study. Lancet 2011;378:2005–12.
43. Yao JC, Hainsworth JD, Wolin EM, et al. Multivariate analysis including biomarkers in the phase III RADIANT-2 study of octreotide LAR plus everolimus (E+O) or placebo (P+O) among patients with advanced neuroendocrine tumors (NET). J Clin Oncol 2012;30 [abstract: 4014].
44. Yao J, Fazio, N, Singh, S, et al. Everolimus in advanced nonfunctional neuroendocrine tumors (NET) of lung or gastrointestinal (GI) origin: efficacy and safety results from the placebo-controlled, double-blind, multicenter, Phase 3 RADIANT-4 study. European Cancer Congress 2015. Abstr 5LBA.
45. Zhang J, Jia Z, Li Q, et al. Elevated expression of vascular endothelial growth factor correlates with increased angiogenesis and decreased progression-free survival among patients with low-grade neuroendocrine tumors. Cancer 2007;109: 1478–86.
46. Inoue M, Hager JH, Ferrara N, et al. VEGF-A has a critical, nonredundant role in angiogenic switching and pancreatic beta cell carcinogenesis. Cancer Cell 2002; 1:193–202.
47. Yao JC, Phan A, Hoff PM, et al. Targeting vascular endothelial growth factor in advanced carcinoid tumor: a random assignment phase II study of depot octreotide with bevacizumab and pegylated interferon alpha-2b. J Clin Oncol 2008;26: 1316–23.
48. Yao J, Guthrie K, Moran C, et al. SWOG S0518: Phase III prospective randomized comparison of depot octreotide plus interferon 2b versus depot octreotide plus bevacizumab (NSC #704865) in advanced, poor prognosis carcinoid patients (NCT00569127). J Clin Oncol 2015;33 [abstract: 4004].
49. Kunz PL, Kuo T, Zahn JM, et al. A phase II study of capecitabine, oxaliplatin, and bevacizumab for metastatic or unresectable neuroendocrine tumors. J Clin Oncol 2010;28:15s(suppl; abstr 4104).
50. Venook AP, Ko AH, Tempero MA, et al. Phase II trial of FOLFOX plus bevacizumab in advanced, progressive neuroendocrine tumors. J Clin Oncol 2008; 26(15s):15545.
51. Berruti A, Fazio N, Ferrero A, et al. Bevacizumab plus octreotide and metronomic capecitabine in patients with metastatic well-to-moderately differentiated neuroendocrine tumors: the XELBEVOCT study. BMC Cancer 2014;14:184.
52. Raymond E, Dahan L, Raoul JL, et al. Sunitinib malate for the treatment of pancreatic neuroendocrine tumors. N Engl J Med 2011;364:501–13.
53. Kulke MH, Lenz HJ, Meropol NJ, et al. Activity of sunitinib in patients with advanced neuroendocrine tumors. J Clin Oncol 2008;26:3403–10.
54. Ahn HK, Choi JY, Kim KM, et al. Phase II study of pazopanib monotherapy in metastatic gastroenteropancreatic neuroendocrine tumours. Br J Cancer 2013;109: 1414–9.
55. Phan AT, Halperin DM, Chan JA, et al. Pazopanib and depot octreotide in advanced, well-differentiated neuroendocrine tumours: a multicentre, single-group, phase 2 study. Lancet Oncol 2015;16(6):695–703.

56. Cives M, Strosberg J, Campos T, et al. A phase II study of axitinib in advanced carcinoid tumors: preliminary analysis. J Clin Oncol 2015;33 [abstract: 4100].

57. Medley L, Morel AN, Farrugia D, et al. Phase II study of single agent capecitabine in the treatment of metastatic non-pancreatic neuroendocrine tumours. Br J Cancer 2011;104:1067–70.

58. Ansell SM, Pitot HC, Burch PA, et al. A Phase II study of high-dose paclitaxel in patients with advanced neuroendocrine tumors. Cancer 2001;91:1543–8.

59. Ansell SM, Mahoney MR, Green EM, et al. Topotecan in patients with advanced neuroendocrine tumors: a phase II study with significant hematologic toxicity. Am J Clin Oncol 2004;27:232–5.

60. Kulke MH, Kim H, Clark JW, et al. A Phase II trial of gemcitabine for metastatic neuroendocrine tumors. Cancer 2004;101:934–9.

61. Engstrom PF, Lavin PT, Moertel CG, et al. Streptozocin plus fluorouracil versus doxorubicin therapy for metastatic carcinoid tumor. J Clin Oncol 1984;2:1255–9.

62. Sun W, Lipsitz S, Catalano P, et al. Phase II/III study of doxorubicin with fluorouracil compared with streptozocin with fluorouracil or dacarbazine in the treatment of advanced carcinoid tumors: Eastern Cooperative Oncology Group Study E1281. J Clin Oncol 2005;23:4897–904.

63. Moertel CG, Hanley JA. Combination chemotherapy trials in metastatic carcinoid tumor and the malignant carcinoid syndrome. Cancer Clin Trials 1979;2: 327–34.

64. Bukowski RM, Tangen CM, Peterson RF, et al. Phase II trial of dimethyltriazenoimidazole carboxamide in patients with metastatic carcinoid. A Southwest Oncology Group study. Cancer 1994;73:1505–8.

65. Kulke MH, Hornick JL, Frauenhoffer C, et al. O6-methylguanine DNA methyltransferase deficiency and response to temozolomide-based therapy in patients with neuroendocrine tumors. Clin Cancer Res 2009;15:338–45.

66. Chan JA, Stuart K, Earle CC, et al. Prospective study of bevacizumab plus temozolomide in patients with advanced neuroendocrine tumors. J Clin Oncol 2012; 30:2963–8.

67. Fine RL, Gulati AP, Krantz BA, et al. Capecitabine and temozolomide (CAPTEM) for metastatic, well-differentiated neuroendocrine cancers: The Pancreas Center at Columbia University experience. Cancer Chemother Pharmacol 2013;71: 663–70.

68. Fine RL, Gulati AP, Tsushima D, et al. Prospective phase II study of capecitabine and temozolomide (CAPTEM) for progressive, moderately, and well-differentiated metastatic neuroendocrine tumors. Gastrointestinal Cancer Symposium. J Clin Oncol 2014;32(suppl 3; abstr 179).

69. Kwekkeboom DJ, de Herder WW, Kam BL, et al. Treatment with the radiolabeled somatostatin analog [177 Lu-DOTA 0,Tyr3]octreotate: toxicity, efficacy, and survival. J Clin Oncol 2008;26:2124–30.

70. Bushnell DL Jr, O'Dorisio TM, O'Dorisio MS, et al. 90Y-edotreotide for metastatic carcinoid refractory to octreotide. J Clin Oncol 2010;28:1652–9.

71. Kulke MH, Siu LL, Tepper JE, et al. Future directions in the treatment of neuroendocrine tumors: consensus report of the National Cancer Institute Neuroendocrine Tumor clinical trials planning meeting. J Clin Oncol 2011;29:934–43.

72. Bushnell D. Treatment of metastatic carcinoid tumors with radiolabeled biologic molecules. J Natl Compr Canc Netw 2009;7:760–4.

73. Kennedy A, Coldwell D, Sangro B, et al. Integrating radioembolization into the treatment paradigm for metastatic neuroendocrine tumors in the liver. Am J Clin Oncol 2012;35:393–8.

74. Ruszniewski P, et al. [177]-Lu-Dotatate significantly improves progression-free survival in patients with midgut neuroendocrine tumours: Results of the phase III NETTER-1 trial. European Cancer Congress 2015. Abstr 6LBA.

75. Alonso-Gordoa T, Capdevila J, Grande E. GEP-NETs update: biotherapy for neuroendocrine tumours. Eur J Endocrinol 2015;172:R31–46.

76. Capdevila J, Salazar R. Molecular targeted therapies in the treatment of gastro-enteropancreatic neuroendocrine tumors. Target Oncol 2009;4:287–96.

77. Mita M, Wolin E, Meyer T, et al. Phase I expansion trial of an oral TORC1/TORC2 inhibitor (CC-223) in nonpancreatic neuroendocrine tumors (NET). J Clin Oncol 2013;31 [abstract: e15004].

Bronchial and Thymic Carcinoid Tumors

Anya Litvak, MD[a], M. Catherine Pietanza, MD[b],*

KEYWORDS

- Bronchial • Thymic • Neuroendocrine • Typical carcinoid • Atypical carcinoid

KEY POINTS

- Bronchial carcinoids are well-differentiated neuroendocrine tumors that account for approximately 2% of all lung tumors.
- Bronchial carcinoids are usually sporadic, but may be associated with multiple endocrine neoplasia type 1 (MEN-1) syndrome, and are classified into typical and atypical carcinoids.
- MEN-1 syndrome is associated with up to 25% of cases of thymic carcinoids.
- Small biopsies and cytology cannot distinguish between atypical and typical carcinoid; surgical specimens are often required for classification.
- Surgery is the primary treatment modality for patients with localized disease and is the only curative option; while in Stage IV disease, there are few recommendations as to the approach to care.

INTRODUCTION

Carcinoid tumors arising in the lung and thymus are rare foregut neuroendocrine tumors (NETs) characterized by neuroendocrine morphology and differentiation and are classified using the World Health Organization (WHO) criteria, first described in 2004 and recently updated in 2015 (**Table 1**).[1] At one end of the spectrum are typical carcinoids (TC), which are low-grade, well-differentiated tumors that often present in early stage, rarely metastasize after surgical resection, and are generally relatively resistant to chemotherapy. At the other end of the spectrum are high-grade, poorly differentiated tumors such as small cell or large cell neuroendocrine carcinomas,

Disclosure Statement: The authors have nothing to disclose.
[a] Thoracic Oncology Service, Division of Solid Tumor Oncology, Department of Medicine, Memorial Sloan Kettering Cancer Center, 300 East 66th Street, New York, NY 10065, USA;
[b] Thoracic Oncology Service, Division of Solid Tumor Oncology, Department of Medicine, Memorial Sloan Kettering Cancer Center, Weill Cornell Medical College, 300 East 66th Street, New York, NY 10065, USA
* Corresponding author.
E-mail address: pietanzm@mskcc.org

Hematol Oncol Clin N Am 30 (2016) 83–102
http://dx.doi.org/10.1016/j.hoc.2015.09.003
0889-8588/16/$ – see front matter © 2016 Elsevier Inc. All rights reserved.

Table 1
WHO 2015 classification for bronchial and thymic NETs

Nomenclature	Grade	Histopathologic Characteristics	Differentiation
Typical carcinoid	Low	Carcinoid morphology, <2 mitosis/2 mm^2, no necrosis, >0.5 cm diameter	Well differentiated
Atypical carcinoid	Intermediate	Carcinoid morphology, 2–10 mitosis/2 mm^2, or foci of necrosis	Well differentiated
Large cell carcinoma	High	NE structure, >10 mitosis/2 mm^2, necrosis (may be extensive), cytology resembling NSCLC, IHC positive for NE markers and/or NE granules by electron microscopy	Poorly differentiated
Small cell carcinoma		Small cell size, scant cytoplasm, nuclei with finely granular chromatin and absent or faint nucleoli, >11 mitoses/2 mm^2, extensive necrosis	

Abbreviations: IHC, immunohistochemistry; NE, neuroendocrine; NET, neuroendocrine tumors; NSCLC, non–small cell lung cancer; WHO, World Health Organization.

Adapted from Travis WD, Brambilla E, Nicholson AG, et al. The 2015 World Health Organization classification of lung tumors. Impact of genetic, clinical and radiologic advances since the 2004 classification. J Thorac Oncol 2015;10:1243–60.

which behave aggressively, often present with distant metastasis, and are sensitive to chemotherapy. Atypical carcinoids (AC) are considered to be well differentiated NETs, although they are intermediate grade and represent a more aggressive phenotype when compared with TC. In this review, the epidemiology and risk factors, as well as diagnostic and treatment paradigms, for typical and AC tumors of the lung and thymus are discussed. Owing to the rarity of these malignancies, treatment approaches have not been validated in large studies.

INCIDENCE, ETIOLOGY, AND PREDISPOSING GENETIC FACTORS
Bronchial Carcinoids

Bronchial carcinoids account for approximately 2% of all primary lung tumors and roughly 25% of all well differentiated NETs with an incidence rate ranging from 0.2 to 2 per 100,000 per year.[2–8] Over the past 30 years, the age-adjusted incidence rate of bronchial carcinoids has increased significantly, by approximately 6% per year.[3,4,8] This trend may represent the improvement in classification of these tumors, as well as the increase in use of imaging techniques that are able to detect asymptomatic disease. In the United States, there are nearly 6000 new cases per year.[9]

Most carcinoids of the lung are TC, with only 10% to 30% of bronchial carcinoids classified as AC.[6,10,11] Patients diagnosed with TC are approximately 10 years younger than those with AC, which occur in the sixth decade of life.[12,13] In children and adolescents, bronchial carcinoids are the most common primary lung neoplasm. These malignancies are found more commonly in women as compared with men and whites as compared with blacks.[8,12]

Currently, there are no clearly defined risk factors for bronchial carcinoids. Based on case series, patients with AC are more likely to be smokers as compared with patients with TC.[6,12,14] No other carcinogen or environmental exposure is implicated in the development of these malignancies.

Most bronchial carcinoids are sporadic tumors, although rare familial cases have been reported. In less than 5% to 10% of cases, bronchial carcinoids are associated with the autosomal dominant syndrome of multiple endocrine neoplasia type 1 (MEN-1), a rare disorder characterized by a predisposition to neoplasms of the pituitary, parathyroid glands, and pancreas. Furthermore, some sporadic bronchial carcinoid tumors demonstrate inactivation of the *MEN-1* gene located on chromosome 11q13.[15] If MEN-1 syndrome is suspected based on family history, an ionized calcium level, intact parathyroid hormone, and prolactin should be sent and the patient should be referred to a geneticist for *MEN-1* mutation analysis.

Thymic Carcinoids

Thymic carcinoids are the least common NETs, accounting for approximately 2% to 5% of all thymic tumors and 0.4% of all carcinoid tumors with an incidence rate of approximately 0.2 per 1,000,000 population per year.[8,16–18] The largest reported series of thymic carcinoid tumors included 205 patients identified from databases of the International Thymic Malignancy Interest Group and the European Society of Thoracic Surgeons.[19] In this series, the median age was 54 years, the male to female ratio was 3:1, and the majority of patients presented with advanced disease.[19] Tumors were classified as TC, AC, or large cell/small cell neuroendocrine carcinomas in 28%, 40%, and 28% of cases, respectively.

MEN-1 syndrome is associated with up to 25% of thymic carcinoid cases, and approximately 8% of patients with MEN-1 syndrome develop thymic NETs.[15,20,21] Because these patients tend to present with advanced disease at diagnosis, prophylactic thymectomy with complete resection of all the anterior mediastinal tissue should be considered, although the benefit of this procedure is controversial. Some experts advocate that males over the age of 25 with MEN-1 syndrome should undergo annual screening to evaluate for thymic NETs; however, there is no consensus on this issue, because there is no study that demonstrates a survival benefit with early diagnosis.[22,23]

PATHOLOGY
Bronchial Carcinoids

The histologic appearance of TC and AC is similar with a uniform population of tumor cells arranged in organoid nests with a moderate amount of cytoplasm with an eosinophilic hue. The finely granular nuclear chromatin frequently has a salt-and-pepper appearance. Necrosis and mitotic activity are used to distinguish TC from AC, as per the WHO criteria detailed herein (**Fig. 1**).[1] Immunohistochemistry stains for chromogranin A, synaptophysin, and CD56 help to confirm neuroendocrine differentiation. Additional immunohistochemistry stains, including CDX-2, Islet1, TTF-1, or specific hormones and biogenic amines, are useful to separate pulmonary NETs from lung metastasis of well differentiated NETs of other organs.

Tumorlets are separated from carcinoid tumors by size, yet the morphology of cells is identical. Nodular neuroendocrine proliferations 0.5 cm or larger are called carcinoid tumors, whereas those measuring less than 0.5 cm are termed tumorlets. Tumorlets are incidental findings in approximately 25% of excised carcinoid tumors and are thought to have no clinical significance, although they can be seen in interstitial or airway inflammatory and fibrosing conditions. Typically no mitoses, no necrosis, and low Ki-67 labeling index are found. A very rare condition called diffuse idiopathic pulmonary neuroendocrine cell hyperplasia is regarded as a preinvasive condition for pulmonary carcinoids. Patients with diffuse idiopathic pulmonary neuroendocrine cell hyperplasia have widespread neuroendocrine cell hyperplasia and tumorlets in their airways, can develop multiple carcinoid tumors, and demonstrate unique findings

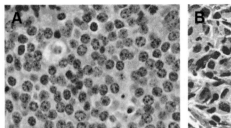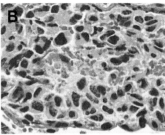

Fig. 1. Histologic appearance of bronchial carcinoid tumors. (*A*) Photomicrograph of typical carcinoid (original magnification ×40). Tumor cells are medium sized polygonal cells with lightly eosinophilic cytoplasm, round to oval finely granular nuclei and inconspicuous mitosis arranged in nests without evidence of necrosis. Mitosis of less than 1/2 mm^2. (*B*) Photomicrograph of atypical carcinoid (original magnification ×40). Tumor cells with eosinophilic cytoplasm, nuclear pleomorphism, and hyperchromasia. The nuclear contours are irregular and angulated with a coarsely granular to punctate chromatin pattern. Punctate areas of necrosis. Mitosis of 14/2 mm^2.

on computed tomography (CT), with multiple nodules, ground glass attenuation, bronchiectasis, and air trapping owing to small airway obstruction.[24]

Recently, gene copy analysis, genome/exome, and transcriptome sequencing of bronchial carcinoids has been performed. The molecular alterations of bronchial carcinoids are distinct from high-grade NETs in that they have a lower rate of mutations (approximately 0.4 mutations per megabase), lack *TP53* and *RB1* loss, and contain frequent mutations in chromatin remodeling genes, such as *MEN1*, *PSIP1*, and *ARID1A*.[25]

Thymic Carcinoids

For thymic carcinoid tumors, the criteria used to separate TC from AC are the same as those applied to bronchial NETs. These tumors are included in the thymic carcinoma group according to the WHO classification of tumors. Among reported cases of well-differentiated thymic NET, the majority are AC. To make the diagnosis of primary thymic NET, metastasis from another site should be excluded.

THE CHALLENGE OF SMALL BIOPSIES

Although carcinoid tumors can be diagnosed by small biopsies or cytology, it is difficult to separate TC from AC. This distinction usually requires a surgical biopsy or resection specimen. AC may be suspected if mitosis or necrosis is present. In small crushed specimens where mitotic figures are difficult to demonstrate, it may be helpful to use Ki-67 staining because most TC show less than 5% staining, AC are usually 10% to 30%, and most large cell neuroendocrine lung carcinoma or small cell lung cancer (SCLC) usually have a very high proliferation index of 80% to 100%.[26]

SYMPTOMS, APPROACH TO MAKING THE DIAGNOSIS, AND STAGING
Symptoms

Bronchial carcinoids

Two-thirds of bronchial carcinoids develop in the major bronchi. As a result, the most common presenting symptoms include obstructive pneumonia, pleuritic pain, atelectasis, dyspnea, cough, and hemoptysis.[6,27] Up to 30% of patients with pulmonary carcinoid tumors are asymptomatic at presentation. Carcinoid syndrome (facial flushing, diarrhea, wheezing) is found in 2% to 5% of bronchial carcinoids, most often when liver metastases are present. The syndrome is rare in well-differentiated pulmonary NETs, especially in localized disease, because foregut carcinoids lack aromatic amino acid decarboxylase and cannot make serotonin and its metabolites.[6,27] Rarely, paraneoplastic syndromes are associated with pulmonary carcinoids (**Table 2**).

Thymic carcinoids

Thymic tumors generally occur in the anterior mediastinal compartment, often infiltrating adjacent structures, with approximately 50% of patients presenting with locally invasive disease or mediastinal lymph node metastasis. Symptoms range according to disease extent, from cough, dyspnea, and chest pain to SVC syndrome and hoarseness, secondary to invasion of the recurrent laryngeal nerve.[28–32] Almost 50% of tumors are complicated by a paraneoplastic endocrinopathy, most commonly Cushing's syndrome (see **Table 2**).[33,34]

Table 2
Paraneoplastic syndromes associated with bronchial and thymic carcinoid tumors

Syndrome	Symptoms	Biochemical Assessment
Carcinoid syndrome *Cause:* Secretion of serotonin and other vasoactive substances into the systemic circulation *Incidence:* 2% of bronchial carcinoids; rare in thymic carcinoids	Flushing, diarrhea, and bronchoconstriction; long-term sequelae of cardiac valvular fibrosis (both right and left), fibrosis in the retroperitoneum, and venous telangiectasias	24-h urine 5-HIAA
Cushing syndrome *Cause:* Ectopic ACTH production *Incidence:* 2% of bronchial carcinoids; up to 50% of thymic carcinoids	Central weight gain, striae, hypertension, hyperglycemia, depression, hirsutism	Should be confirmed with 1 of the following 3 tests: • 1 mg overnight dexamethasone suppression test • 2–3 midnight salivary cortisol levels • 24-h urinary free cortisol If cortisol is elevated, should check serum ACTH
Acromegaly *Cause:* Ectopic GHRH production *Incidence:* Rare in both bronchial and thymic carcinoids	Swelling and enlargement of the hands, feet, nose, lips, and ears, acrochordon, carpel tunnel syndrome	GH; GHRH; and IGF-1
Hyponatremia *Cause:* SIADH secretion or atrial natriuretic peptide production *Incidence:* Rare in both bronchial and thymic carcinoids	Anorexia, nausea, muscle aches, myoclonus, ataxia, tremors, altered mental status, seizures, cerebral edema	Urine osmolality, urine sodium, serum sodium

Abbreviations: 5-HIAA, 5-hydroxyindoleacetic acid; ACTH, adrenocorticotropic hormone; GH, growth hormone; GHRH, growth hormone releasing hormone; IGF-1, insulin-like growth factor-1; SIADH, syndrome of inappropriate antidiuretic hormone.

Diagnosis

Biopsy

Biopsy is necessary for tissue confirmation of carcinoids. Central, bronchial tumors can easily be sampled by bronchoscopy, preferably with flexible bronchoscopy, whereas peripheral lesions can be biopsied by core needle; however, a definitive diagnosis may be difficult to ascertain in small cytology samples, as discussed. For thymic carcinoids, lymphoma or mediastinal germ cell tumor should be ruled out because these diseases are treated medically rather than surgically. Primary resection can be considered for a small, encapsulated thymic mass, along with the thymus, to establish the diagnosis and as definitive treatment. A larger thymic mass with indistinct margins should ideally be biopsied before resection to establish a diagnosis and to determine treatment recommendations. CT-guided core needle biopsy often is performed for the evaluation of thymic masses, although endoscopic or transbronchial ultrasound-guided fine needle aspiration biopsy or mediastinoscopy are helpful to assess the mediastinum.

Imaging

A CT scan of the chest is the recommended imaging for both bronchial and thymic carcinoids, which, in particular, may additionally necessitate mediastinal multiphase CT.[35] Liver and bone metastases are the most common sites of spread. As such, a multiphase CT or MRI with dynamic acquisition and diffuse weighted sequencing of the liver should be used. MRI also can be used to detect and characterize bone metastasis, especially the spine.

Owing to the overexpression of somatostatin receptors, immunoscintigraphy by somatostatin analogs such as octreotide has been approved since 1994 for imaging of patients with NETs. In one series, the sensitivity and specificity were 90% and 83%, respectively.[36] Most octreotide scans are performed with single photon emission CT imaging that enables 3-dimensional scanning or single photon emission CT–CT, which facilitates the display of cross-sectional imaging. However, over the last 15 years, the quality of CT and MRI imaging has improved significantly. In a review that compared modern octreotide scans with CT or MRI scans, multiphase contrast-enhanced CT or MRI scans detected more pathologic lesions than did single photon emission CT–octreotide scanning, and octreotide scans failed to identify any soft tissue lesions or primary tumors that were not seen on CT or MRI scans.[37] These data suggest that routine octreotide scans should not be added to CT scans regularly for surveillance after resection. Furthermore, the need for an octreotide scan preoperatively in patients with resectable disease is debatable, because extrathoracic metastatic disease is rare and cross-sectional imaging with CT scan may be better for detecting such lesions. Baseline octreotide scans are useful in patients with carcinoid syndrome or metastatic disease to determine somatostatin receptor status and the therapeutic utility of somatostatin analogs.

Fluorine 18-fluorodeoxyglucose (FDG) PET scanning may be less accurate because these indolent tumors generally have a low standard uptake value, although some authors still advocate for its potential use.[38,39] Recent series have shown that FDG-PET is useful for the assessment of intermediate- and high-grade NETs and may have prognostic value.[40,41] In the preoperative setting, the need for a PET scan is debatable as demonstrated by the findings of a recent, large retrospective study where the sensitivity of 18F-FDG PET/CT for mediastinal lymph node metastasis was considerably poorer for patients with bronchial carcinoid than that for non-SCLC (NSCLC; 33% vs 84% for NSCLC), but the specificity was comparable (94% vs 89% for NSCLC), suggesting that lymph node metastases accurately cannot be ruled out with a negative PET/CT.[42,43] As such, in the preoperative setting, if treatment decisions are based on N2 status, mediastinal staging is required with either endobronchial ultrasonography or mediastinoscopy.

Echocardiogram should be performed at diagnosis and during follow-up for patients with carcinoid syndrome to evaluate for the presence of carcinoid heart disease, which is characterized by plaquelike deposits of fibrous tissue in the right and left valves and endocardium and occurs in more than 50% of patients with carcinoid syndrome.[44,45]

Biochemical assessment

Increased chromogranin A levels have been measured in serum or plasma, although they have been found to be lower in pulmonary carcinoids compared with gastroenteropancreatic NETs.[46–48] In the setting of advanced or metastatic disease, chromogranin A levels can be useful to follow disease activity.[46] Although rare in bronchial and thymic carcinoids, if carcinoid syndrome is suspected, a 24-hour urinary excretion of 5-hydroxyindoleacetic acid should be measured (see **Table 2**). Serotonin levels should not be followed because there are several assays with variable sensitivity and specificity, and levels can be affected by release of platelet serotonin and tryptophan and serotonin-rich foods. Patients with sporadic, non–MEN-1–associated thymic carcinoids should undergo evaluation for Cushing's syndrome, because its incidence is high in this population.[33,34] Acromegaly and hyponatremia secondary to syndrome of inappropriate antidiuretic hormone are rare and usually are seen only in sporadic cases (see **Table 2**).[49,50]

Staging and Prognosis

Bronchial carcinoids

Bronchial carcinoid tumors are staged according to the TNM classification used for NSCLC in the seventh edition of the American Joint Committee on Cancer staging system. The International Association for the Study of Lung Cancer proposed and approved this staging in 2009 when it was determined that the TNM staging system was helpful in predicting prognosis for bronchial carcinoids.[51] Applying this staging system to cases in the National Cancer Institute Surveillance, Epidemiology, and End Results registry and cases submitted to the International Association for the Study of Lung Cancer database, it was determined that 5-year overall survival (OS) for patients with stage I, II, III, and IV disease were 93%, 74% to 85%, 67% to 75%, and 57%, respectively.[51]

Survival is significantly better for TC than for AC. The 5- and 10-year survival rates have been reported as 87% to 100% and 82% to 87%, respectively, for TC, and 30% to 90% and 35% to 56%, respectively, for AC.[12,52–65] Other predictors of survival include tumor size, nodal involvement, higher mitotic rates (ie, atypical subtype), and age older than 60.[12,13,51] Importantly, patients with multiple nodules have a very favorable prognosis, likely because these individuals tend to have the underlying preinvasive lesion, diffuse idiopathic pulmonary neuroendocrine cell hyperplasia, and multiple synchronous primaries rather than intrapulmonary metastasis.[24,51]

Thymic carcinoids

A formal staging classification has not been developed for thymic carcinoids and therefore Masaoka-Koga system, Masaoka system, or the terms "local," "locally advanced," and "metastatic" are used commonly (**Table 3**). Thymic carcinoids are felt to have a more aggressive behavior, recur locally, and metastasize more frequently, as compared with other NETs arising elsewhere. In the largest series of thymic carcinoids to date, median survival was 13.5 years for Masaoka stages I and

Table 3	
Masaoka staging system	
Stage	Description
I	Macroscopically encapsulated with no microscopically detectable capsular invasion
II	Macroscopic invasion of mediastinal fatty tissue or mediastinal pleura or microscopic invasion into the capsule
III	Macroscopic invasion into surrounding structures (pericardium, great vessels, lung)
IVa	Pleural or pericardial dissemination
IVb	Lymphogenous or hematogenous metastasis

II, 7.3 years for stage II, 3.8 years for stage IVa, and 4.2 years for stage IVb.[19] Masaoka stage and R0 resection was a significant prognostic factor for survival, although histologic subtype did not show any effect on survival.[19] Another study did show that histologic subtype effects survival. In a group of 50 patients with long-term clinical follow-up, disease-free survival correlated with tumor grade; low-grade tumors had 5- and 10-year disease-free survivals of 50% and 9%, intermediate-grade tumors had a disease-free survival of 20% at 5 years, and none were disease free at 10 years. None of the patients with high-grade tumors were disease free at 5 years.[31]

TREATMENT OF BRONCHIAL CARCINOIDS
Stages I, II, and III

Surgery
Surgery is the primary treatment modality and the best curative option for patients with bronchial carcinoids. Because carcinoids often present centrally, pneumonectomy or bilobectomy are used frequently. However, lung parenchymal-sparing surgery such as bronchial sleeve, or wedge resection is favored in view of the low recurrence potential, especially for TC.[14,66] Because carcinoids generally do not spread submucosally, a surgical margin as close as 5 mm is considerate adequate. If positive margins are reported and the patient can tolerate a repeat surgery, repeat resection with wider margins can be considered. For patients with favorable prognostic features, such as typical histology and absence of lymph node involvement, a more limited resection has been proposed.[27,67] Patients with AC should be resected using the same principles guiding surgery for NSCLC.[68]

Because mediastinal lymph node metastases occur in up to 20% of cases of TC and 30% to 70% of cases of AC, complete mediastinal lymph node dissection is advocated, with surgical resection of nodal metastases when feasible.[13,57,65,69–72] Multiple series have found decreased incidence of local recurrence and improved survival when complete mediastinal lymph node dissection is performed.[11,65,69,70]

Adjuvant therapy
Currently, there is no consensus on adjuvant therapy in bronchial carcinoids after resection; trials in the adjuvant setting are lacking. For this reason, it is important to establish appropriate management and treatment plans within a multidisciplinary tumor board. In general, adjuvant chemotherapy after surgical resection for patients with TC with or without regional lymph node metastases (stages I, II, and III) is not recommended because the risk of recurrence has been shown to be low. In a series of 291 resected TC, only 3% of patients developed recurrence.[73] Similarly, after surgical resection, patients with stage I AC are followed expectantly. However, because systemic recurrence occurs more frequently in patients with AC with N1 or N2

involvement (stages II and III disease), adjuvant chemotherapy has been advocated by some based on retrospective literature.[73,74] Nonetheless, the optimal adjuvant regimen in this setting currently is unknown. Owing to the similarities with SCLC, etoposide and cisplatin or carboplatin generally are used.[74] Although the benefit is uncertain, multiple small retrospective reviews demonstrate that AC patients with N1 or N2 involvement who receive adjuvant platinum-based therapies still experience distal recurrences and die of disease within 10 years of treatment.[73,75] Prospective clinical trials in this setting are clearly needed to determine the best regimen for adjuvant treatment to reduce recurrence rates and improve OS.

Radiation therapy

The use of radiation therapy for carcinoid tumors is most similar to its pattern of use in NSCLC, although there is a lack of data and uncertainty of benefit. For tumors that are resectable, adjuvant radiation therapy may be offered in situations of residual disease (R1 resection) and mediastinal lymphadenopathy (N2 disease). The use of adjuvant radiation therapy for nodal disease is probably of greater utility in the more aggressive AC. However, carcinoid tumors generally are thought to be less responsive to radiation therapy than SCLC.[74,76]

Locally Advanced Unresectable Disease

Definitive radiation therapy can provide effective treatment for a locally unresectable primary tumor.[76,77] The addition of chemotherapy, such as a platinum-based regimen used in SCLC, is used occasionally, although response rates seem lower; whether this approach improves results as compared with radiation therapy alone remains uncertain. Data to guide optimal treatment are limited secondary to the rarity of these tumors and lack of prospective clinical trials.

Surveillance of Resected Bronchial Carcinoids

Local and distant disease recurrence can occur years after surgical resection and, for this reason, long-term follow-up of patients with bronchial carcinoids is warranted. The optimal surveillance strategy is not defined currently. The National Comprehensive Cancer Network guidelines recommend reevaluation every 3 to 12 months after resection and then every 6 to 12 months for up to 10 years.[35] However, this may not be necessary in patients with node-negative TC, because recurrence is rare in this population.[73] Somatostatin receptor scintigraphy is not recommended routinely during surveillance after curative resection unless metastatic disease is suspected. Biochemical evaluations with chromogranin A and 5-hydroxyindoleacetic acid may also be helpful to monitor disease activity in the setting of metastatic disease, but do not need to be monitored postoperatively.

Stage IV Disease

Overview

Because carcinoid tumors can be relatively indolent and there are no curative therapeutic options in the metastatic setting, quality of life is a critical consideration in deciding on a treatment plan. In asymptomatic patients with TC and AC and a low tumor burden, a watch and wait policy with regular follow-up and imaging every 3 to 6 months can be pursued. Key factors in deciding when to initiate treatment include how quickly the patient progresses off treatment, the burden of disease, and the presence of hormone-related symptoms. In patients who have clinically significant tumor burden and/or carcinoid syndrome, somatostatin analogs as first-line treatment should be considered, in the setting of a positive octreotide scan.[78,79] Chemotherapy or targeted therapy, such as everolimus, should be considered for those patients with more rapidly progressing tumors or those who have progressed on less toxic treatments.[80–82] Additional prospective, randomized studies are needed for both traditional cytotoxic and molecularly targeted agents because treatment principles generally are extrapolated from the experience with the more common gastrointestinal carcinoids. Palliative local therapy such as local resection, radiation therapy, radioablation, or cryoablation can be used for symptomatic lesions.[76]

Somatostatin analogs

Retrospective reviews including small numbers of patients with pulmonary carcinoids have reported on the use of somatostatin analogs with improvement in carcinoid syndrome symptoms, as well as prolonged disease control and survival, with very few individuals achieving a tumor response.[79,83,84] These results are similar to the experience with octreotide in gastrointestinal carcinoids. In the Placebo Controlled, Double Blind, Prospective, Randomized Study on the Effect of Octreotide LAR in the Control of Tumor Growth in Patients with Metastatic Neuroendocrine Midgut Tumors (PROMID) study, long-acting release (LAR) octreotide acetate significantly prolonged time to tumor progression compared with placebo in patients with newly diagnosed functionally active or inactive well-differentiated midgut NETs (14.3 vs 6 months; hazard ratio [HR], 0.34; 95% CI, 0.20–0.59; P = .000072) without an improvement in OS.[85] Additionally, in the phase III, randomized, placebo-controlled Controlled Study of Lanreotide Antiproliferative Response In NeuroEndocrine Tumors (CLARINET) study, lanreotide autogel significantly prolonged time to tumor progression compared with placebo in 204 patients with nonfunctional enteropancreatic NETs (median not reached versus a median of 18 months; HR, 0.47; 95% CI, 0.30–0.73; P<.001).[86] Neither of these studies have shown a benefit in OS,[85,86] likely owing to the high rate of somatostatin analog use in each of the placebo arms after progression.

Although neither of the prospective studies included foregut NETs, somatostatin analogs should be considered as first-line systemic treatment for patients with advanced bronchial carcinoids of low proliferative index, who have positive octreotide scans, owing to their excellent safety profile. Caution should be used in patients with lesions that have a high mitotic index, a high tumor burden, or rapidly progressing disease; and first imaging should be performed relatively soon after administration of the somatostatin analog to monitor response to therapy.

Peptide receptor radionuclide therapy

In patients with advanced disease that is resistant to octreotide, peptide receptor radionuclide therapy with radiolabeled somatostatin analogs is being evaluated in several centers.[87] Indium-111, yttrium-90, and lutetium-177 are linked to somatostatin analogs and then internalized by tumor cells. [90Y-DOTA]-DPhe1-Tyr3-octreotide (yttrium-90 DOTATOC) and lutetium-177 DOTATOC show particular promise in selected patients. An early phase II study of yttrium-90 DOTATOC found the response rate to be as high as 29% in 7 bronchial carcinoids.[88] In a large retrospective study of 1109 metastatic NETs, which included 84 bronchial carcinoids, a 29% partial response and median survival of 40 months from diagnosis were demonstrated.[89] Grade 3 to 4 adverse events were reported in 13% of patients, including mainly renal or hematologic toxicities.[89] Although these are promising results, peptide receptor radionuclide therapy remains experimental, at least in the United States, and can be only be administered in the setting of a clinical trial.

Cytotoxic therapy

Data regarding the efficacy of chemotherapy specifically in bronchial carcinoid (as opposed to gastrointestinal carcinoids) are lacking, because this tumor type has not been studied independent of other NETs and has been omitted occasionally from such trials. Furthermore, many of the older studies have used outdated classification systems for carcinoids and different criteria for response. Various chemotherapeutic agents have been used, including doxorubicin, 5-fluorouracil, dacarbazine, cisplatin, carboplatin, etoposide, streptozocin, and interferon-alpha.[46,82] Newer agents are being studied actively in neuroendocrine carcinoma. Results from larger retrospective and prospective studies are summarized in **Table 4**.

Etoposide–Platinum Regimens

Regimens typically used for SCLC are often recommended if cytotoxic therapy is used.[74,90] However, TC and AC clearly are less chemosensitive than SCLC. In 3 small retrospective series that included 38 patients treated with cisplatin and etoposide the

Table 4
Systemic therapy for stage IV bronchial carcinoids

Study	Treatment Arms	No. of Patients	Response[a]	Median PFS (mo)	Median OS (mo)
Prospective					
Moertel & Hanley,[82] 1979	Streptozocin/cytoxan streptozocin/5-FU	17	12%	NR	15
Fazio et al,[98] 2013	Octreotide LAR plus everolimus (n = 33)	44 (33 TC, 9 AC, 2 NOS)	0% (67% had minor response)	14	NR
	Octreotide LAR (n = 11)		0% (27% had minor response)	6	
Fjällskog et al,[91] 2001	Cisplatin/etoposide	18	NR (56% responded radiologically and/or biochemically)	9	NR
Retrospective					
Ekeblad et al,[92] 2007	Temozolomide	31 (14 TC, 15 AC, 2 NOS)	14%	7	16
Wirth et al,[75] 2004	Platinum/etoposide based	18 (8 TC, 10 AC)	23%	NR	20
Forde et al,[84] 2014	Platinum/etoposide based	17	24%	7	NR
Granberg et al,[46] 2001	Interferon based ± Octreotide LAR (n = 27)	31 (27 TC, 4 AC)	4%	NR	76
	Cisplatin/etoposide (n = 8)		25%		
	Streptozocin + 5-FU or doxorubicin		0%		

Abbreviations: 5-FU, 5-fluorouracil; AC, atypical carcinoid; LAR, long-acting release; NOS, not otherwise specified; NR, not reported; OS, overall survival; PFS, progression-free survival; TC, typical carcinoid.
[a] Response includes complete and partial response.
Data from Refs.[46,75,82,84,91,92,98]

response rates were between 20% and 25%.[46,73,84] Cisplatin and etoposide were administered to 18 patients with foregut carcinoids (lung and thymus) who had progressed after first- or second-line treatment in a prospective study. Radiographic response was noted in 2 of the 5 patients with AC (40%) and in 5 of the 13 with TC (39%). The median response duration was 9 months (range, 6–30).[91]

Temozolomide-Based Therapies

Temozolomide, a nonclassical oral alkylating agent, has been evaluated either alone or in combination with other agents. In a retrospective study of 31 patients treated with temozolomide, which included both bronchial TC and AC, a partial response to treatment was noted in 3 patients (14%), and stable disease was observed in 11 patients (52%), with a median progression-free survival (PFS) of 7 months.[92] Eighteen patients with carcinoid and pancreatic NETs metastatic to the liver who received capecitabine and temozolomide were evaluated for response and outcome.[93] Overall response rate was 61%, and 3 of the 4 carcinoid patients attained clinical benefit (complete response, n = 1; partial response, n = 1, stable disease, n = 1). From the time of liver metastases, median PFS and OS were 14 months (range, 4–18) and 83 months (range, 18.5–140), respectively. These results suggest that the regimen of capecitabine and temozolomide is active and may prolong survival in this malignancy. In contrast, in 2 prospective trials that included patients with carcinoid tumors, a 7% response rate was noted using temozolomide with thalidomide and no response was observed using temozolomide and bevacizumab.[94,95] Because some studies have shown promising results for temozolomide, either alone or in combination with other agents in metastatic bronchial carcinoids, larger, prospective studies should be developed. Further, analysis of methyl-guanine DNA methyltransferase expression in NETs may be helpful to select responders.[96]

Mammalian Target of Rapamycin Inhibitors

The mammalian target of rapamycin pathway, which regulates cell growth, proliferation, and metabolism, has been implicated in the pathogenesis of NETs. In the randomized, placebo-controlled phase III study of everolimus plus octreotide LAR (RADIANT-2) that included 429 patients with low-grade or intermediate-grade carcinoids with prior history of carcinoid syndrome, of which 44 were of pulmonary histology, the median PFS was 16.4 months (95% CI, 13.7–21.2) for the group receiving the combination of everolimus and octreotide LAR compared with 11.3 months (95% CI, 8.4–14.6) in the octreotide LAR only group (HR, 0.77; 95% CI, 0.59–1.0; P = .026), thus achieving the primary endpoint of the study.[97] For the 44 bronchial carcinoid patients included in the study, median PFS was 13.6 and 5.6 months in the everolimus plus octreotide LAR group versus the octreotide LAR only group, respectively.[97,98] Side effects were common, with nearly one-half of patients treated with everolimus experiencing grade 3 or 4 adverse events, including diarrhea, stomatitis, and thrombocytopenia. RADIANT-4, the double-blind, phase III study comparing everolimus to placebo (NCT01524783) has met its primary endpoint of improvement in PFS. By central review, the PFS of everolimus was found to be 11 months compared to 3.9 months in the placebo arm [HR: 0.48 (95% CI, 0.35–0.67); P<.00001]. These data further support the use of the agent in bronchial carcinoids.[99] Details from this study will be reported, in full, in the near future. We are awaiting results from the 3-arm Trial to Evaluate Pasireotide LAR/Everolimus Alone/in Combination in Patients With Lung/Thymus NET (LUNA), a phase II study of everolimus versus pasireotide, a long-acting somatostatin analog, versus the combination in advanced bronchial carcinoids, which also allows for patients with thymic carcinoids (NCT01563354).

Vascular Endothelial Growth Factor Receptor Inhibitors

Well-differentiated carcinoid tumors are highly vascularized and extensively express vascular endothelial growth factor, hypoxia inducible factor 1α, and microvessel density.[100] As such, angiogenesis inhibitors have been investigated in this disease. In a phase II study in low to intermediate-grade NETs, patients were randomized to receive either bevacizumab or pegylated interferon-alfa-2b. Only 4 patients with pulmonary carcinoids were included in this trial, where an 18% partial response rate was observed in the bevacizumab group compared with no responses in the pegylated interferon-alfa-2b arm.[101] Fourteen patients with foregut carcinoids of the lung and stomach were included in a phase II study using sunitinib, a multitargeted oral tyrosine kinase inhibitor of VEGF receptor and platelet-derived growth factor receptor. The overall response rate for patients with carcinoid tumors was only 2.4%, although 83% of patients had stable disease with a median time to tumor progression of 10.2 months and a 1-year survival rate of 83.4%.[102] These results were even more impressive in patients with pancreatic neuroendocrine carcinoma, where a randomized phase III trial of sunitinib versus placebo demonstrated a significant improvement in PFS (11.4 vs 5.5 months, respectively; HR, 0.42; 95% CI, 0.26–0.66; $P<.001$).[103] A phase II study analyzed the antitumor efficacy of the combination of sorafenib plus bevacizumab in 44 NETs, including 9 foregut NETs, with a 10% overall response rate noted in carcinoid tumors.[104] The Pazopanib as a Single Agent in Advanced NETs (PAZONET) study, used pazopanib, an oral tyrosine kinase inhibitor of VEGF receptor, platelet-derived growth factor receptor, and KIT, as a sequencing treatment in progressive metastatic NET and showed a clinical benefit (defined as complete response, partial response, and stable disease at 6 months) in 85% of patients, including patients with bronchial carcinoids.[105] Based on these results, additional studies evaluating antiangiogenic activity in bronchial carcinoids are required.

Localized therapy in the setting of metastatic disease

There is little evidence to guide on local therapies for the management of patients with metastatic disease. The consensus is to reserve surgery with curative intent for patients with limited sites of disease where radical treatment is possible for all involved lesions. Such surgeries can be performed in patients with slowly progressive TC and possibly low proliferative AC. This is best illustrated in a series of well-selected patients who underwent complete resection of liver metastases and were shown to have an increased 5-year OS rate of greater than 70%.[106] Locoregional therapies including surgery, radiofrequency ablation, and cryoablation also can be used to decrease tumor burden and symptoms from bronchial primary sites or at metastatic disease sites.

In addition to surgical resection, patients with liver metastases can undergo hepatic artery embolization, with or without intraarterial chemotherapy, because these procedures have been associated with responses and improved outcomes in patients with carcinoid tumors.[107] Nine patients with pulmonary carcinoids who developed liver metastases underwent hepatic artery chemoembolization in a recently reported single institution retrospective review. Prolonged stable disease lasting up to 19 months was noted in 8 of these patients, with 3 achieving a partial response.[84] A newer embolization method using injectable particles conjugated to yttrium-90 permits delivery of internal radiation into hepatic arteries that supply carcinoid liver metastases.[100] Because randomized trials in embolization methods are lacking and some patients do experience treatment-related toxicities, patients must be selected carefully for these procedures. Furthermore, as of this writing, there is no clear evidence to suggest beneficial response of chemoembolization over particle embolization alone.

TREATMENT OF THYMIC CARCINOIDS

Because thymic carcinoids are incredibly rare with only a few hundred cases described in the literature, data on the optimal treatment are limited. For resectable disease, surgery remains the mainstay of therapy with a goal of R0 resection, because this is a strong prognostic factor for OS.[19] Unfortunately, even after complete surgical resection, there is a high rate of local recurrence. As such, perioperative chemotherapy, adjuvant radiation, or both frequently are considered. However, the evidence to support such therapy is extremely limited. For instance, case reports have demonstrated that radiation therapy with or without chemotherapy in the adjuvant setting may improve local control, although no survival benefit has been shown to date.[18,19,108]

In the metastatic setting, similar systemic therapies used for bronchial carcinoids can be applied, although the evidence for the effectiveness of these treatments is much more limited.[108] Palliative surgical resection or debulking of a large tumor to relieve compressive or hormonal symptoms may also be used to improve symptoms in highly selected patients.

SUMMARY

Bronchial and thymic carcinoids are foregut NETs that occur rarely, although the incidence has been increasing in recent years. These tumors are characterized by neuroendocrine morphology and differentiation and are classified using the WHO criteria, which separates TC and AC predominantly based on the presence of necrosis and number of mitosis. However, diagnostically it is difficult to differentiate between the two when small biopsies are available. In contrast with bronchial carcinoids, thymic carcinoid patients are more often men, of atypical histology, associated with MEN-1 syndrome, and demonstrate paraneoplastic syndromes. The evaluation of patients who present with these cancers include cross-sectional imaging with CT scans or MRI with a specific analysis of the liver, as it is a common metastatic site. Notably, both bronchial and thymic carcinoids follow staging systems of their site of origin.

Surgery is the only curative option in these malignancies. Although adjuvant therapy is advocated in resected disease, the best regimens are unknown and data showing evidence of benefit are lacking. For asymptomatic patients with metastatic disease, initial expectant observation can be pursued. In patients who have a clinically significant tumor burden, treatment can be approached in a stepwise fashion, using somatostatin analogs for those with positive octreotide scans initially; systemic therapies such as temozolomide, sunitinib or everolimus, subsequently; and chemotherapy at the time of more rapidly progressing disease. Liver-directed treatment can be administered when necessary, and for those with symptomatic lesions, local resection, radiation therapy, radioablation, or cryoablation can be considered. Additional prospective, randomized studies that include bronchial and thymic carcinoid patients are warranted.

REFERENCES

1. Travis WD, Brambilla E, Nicholson AG, et al. The 2015 World Health Organization classification of lung tumors. Impact of genetic, clinical and radiologic advances since the 2004 classification. J Thorac Oncol 2015;10:1243–60.
2. Quaedvlieg PF, Visser O, Lamers CB, et al. Epidemiology and survival in patients with carcinoid disease in The Netherlands. An epidemiological study with 2391 patients. Ann Oncol 2001;12:1295–300.

3. Hauso O, Gustafsson BI, Kidd M, et al. Neuroendocrine tumor epidemiology: contrasting Norway and North America. Cancer 2008;113:2655–64.
4. Modlin IM, Lye KD, Kidd MA. 5-decade analysis of 13,715 carcinoid tumors. Cancer 2003;97:934–59.
5. Hemminki K, Li X. Incidence trends and risk factors of carcinoid tumors: a nationwide epidemiologic study from Sweden. Cancer 2001;92:2204–10.
6. Fink G, Krelbaum T, Yellin A, et al. Pulmonary carcinoid: presentation, diagnosis, and outcome in 142 cases in Israel and review of 640 cases from the literature. Chest 2001;119:1647–51.
7. Gatta G, Ciccolallo L, Kunkler I, et al. Survival from rare cancer in adults: a population-based study. Lancet Oncol 2006;7:132–40.
8. Yao JC, Hassan M, Phan A, et al. One hundred years after "carcinoid": epidemiology of and prognostic factors for neuroendocrine tumors in 35,825 cases in the United States. J Clin Oncol 2008;26:3063–72.
9. Oberg K, Hellman P, Kwekkeboom D, et al. Neuroendocrine bronchial and thymic tumours: ESMO clinical practice guidelines for diagnosis, treatment and follow-up. Ann Oncol 2010;21:v220–2.
10. Kulke MH, Mayer RJ. Carcinoid tumors. N Engl J Med 1999;340:858–68.
11. Davini F, Gonfiotti A, Comin C, et al. Typical and atypical carcinoid tumours: 20-year experience with 89 patients. J Cardiovasc Surg 2009;50:807–11.
12. Asamura H, Kameya T, Matsuno Y, et al. Neuroendocrine neoplasms of the lung: a prognostic spectrum. J Clin Oncol 2006;24:70–6.
13. Thomas CF Jr, Tazelaar HD, Jett JR. Typical and atypical pulmonary carcinoids: outcome in patients presenting with regional lymph node involvement. Chest 2001;119:1143–50.
14. McCaughan BC, Martini N, Bains MS. Bronchial carcinoids. Review of 124 cases. J Thorac Cardiovasc Surg 1985;89:8–17.
15. Debelenko LV, Brambilla E, Agarwal SK, et al. Identification of MEN1 gene mutations in sporadic carcinoid tumors of the lung. Hum Mol Genet 1997;6:2285–90.
16. Strollo DC, Rosado de Christenson ML, Jett JR. Primary mediastinal tumors. Part 1: tumors of the anterior mediastinum. Chest 1997;112:511–22.
17. Chaer R, Massad MG, Evans A, et al. Primary neuroendocrine tumors of the thymus. Ann Thorac Surg 2002;74:1733–40.
18. Gaur P, Leary C, Yao JC. Thymic neuroendocrine tumors: a SEER database analysis of 160 patients. Ann Surg 2010;251:1117–21.
19. Filosso PL, Yao X, Ahmad U, et al. Outcome of primary neuroendocrine tumors of the thymus: a joint analysis of the International Thymic Malignancy Interest Group and the European Society of Thoracic Surgeons databases. J Thorac Cardiovasc Surg 2015;149:103–9.
20. Gibril F, Chen YJ, Schrump DS, et al. Prospective study of thymic carcinoids in patients with multiple endocrine neoplasia type 1. J Clin Endocrinol Metab 2003;88:1066–81.
21. Ferolla P, Falchetti A, Filosso P, et al. Thymic neuroendocrine carcinoma (carcinoid) in multiple endocrine neoplasia type 1 syndrome: the Italian series. J Clin Endocrinol Metab 2005;90:2603–9.
22. Powell AC, Alexander HR, Pingpank JF, et al. The utility of routine transcervical thymectomy for multiple endocrine neoplasia 1-related hyperparathyroidism. Surgery 2008;144:878–83.
23. Goudet P, Murat A, Cardot-Bauters C, et al. Thymic neuroendocrine tumors in multiple endocrine neoplasia type 1: a comparative study on 21 cases among

a series of 761 MEN1 from the GTE (Groupe des Tumeurs Endocrines). World J Surg 2009;33:1197–207.

24. Davies SJ, Gosney JR, Hansell DM, et al. Diffuse idiopathic pulmonary neuroendocrine cell hyperplasia: an under-recognised spectrum of disease. Thorax 2007;62:248–52.

25. Fernandez-Cuesta L, Peifer M, Lu X, et al. Frequent mutations in chromatin remodeling genes in pulmonary carcinoids. Nat Commun 2014;5:3518.

26. Pelosi G, Rodriguez J, Viale G, et al. Typical and atypical pulmonary carcinoid tumor overdiagnosed as small-cell carcinoma on biopsy specimens: a major pitfall in the management of lung cancer patients. Am J Surg Pathol 2005;29:179–87.

27. Chughtai TS, Morin JE, Sheiner NM, et al. Bronchial carcinoid–twenty years' experience defines a selective surgical approach. Surgery 1997;122:801–8.

28. de Montpréville VT, Macchiarini P, Dulmet E. Thymic neuroendocrine carcinoma (carcinoid): a clinicopathologic study of fourteen cases. J Thorac Cardiovasc Surg 1996;111:134–41.

29. Fukai I, Masaoka A, Fujii Y, et al. Thymic neuroendocrine tumor (thymic carcinoid): a clinicopathologic study in 15 patients. Ann Thorac Surg 1999;67:208–11.

30. Wick MR, Carney JA, Bernatz PE, et al. Primary mediastinal carcinoid tumors. Am J Surg Pathol 1982;6:195–205.

31. Moran CA, Suster S. Neuroendocrine carcinomas (carcinoid tumor) of the thymus. A clinicopathologic analysis of 80 cases. Am J Clin Pathol 2000;114:100–10.

32. Wang DY, Chang DB, Kuo SH, et al. Carcinoid tumours of the thymus. Thorax 1994;49:357–60.

33. Wick MR, Rosai J. Neuroendocrine neoplasms of the thymus. Pathol Res Pract 1988;183:188–99.

34. de Perrot M, Spiliopoulos A, Fischer S, et al. Neuroendocrine carcinoma (carcinoid) of the thymus associated with Cushing's syndrome. Ann Thorac Surg 2002;73:675–81.

35. National Comprehensive Cancer Network (NCCN). NCCN Clinical practice guidelines in oncology. Available at: http://www.nccn.org/professionals/physician_gls/f_guidelines.asp. Accessed June 01, 2015.

36. Yellin A, Zwas ST, Rozenman J, et al. Experience with somatostatin receptor scintigraphy in the management of pulmonary carcinoid tumors. Isr Med Assoc J 2005;7:712–6.

37. Reidy-Lagunes DL, Gollub MJ, Saltz LB. Addition of octreotide functional imaging to cross-sectional computed tomography or magnetic resonance imaging for the detection of neuroendocrine tumors: added value or an anachronism? J Clin Oncol 2011;29:e74–5.

38. Erasmus JJ, McAdams HP, Patz EF Jr, et al. Evaluation of primary pulmonary carcinoid tumors using FDG PET. Am J Roentgenol 1998;170:1369–73.

39. Daniels CE, Lowe VJ, Aubry MC, et al. The utility of fluorodeoxyglucose positron emission tomography in the evaluation of carcinoid tumors presenting as pulmonary nodules. Chest 2007;131:255–60.

40. Kayani I, Bomanji JB, Groves A, et al. Functional imaging of neuroendocrine tumors with combined PET/CT using 68Ga-DOTATATE (DOTA-DPhe1,Tyr3-octreotate) and 18F-FDG. Cancer 2008;112:2447–55.

41. Binderup T, Knigge U, Loft A, et al. 18F-fluorodeoxyglucose positron emission tomography predicts survival of patients with neuroendocrine tumors. Clin Cancer Res 2010;16:978–85.

42. Lim E, Baldwin D, Beckles M, et al. Guidelines on the radical management of patients with lung cancer. Thorax 2010;65:iii1–27.
43. Pattenden H, Leung M, Beddow E. Test performance of PET-CT for mediastinal lymph node staging of pulmonary carcinoid tumours. Thorax 2015;70:379–81. Available at: http://thorax.bmj.com/content/70/4/379.long - aff-1.
44. Pellikka PA, Tajik AJ, Khandheria BK, et al. Carcinoid heart disease. Clinical and echocardiographic spectrum in 74 patients. Circulation 1993;87:1188–96.
45. Lundin L, Norheim I, Landelius J, et al. Carcinoid heart disease: relationship of circulating vasoactive substances to ultrasound-detectable cardiac abnormalities. Circulation 1988;77:264–9.
46. Granberg D, Eriksson B, Wilander E, et al. Experience in treatment of metastatic pulmonary carcinoid tumors. Ann Oncol 2001;12:1383–91.
47. Campana D, Nori F, Piscitelli L, et al. Chromogranin A: is it a useful marker of neuroendocrine tumors? J Clin Oncol 2007;25:1967–73.
48. Soga J, Yakuwa Y, Osaka M. Evaluation of 342 cases of mediastinal/thymic carcinoids collected from literature: a comparative study between typical carcinoids and atypical varieties. Ann Thorac Cardiovasc Surg 1999;5:285–92.
49. Jansson JO, Svensson J, Bengtsson BA, et al. Acromegaly and Cushing's syndrome due to ectopic production of GHRH and ACTH by a thymic carcinoid tumour: in vitro responses to GHRH and GHRP-6. Clin Endocrinol 1998;48: 243–50.
50. Okada S, Ohshima K, Mori M. The Cushing syndrome induced by atrial natriuretic peptide-producing thymic carcinoid. Ann Intern Med 1994;121:75–6.
51. Travis WD, Giroux DJ, Chansky K, et al. The IASLC Lung Cancer Staging Project: proposals for the inclusion of broncho-pulmonary carcinoid tumors in the forthcoming (seventh) edition of the TNM Classification for Lung Cancer. J Thorac Oncol 2008;3:1213–23.
52. Ferguson MK, Landreneau RJ, Hazelrigg SR, et al. Long-term outcome after resection for bronchial carcinoid tumors. Eur J Cardiothorac Surg 2000;18: 156–61.
53. Gustafsson BI, Kidd M, Chan A, et al. Bronchopulmonary neuroendocrine tumors. Cancer 2008;113:5–21.
54. Filosso PL, Oliaro A, Ruffini E, et al. Outcome and prognostic factors in bronchial carcinoids: a single-center experience. J Thorac Oncol 2013;8:1282–8.
55. Skuladottir H, Hirsch FR, Hansen HH, et al. Pulmonary neuroendocrine tumors: incidence and prognosis of histological subtypes. A population-based study in Denmark. Lung Cancer 2002;37:127–35.
56. Divisi D, Crisci R. Carcinoid tumors of the lung and multimodal therapy. Thorac Cardiovasc Surg 2005;53:168–72.
57. Cardillo G, Sera F, Di Martino M, et al. Bronchial carcinoid tumors: nodal status and long-term survival after resection. Ann Thorac Surg 2004;77:1781–5.
58. Ducrocq X, Thomas P, Massard G, et al. Operative risk and prognostic factors of typical bronchial carcinoid tumors. Ann Thorac Surg 1998;65:1410–4.
59. Soga J, Yakuwa Y. Bronchopulmonary carcinoids: an analysis of 1,875 reported cases with special reference to a comparison between typical carcinoids and atypical varieties. Ann Thorac Cardiovasc Surg 1999;5:211–9.
60. Matilla Gonzalez J, Garcia-Yuste M, Moreno-Mata N, et al. Typical and atypical carcinoid tumors (NEC grades 1 and 2): prognostic factors in metastases and local recurrence. Lung Cancer 2005;49:S60. Available at: http://www.uptodate.com/contents/bronchial-carcinoid-tumors-treatment-and-prognosis/abstract/22.

61. Fiala P, Petrásková K, Cernohorský S, et al. Bronchial carcinoid tumors: long-term outcome after surgery. Neoplasma 2003;50:60–5.
62. Gould PM, Bonner JA, Sawyer TE, et al. Bronchial carcinoid tumors: importance of prognostic factors that influence patterns of recurrence and overall survival. Radiology 1998;208:181–5.
63. Filosso PL, Rena O, Donati G, et al. Bronchial carcinoid tumors: surgical management and long-term outcome. J Thorac Cardiovasc Surg 2002;123:303–9.
64. García-Yuste M, Matilla JM, Alvarez-Gago T, et al. Prognostic factors in neuroendocrine lung tumors: a Spanish Multicenter Study. Spanish Multicenter Study of Neuroendocrine Tumors of the Lung of the Spanish Society of Pneumonology and Thoracic Surgery (EMETNE-SEPAR). Ann Thorac Surg 2000;70:258–63.
65. Rea F, Rizzardi G, Zuin A, et al. Outcome and surgical strategy in bronchial carcinoid tumors: single institution experience with 252 patients. Eur J Cardiothorac Surg 2007;31:186–91.
66. Harpole DH Jr, Feldman JM, Buchanan S, et al. Bronchial carcinoid tumors: a retrospective analysis of 126 patients. Ann Thorac Surg 1992;54:50–4.
67. Yendamuri S, Gold D, Jayaprakash V, et al. Is sublobar resection sufficient for carcinoid tumors? Ann Thorac Surg 2011;92:1774–8.
68. Marty-Ane CH, Costes V, Pujol JL, et al. Carcinoid tumors of the lung: do atypical features require aggressive management? Ann Thorac Surg 1995;59:78–83.
69. Garcia-Yuste M, Matilla JM, Cueto A, et al. Typical and atypical carcinoid tumours: analysis of the experience of the Spanish Multi-centric Study of Neuroendocrine Tumours of the Lung. Eur J Cardiothorac Surg 2007;31:192–7.
70. Mineo TC, Guggino G, Mineo D, et al. Relevance of lymph node micrometastases in radically resected endobronchial carcinoid tumors. Ann Thorac Surg 2005;80:428–32.
71. Wurtz A, Benhamed L, Conti M, et al. Results of systematic nodal dissection in typical and atypical carcinoid tumors of the lung. J Thorac Oncol 2009;4:388–94.
72. Ferolla P, Daddi N, Urbani M, et al. Tumorlets, multicentric carcinoids, lymph-nodal metastases, and long-term behavior in bronchial carcinoids. J Thorac Oncol 2009;4:383–7.
73. Lou F, Sarkaria I, Pietanza C, et al. Recurrence of pulmonary carcinoid tumors after resection: implications for postoperative surveillance. Ann Thorac Surg 2013;96:1156–62.
74. Kalemkerian GP, Loo BW, Akerley W, et al. NCCN clinical practice guidelines in oncology: small cell lung cancer version I.2016. Fort Washington (PA): National Comprehensive Cancer Network (NCCN); 2015. Available at: http://www.nccn.org/professionals/physician_gls/pdf/sclc.pdf. Accessed June 1, 2015.
75. Wirth LJ, Carter MR, Janne PA, et al. Outcome of patients with pulmonary carcinoid tumors receiving chemotherapy or chemoradiotherapy. Lung Cancer 2004;44:213–20.
76. Mackley HB, Videtic GM. Primary carcinoid tumors of the lung: a role for radiotherapy. Oncology (Williston Park) 2006;20:1537–43.
77. Chakravarthy A, Abrams RA. Radiation therapy in the management of patients with malignant carcinoid tumors. Cancer 1995;75:1386–90.
78. Granberg D, Sundin A, Janson ET, et al. Octreoscan in patients with bronchial carcinoid tumours. Clin Endocrinol 2003;59:793–9.
79. Filosso PL, Ruffini E, Oliaro A, et al. Long-term survival of atypical bronchial carcinoids with liver metastases, treated with octreotide. Eur J Cardiothorac Surg 2002;21:913–7.

80. Moertel CG, Kvols LK, O'Connell MJ, et al. Treatment of neuroendocrine carcinomas with combined etoposide and cisplatin. Evidence of major therapeutic activity in the anaplastic variants of these neoplasms. Cancer 1991;68:227–32.

81. Sun W, Lipsitz S, Catalano P, et al. Phase II/III study of doxorubicin with fluorouracil compared with streptozocin with fluorouracil or dacarbazine in the treatment of advanced carcinoid tumors: Eastern Cooperative Oncology Group Study E1281. J Clin Oncol 2005;23:4897–904.

82. Moertel CG, Hanley JA. Combination chemotherapy trials in metastatic carcinoid tumor and the malignant carcinoid syndrome. Cancer Clin Trials 1979;2: 327–34.

83. Srirajaskanthan R, Toumpanakis C, Karpathakis A, et al. Surgical management and palliative treatment in bronchial neuroendocrine tumours: a clinical study of 45 patients. Lung Cancer 2009;65:68–73.

84. Forde PM, Hooker CM, Boikos SA, et al. Systemic therapy, clinical outcomes, and overall survival in locally advanced or metastatic pulmonary carcinoid: a brief report. J Thorac Oncol 2014;9:414–8.

85. Rinke A, Muller HH, Schade-Brittinger C, et al. Placebo-controlled, double-blind, prospective, randomized study on the effect of octreotide LAR in the control of tumor growth in patients with metastatic neuroendocrine midgut tumors: a report from the PROMID Study Group. J Clin Oncol 2009;27:4656–63.

86. Caplin ME, Pavel M, Ćwikła JB, et al. Lanreotide in metastatic enteropancreatic neuroendocrine tumors. N Engl J Med 2014;371:224–33.

87. Gridelli C, Rossi A, Airoma G, et al. Treatment of pulmonary neuroendocrine tumours: state of the art and future developments. Cancer Treat Rev 2013;39: 466–72.

88. Waldherr C, Pless M, Maecke HR, et al. The clinical value of [90Y-DOTA]-DPhe1-Tyr3-octreotide (90Y-DOTATOC) in the treatment of neuroendocrine tumours: a clinical phase II study. Ann Oncol 2001;12:941–5.

89. Imhof A, Brunner P, Marincek N, et al. Response, survival, and long-term toxicity after therapy with the radiolabeled somatostatin analogue [90Y-DOTA]-TOC in metastasized neuroendocrine cancers. J Clin Oncol 2011;29:2416–23.

90. Detterbeck FC. Management of carcinoid tumors. Ann Thorac Surg 2010;89(3): 998–1005.

91. Fjällskog ML, Granberg DP, Welin SL, et al. Treatment with cisplatin and etoposide in patients with neuroendocrine tumors. Cancer 2001;92:1101–7.

92. Ekeblad S, Sundin A, Janson ET, et al. Temozolomide as monotherapy is effective in treatment of advanced malignant neuroendocrine tumors. Clin Cancer Res 2007;13:2986–91.

93. Fine RL, Gulati AP, Krantz BA, et al. Capecitabine and temozolomide (CAPTEM) for metastatic, well-differentiated neuroendocrine cancers: the Pancreas Center at Columbia University experience. Cancer Chemother Pharmacol 2013;71: 663–70.

94. Kulke MH, Stuart K, Enzinger PC, et al. Phase II study of temozolomide and thalidomide in patients with metastatic neuroendocrine tumors. J Clin Oncol 2006;24:401–6.

95. Chan JA, Stuart K, Earle CC, et al. Prospective study of bevacizumab plus temozolomide in patients with advanced neuroendocrine tumors. J Clin Oncol 2012;30:2963–8.

96. Kulke MH, Scherubl H. Accomplishments in 2008 in the management of gastrointestinal neuroendocrine tumors. Gastrointest Cancer Res 2009;3(5 Suppl 2): S62–6.

97. Pavel ME, Hainsworth JD, Baudin E, et al. Everolimus plus octreotide long-acting repeatable for the treatment of advanced neuroendocrine tumours associated with carcinoid syndrome (RADIANT-2): a randomised, placebo-controlled, phase 3 study. Lancet 2011;378:2005–12.

98. Fazio N, Granberg D, Grossman A, et al. Everolimus plus octreotide long-acting repeatable in patients with advanced lung neuroendocrine tumors: analysis of the phase 3, randomized, placebo-controlled RADIANT-2 study. Chest 2013; 143:955–62.

99. Yao J, Fazio N, Singh S, et al. Everolimus in advanced nonfunctional neuroendocrine tumors of lung or gastrointestinal origin: efficacy and safety results from the placebo-controlled, double-blind, multicenter, Phase 3 RADIANT-4 Study. 18th ECCO-40th ESMO Congress, September 25–29, 2015, Vienna, Austria. Abstract 5LBA.

100. Reidy-Lagunes D, Thornton R. Pancreatic neuroendocrine and carcinoid tumors: what's new, what's old, and what's different? Curr Oncol Rep 2012;14: 249–56.

101. Yao JC, Phan A, Hoff PM, et al. Targeting vascular endothelial growth factor in advanced carcinoid tumor: a random assignment phase II study of depot octreotide with bevacizumab and pegylated interferon alpha-2b. J Clin Oncol 2008;26:1316–23.

102. Kulke MH, Lenz HJ, Meropol NJ, et al. Activity of sunitinib in patients with advanced neuroendocrine tumors. J Clin Oncol 2008;26:3403–10.

103. Raymond E, Dahan L, Raoul JL, et al. Sunitinib malate for the treatment of pancreatic neuroendocrine tumors. N Engl J Med 2011;364:501–13.

104. Castellano D, Capdevila J, Sastre J, et al. Sorafenib and bevacizumab combination targeted therapy in advanced neuroendocrine tumour: a phase II study of Spanish Neuroendocrine Tumour Group (GETNE0801). Eur J Cancer 2013; 49:3780–7.

105. Pulido E, Castellano D, Garcia-Carbonero R, et al. PAZONET: results of a phase II trial of pazopanib as a sequencing treatment in progressive metastatic neuroendocrine tumors (NETs) patients (pts), on behalf of the Spanish task force for NETs (GETNE)—NCT01280201. J Clin Oncol 2012;30(Suppl) [abstract: 4119].

106. Glazer ES, Tseng JF, Al-Refaie W, et al. Long-term survival after surgical management of neuroendocrine hepatic metastases. HPB (Oxford) 2010;12:427–33.

107. Gupta S, Johnson MM, Murthy R, et al. Hepatic arterial embolization and chemoembolization for the treatment of patients with metastatic neuroendocrine tumors: variables affecting response rates and survival. Cancer 2005;104: 1590–602.

108. Crona J, Björklund P, Welin S, et al. Treatment, prognostic markers and survival in thymic neuroendocrine tumours. a study from a single tertiary referral centre. Lung Cancer 2013;79:289–93.

Surgical Management of Pancreatic Neuroendocrine Tumors

Thomas E. Clancy, MD

KEYWORDS

- Neuroendocrine • Pancreas • Pancreatectomy • Surgery • Enucleation

KEY POINTS

- Pancreatic neuroendocrine tumors are relatively rare and make up approximately 1% to 2% of all solid pancreatic tumors.
- They include a diverse group of neoplasms, with clinical behavior ranging from small indolent tumors to widely metastatic disease.
- A minority are associated with hormone secretion and syndromes of hormone excess.
- Surgery is the treatment of choice for localized disease and may include formal pancreatic resection or parenchyma-preserving enucleation in some cases.
- Surgical care must be individualized to tumor characteristics and clinical symptoms.

Pancreatic neuroendocrine tumors (PNETs) are relatively rare, constituting approximately 1% to 2% of all pancreatic neoplasms and with an overall incidence of approximately 5 cases per million annually.[1] Despite sharing histologic characteristics with neuroendocrine tumors from other sites, PNETs have unique biology and clinical behavior from other neuroendocrine neoplasms.[2] These tumors include a heterogeneous group of neoplasms that have long been held in unique fascination by physicians and surgeons because of the ability of some tumors to secrete specific hormones and their association with well-described clinical syndromes. Most PNETs, however, do not secrete specific hormones and are often referred to as nonfunctioning PNET. Recent years have seen an increased understanding of the origin[3] and biological basis of PNETs[2] as well as in new targeted therapies for advanced PET.[4–6] Surgical resection remains the mainstay of therapy for localized and occasionally metastatic disease.

Disclosure Statement: The author has nothing to disclose.
Division of Surgical Oncology, Brigham and Women's Hospital, 75 Francis Street, Boston, MA 02115, USA
E-mail address: tclancy@partners.org

Hematol Oncol Clin N Am 30 (2016) 103–118
http://dx.doi.org/10.1016/j.hoc.2015.09.004
0889-8588/16/$ – see front matter

In addition to their relatively rare incidence and diverse clinical manifestations, PNETs have a wide range of biological behavior and associated prognosis. Although many PNETs are relatively slow growing and have a favorable long-term prognosis,[7] others may present with locally invasive or metastatic disease.[8] Furthermore, some PNETs may present in association with genetic syndromes, such as multiple endocrine neoplasia type I (MEN1),[9] that will influence rates of recurrence. This variability in biological behavior and recurrence risk precludes a unified treatment strategy for all PNETs. Unique surgical considerations for functioning and nonfunctioning PNETs, both localized and metastatic, are considered.

CLINICAL PRESENTATION AND DIAGNOSIS
Functioning Pancreatic Neuroendocrine Tumors

PNETs are classified as functional based on secretion of one of a variety of hormones, including insulin, gastrin, glucagon, vasoactive intestinal peptide (VIP), and rarely somatostatin.[10] The clinical presentation and evaluation of these are specific to each type of tumor.

Insulinoma

Given the unregulated production of insulin, patients with insulinoma will typically present with signs and symptoms of hypoglycemia, including neuroglycopenic or sympathetic effects. Neuroglycopenic symptoms may include headaches, blurred vision, forgetfulness, and difficulties with speech. Activation of the sympathetic nervous system can result in sweating, tachycardia, tremors, and weakness. Both neuroglycopenic and sympathetic symptoms may be relieved with eating. Excess caloric intake coupled with the anabolic effects of insulin often leads to weight gain in these patients.

Diagnosis of insulinoma is traditionally suspected based on the combination of clinical signs, known as Whipple's triad in recognition of the original description of these tumors by Whipple and Frantz[11] in 1935. This triad consists of the presence of symptomatic hypoglycemia with fasting, documented plasma glucose of less than 50 mg/dL with symptoms, and the relief of symptoms with glucose administration. Diagnosis is confirmed by assessment of serum insulin, proinsulin, C-peptide, and glucose to establish hyperinsulinism[12]; the absence of ketosis or sulfonylurea metabolites in blood or urine is important to rule out factitious hyperinsulinism. Within 48 hours of an observed fast, between 90% and 95% of patients will develop hypoglycemia, with a diagnostic insulin-to-glucose ration of more than 0.4. Although far less common than insulinoma, adult nesidioblastosis or beta cell hyperplasia will occasionally present with similar laboratory and clinical findings.[13] This syndrome has been described in a population of patients after bariatric surgery.[14,15]

In the absence of a clinical syndrome such as MEN1, most insulinomas occur as small, solitary, benign lesions.[16] Although tumors may range in size, most are less than 2 cm in size and can be found with relatively equal distribution throughout the pancreas.[17] Very few patients with insulinoma develop metastatic spread, with a rate of less than 10%, far less than other pancreatic islet cell tumors.[18]

Although selective pancreatic angiography with calcium stimulation and hepatic venous sampling was traditionally used to detect these small lesions,[19] contrast-enhanced computed tomography (CT) can localize most lesions[20] (**Fig. 1**). Endoscopic ultrasound (EUS) is quite sensitive for the detection of insulinoma, and the combination of EUS with CT can identify nearly all lesions.[21] Conventional MRI is similarly sensitive in this setting.[22] The use of somatostatin receptor scintigraphy is limited given the low expression of type 2 somatostatin receptors on insulinomas.[23]

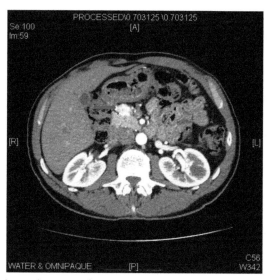

Fig. 1. Contrast-enhanced CT scan of insulinoma in pancreatic head (*arrow*). Tumor demonstrates arterial enhancement and is thereby distinguished from the remaining pancreatic parenchyma.

Gastrinoma

The identification of patients with severe ulcer disease and associated non–insulin-producing islet cell tumors led to the description of gastrinomas by Zollinger and Ellison[24] in 1955. Gastrinomas are associated with MEN1 in approximately 25% of cases[25] and develop metastatic disease in 60% to 90%.[26,27] Patients may present with disabling pain, diarrhea, reflux, and duodenal ulcers.

Hypergastrinemia in the setting of excess gastric acid secretion is important to rule out atrophic gastritis or proton pump inhibitor use. Secretin stimulation causes a paradoxic increase in serum gastrin in the setting of a gastrinoma, which can be used to diagnose the tumors.[28]

Gastrinomas are frequently multifocal, with a higher propensity for local or distant spread than insulinoma. Most are localized in an area referred to as the gastrinoma triangle, delineated by the junction of the cystic duct and common bile duct, the body and neck of the pancreas, and the second and third portion of the duodenum.[29] Localization of tumors may be challenging with traditional cross-sectional imaging, though somatostatin receptor scintigraphy has a sensitivity of approximately 60%.[30] In some cases, operative exploration can be required to identify lesions using palpation, intraoperative ultrasound, duodenotomy, and transillumination of the duodenum[31] (**Fig. 2**).

Glucagonoma

Glucagonoma is a rare functioning pancreatic neuroendocrine tumor associated with a range of signs, most characteristically a rash known as necrolytic migratory erythema, a vesicular, erythematous necrotic dermatitis. Patients present with diabetes, glossitis, weight loss, and weakness. Deep vein thrombosis can occur in 30% of patients, and patients present with anemia and a decreased level of amino acids due to gluoneogensis.[32] These tumors are often large at diagnosis, and contrast-enhanced CT scan is often sufficient for localization. Patients often present with advanced and metastatic disease.

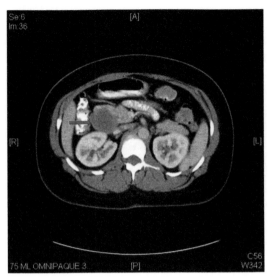

Fig. 2. Contrast-enhanced CT scan of a patient with metastatic gastrinoma to the periduodenal space. A 5-cm lesion adjacent to the duodenum was identified (*arrow*); biopsy was consistent with neuroendocrine tumor, and the lesion was the only site localized on octreotide scan. On surgical exploration, a primary tumor measuring 5 mm was identified in the duodenal wall.

VIPoma

Vasoactive intestinal peptide (VIPoma) are exceedingly rare tumors associated with secretion of the hormone VIP. The syndrome of copious watery diarrhea, hypokalemia, and achlorhydria is also described as pancreatic cholera. These tumors are characteristically large and are often metastatic to the liver at the time of diagnosis. Most are easily visualized by contrast-enhanced CT or somatostatin receptor scintigraphy.

Nonfunctioning Pancreatic Neuroendocrine Tumors

Approximately 70% of PNETs do not secrete a specific hormone and are not associated with specific clinical syndromes. These tumors are often asymptomatic in the absence of vague abdominal pain. Although symptoms may include abdominal pain, jaundice, pancreatic insufficiency, a palpable mass, and anorexia, tumors are often detected before symptoms as incidental finding on imaging studies performed for an unrelated indication.[33] In one 20-year cohort of nonfunctioning PNET, 35% of patients were asymptomatic with an incidental diagnosis.[34] Patients with advanced disease may present with locally advanced disease involving the mesenteric vessels or with widespread metastases.

PNETs typically appear as hypervascular lesions on CT, as opposed to the often hypovascular appearance of adenocarcinoma. MRI has a comparable sensitivity and specificity (**Fig. 3**). Somatostatin-receptor scintigraphy has excellent sensitivity and specificity and is particularly important for evaluating the presence of occult metastatic disease.[35] Definitive diagnosis can often be obtained with EUS-guided fine-needle aspiration. Serum chromogranin A is a valuable tumor marker in the management of well-differentiated PNETS, and levels can be used in determining response to therapy and for serial follow-up of patients.

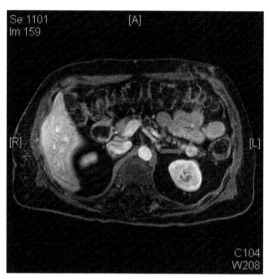

Fig. 3. MRI demonstrates a 2-cm enhancing mass in the pancreatic tail (*arrow*). Resection confirmed PNET.

STAGING

The World Health Organization classifies neuroendocrine tumors into different grades based on histologic characteristics. Well-differentiated tumors include low-grade (G1) tumors with a low mitotic count and Ki-67 proliferative index of less than 3% as well as intermediate-grade (G2) tumors with mitotic counts of 2 to 20 per high-power field (HPF) and Ki-67 rate of 3% to 20%. Poorly differentiated tumors or high-grade (G3) tumors have mitotic rates more than 2 per 10 HPF and Ki-67 rate of greater than 20%.[36] High-grade tumors, often referred to as neuroendocrine carcinomas, display more aggressive clinical behavior[10] and unlike, well-differentiated tumors, are generally not candidates for surgical resection.

Staging systems include variants proposed by the American Joint Committee on Cancer and a second promoted by the European Neuroendocrine Tumor Society.[37,38] Both systems are useful for predicting survival, with overall survival ranging from 90% to 100% at 5 years for stage I tumors to approximately 60% for stage IV tumors.[7,39]

SURGICAL MANAGEMENT
Functioning Pancreatic Neuroendocrine Tumors

Insulinoma
Although surgical resection of localized disease is the mainstay of therapy for all PNETs, insulinomas are unique in their relative lack of metastases and potential for treatment with pancreas-sparing procedures. Unlike formal pancreatic surgery, such as distal pancreatectomy, central pancreatectomy, or pancreaticoduodenectomy, enucleation involves removal of just the tumor and associated capsule, sparing otherwise normal pancreatic parenchyma (**Fig. 4**). In a systematic review of case series with a total of more than 6200 insulinoma patients, Mehrabi and colleagues[17] describe enucleation as the procedure of choice in more than half of insulinomas.

Enucleation is particularly applicable to small, benign, superficial tumors.[40] Tumors closer to the main pancreatic duct will have a higher risk of postoperative pancreatic

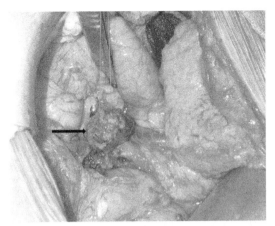

Fig. 4. Enucleation, pancreatic head insulinoma (*arrow*). Patient in **Fig. 1** was taken to the operating room for symptomatic insulinoma. Enucleation was possible as the mass was greater than 3 mm from the pancreatic duct.

fistula after enucleation. Tumors located deeper in the parenchyma, larger tumors, or tumors with any suspicion of malignancy are more appropriately treated with formal resection. Enucleation is also well described using minimally invasive or laparoscopic techniques.[41] The use of intraoperative ultrasound should be routine in either open or laparoscopic cases to identify the distance between the tumor and the main pancreatic duct and to exclude multiple tumors.[42] Given the benign behavior of most insulinomas, lymph node dissection is not required as part of the procedure.[43]

In rare instances, a thorough evaluation has failed to identify the location of an insulinoma; it was thought that blind distal pancreatectomy would remove most occult lesions. This procedure is now rarely performed because of improved localization techniques. In cases of truly undetected lesions, it is more appropriate to stop the operation and seek more accurate localization.[44]

Surgery for insulinoma in the presence of MEN1 is aimed at controlling all excess insulin secretion by removing all possible tumor burden. Preoperative localization is essential given the propensity for multifocal disease (**Box 1**).

Gastrinoma

Although the historical surgical treatment of gastrinoma was total gastrectomy to remove all acid-producing tissue, symptoms are now much more easily managed

---

Box 1
Insulinoma: surgical considerations

- Enucleation preferred for tumors distant (>2–3 mm) from pancreatic duct
- Formal resection indicated if enucleation not possible
- Lymph node dissection not needed
- Laparoscopic resection beneficial
- No indication for blind distal pancreatectomy
- Role for surgery in MEN1 to remove tumor burden

with acid-reducing agents, such as histamine type-2 blockers and proton pump inhibitors. The identification of a causative tumor offers the possibility of biochemical cure, prevention of disease progression, and prolongation of survival. As noted earlier, surgical resection may require operative exploration with ultrasound, direct palpation, duodenal transillumination, or duodenotomy. Surgical resection of the primary tumor and involved lymph nodes is the only potentially curative treatment.[45] Based on the high incidence of lymph node metastases in sporadic gastrinomas and the prognostic importance of nodal metastases, most investigators recommend routine systematic lymph node dissection in the peripancreatic, periduodenal, and pancreaticoduodenal area during surgery for sporadic gastrinoma.[46]

Resection in sporadic cases of gastrinoma may lead to long-term cure in approximately one-third of patients, with disease-specific survival at 10 years of 95%.[25] Enucleation may be applicable for tumors with an adequate margin to the pancreatic duct (3 mm), particularly in pancreatic head tumors in order to avoid pancreaticoduodenectomy, whereas distal pancreatectomy may be required for tumors of the pancreatic body or tail. Tumors larger than 2 cm or involving the pancreatic duct may require pancreaticoduodenectomy. Given the often-difficult localization of duodenal gastrinoma, requiring direct palpation, laparoscopic resection is controversial.

Unlike insulinoma, surgery for gastrinoma in the setting of MEN1 has an extremely high rate of recurrence. Although patients with hyperparathyroidism and gastrinoma with MEN1 require subtotal parathyroidectomy to remove stimulation of gastric acid from hypercalcemia, surgery for the gastrinoma itself is more controversial. Given the favorable prognosis with small (<2 cm) gastrinomas and the multifocal nature of the disease, nonoperative management is generally recommended for small tumors in the setting of MEN1. Surgery to prevent malignant transformation has been recommended by some investigators for larger tumors.[47] More radical surgery to remove the field defect of MEN1 with pancreaticoduodenectomy or total pancreatectomy is supported by some investigators.[48] Given the high recurrence rate and often slow-growing nature of disease, a more targeted surgical approach in MEN1 is advocated.[49] Incomplete resection is not beneficial, and surgery is not indicated with extensive metastases (**Box 2**).

Other functional pancreatic neuroendocrine tumors

Potentially curative surgical resection is recommended if feasible. Glucagonomas frequently present as large tumors and at an advanced stage, precluding safe resection. As most tumors arise in the body and tail, distal pancreatectomy is often possible if resection is feasible. Enucleation is rarely possible and not indicated. Similarly, laparoscopic resection may not be feasible because of the large size of lesions and propensity for liver metastases.[50] VIPomas are very rare and frequently occur in the

---

Box 2
Gastrinoma: surgical considerations

- Enucleation possible in some patients
- Surgical exploration required to identify tumors in the gastrinoma triangle (delineated by cystic duct, junction of body/neck of pancreas), and
- Lymph node dissection indicated
- Laparoscopic resection suboptimal because of difficulty with identification of tumors
- Smaller tumors observed in MEN1; resection of larger tumors controversial

pancreatic tail. Large and metastatic lesions are common, making curative resection challenging. For these and other rare functional PNETs, cytoreductive surgery may be indicated to improve hormonal control; surgery for liver metastases may be performed at the same time as resection of the primary tumor, if possible[51] (**Box 3**).

Nonfunctioning Pancreatic Neuroendocrine Tumors

Unlike functional PNETs, the primary goal of surgical management of nonfunctional PNETs is to prevent metastases and improve long-term survival.[52,53] Surgical resection typically consists of formal anatomic resection of the pancreatic head (pancreaticoduodenectomy) or body/tail (distal pancreatectomy with or without splenectomy). Local invasion of nearby organs or vascular structures is not a contraindication to potentially curative resection if all macroscopic disease can be removed.[54,55] Controversies in operative management include the role of conservative management in small incidentally detected PNETs (<2 cm), the role of pancreas-sparing operations for small PNETs, and the role of resection in MEN1.

Small nonfunctioning pancreatic neuroendocrine tumors

Studies have demonstrated a direct relationship between tumor size and risk of metastases.[56] With increased utilization and improved accuracy of cross-sectional imaging, an increasing number of incidental, small (<2.0 cm) PNETs are now identified.[57,58] Given that only 6% of nonfunctional PNETs less than 2 cm in size will be metastatic at diagnosis, some suggests a conservative strategy; the optimal management of these more indolent neoplasms is debated.

Support for an expectant management approach is supported by 2 recent studies. Gajoux and colleagues[59] described an observational study of 46 patients with small PNETs, with a median follow-up of 34 months. Eight patients underwent surgery for patient preference or for growth of tumors under observation. In the remaining 38 patients, there was no evidence of spread to lymph nodes or distant sites; most patients showed no growth. Lee and colleagues[60] described a series of 133 patients win incidental PNETs; in a group of 77 patients with a median tumor size of 1.0 cm and mean follow-up of 45 months, no patient showed significant growth or disease progression. Based on these data, serial imaging of PNETs less than 2.0 cm in size with MRI every 6 months for 2 years and annually afterward might be considered, with surgery reserved for growth or evidence of nodal metastases.[61]

Other data, however, suggest a more aggressive approach to even small incidental tumors. A retrospective group of 139 incidentally discovered PNETs included 39 patients with tumors 2.0 cm or smaller; in this group, 7.7% had late metastases or recurrence.[62] In a 20-year analysis of the Surveillance, Epidemiology, and End Results database, disease-specific survival at 5, 10, and 15 years for PNETs smaller than 2 cm was 91.5, 84.0, and 76.8%.[57] In a multi-institutional cohort of nonfunctioning PNET who underwent surgery, 3 of 56 patients with tumors less than 2 cm developed distant metastases, with 2 disease-related deaths. The investigators concluded that

---

Box 3
Additional functioning PNETs: surgical considerations

- Tumors usually present as large lesions, and metastases are common.
- Curative resection is rarely possible.
- Enucleation is not indicated.

the decision to proceed to surgical resection should not merely be based on size but also include tumor characteristics, such as grade.[63] In a recent review of 136 surgical patients, Hashim and colleagues[64] suggested a metastatic rate of 8% in tumors as small as 1.5 cm. Given this risk and the inability to accurately predict metastatic potential, resection was advised for small tumors.

Extent of surgery

The extent of surgery required when resecting small lesions is also a matter of debate. Enucleation is proposed for small lesions to avoid pancreatic insufficiency.[65] Tumor recurrence after enucleation is one potential concern; one series demonstrated an 8% risk of recurrence after enucleation of small incidental PNETs with a median follow-up less than 5 years.[66] The precise size threshold whereby enucleation may be safely performed for nonfunctional PNETs is unclear.

Furthermore, enucleation is typically performed at the expense of accurate nodal sampling. Individual series have shown a risk of nodal metastases in tumors smaller than 2 cm between 7.7% and 26.0%.[62,67,68] Although debate exists regarding the value of lymphadenectomy with surgery for PNETs, several large single-institution studies suggest a correlation between nodal metastases and outcome.[64,69,70] Conversely, a review of PNETs in the National Cancer Data Base suggested that tumor grade but not size or nodal metastases was associated with long-term survival.[71] Similarly, the largest single-institutional experience of nonfunctional PNETs reported that overall survival is predicted by tumor grade as determined by the Ki-67 index, without input of tumor size or nodal involvement.[72] The therapeutic value of lymphadenectomy is undefined, though potential prognostic information is gained from nodal sampling. Until the role of lymphadenectomy is better defined, the National Comprehensive Cancer Network's guidelines recommend consideration of lymph node resection for PNETs between 1 and 2 cm in size.[73]

Nonfunctioning pancreatic neuroendocrine tumors in multiple endocrine neoplasia type 1

Management of PNETs in the setting of MEN1 is complicated by the multifocal nature of small tumors, which almost universally behave in an indolent manner. Although the precise incidence of PNETs in MEN1 is unclear, data suggest that, when EUS is used for diagnosis, PNETs are found in between 54% and 93% of asymptomatic patients with MEN1, with most tumors less than 1 cm in size.[74] Evidence suggests that lesions smaller than 1 cm act in an indolent manner, with risk of malignancy increased as tumors exceed 2.0 cm.[75,76] Surveillance data for asymptomatic small PNETs in MEN1 suggest that most small lesions remain stable or decrease in size with a median follow-up of 6 years, though other tumors may develop on surveillance and may grow at a rate faster than earlier lesions.[77] Surgery, when indicated, can include parenchyma-sparing operations to total pancreatectomy with intraoperative ultrasound guidance to avoid leaving occult tumors behind (**Box 4**).[9]

Surgery for Metastatic Pancreatic Neuroendocrine Tumors

Neuroendocrine liver metastases (NELM) may occur in up to half of all patients with PNETs, and metastatic disease has a significant impact on prognosis.[1,70] Liver-directed treatment of NELM can include several modalities, such as surgery, tumor ablation, and transarterial embolization. In addition, new systemic approaches have proven beneficial specifically in metastatic neuroendocrine tumors from the pancreas.[4-6] Although a comprehensive review of NELM is beyond the scope of this article, several salient points about surgical management of liver metastases are relevant for functional and nonfunctional tumors (**Box 5**).

Box 4
Nonfunctioning PNETs: surgical considerations

- All tumors greater than 2 cm should be resected, typically with formal anatomic resection (pancreaticoduodenectomy, distal pancreatectomy) including negative margins and regional lymph nodes.

- Evidence suggests incidental tumors less than 1 cm can be followed with surveillance.

- Some studies with short-term follow-up suggest that all nonfunctioning PNET less than 2 cm might be followed with surveillance, with resection for growth.

- Pancreatic enucleation is most appropriate for small PNETs; lymph node resection should be considered for tumors 1 to 2 cm in size.

- MEN1 is associated with small, multifocal tumors, most of which have a low risk of progression. Surgery is reserved for tumors greater than 1 to 2 cm in size.

Functional pancreatic neuroendocrine tumors

Surgical therapy for metastatic disease in functional PNETs may be considered not only for potential oncologic benefit for control of hormone excess. Cytoreductive surgery including nonanatomic or formal hepatectomy may be considered for metastatic disease if most tumor burden can be removed. Debulking or cytoreductive surgery is potentially beneficial if more than 90% of the tumor burden can be removed,[43,51,78] though the precise means of estimating tumor volume are not clear.[79] Regardless of the potential oncologic benefits, reducing the tumor burden can improve symptom control in many patients with hormonally active tumors if tumors develop resistance to medical therapy.[80] Synchronous resection of primary pancreatic tumors and liver metastases must be undertaken with caution given the increased morbidity of the combined procedures.[81,82]

Nonfunctional pancreatic neuroendocrine tumors

Unlike functional tumors, metastatic nonfunctional PNETs do not lead to symptoms of hormonal excess; surgery is only indicated for potential oncologic benefit. Data supporting metastasectomy with nonfunctional pancreatic primary tumors are often retrospective and nonrandomized, allowing for the strong possibility of selection bias. Numerous single-institutional and retrospective studies suggest a survival benefit to surgical resection of NELM from intestinal or pancreatic primary tumors,[83,84] a benefit confirmed in pooled multi-institutional data as well.[85] This potential benefit is confirmed in studies limited to nonfunctional PNETs.[81,86] In a review of 72 patients, complete resection of all liver metastases led to a 5-year overall survival of 60%, compared with 45% in patients unable to have disease resected.[81]

Box 5
Metastatic PNETs: surgical considerations

- Cytoreductive surgery may be beneficial in metastatic functional PNETs to relieve symptoms of hormonal excess.

- Resection may offer improved overall survival in metastatic nonfunctional PNETs in low-grade or well-differentiated tumors if all disease can be removed or treated.

- Recurrence rates are near universal, with a high rate of occult metastases in the clinically normal liver.

Despite favorable survival data in these series, recurrence rates after metastasectomy are nearly universal, even with microscopically negative resection. Of note, data from a prospective cohort of patients with NELM show that careful thin-slice examination of the liver after resection of NELM reveals a high rate of occult disease.[87] CT scan had only 38% accuracy in determining the extent of disease, with most NELM only detected on the pathology examination. This finding suggests that most potentially curative resections for NELM are actually cytoreductive. In the absence of randomized data, surgery to remove liver metastases can be recommended primarily in low-grade tumors, with metastases limited to the liver, and if all disease can be feasibly resected.[88,89]

SUMMARY

PNETs include a diverse group of neoplasms, including functional and nonfunctional disease. Surgical resection is the mainstay of therapy for localized disease, and precise surgical techniques and goals should be tailored to clinical presentation and biological behavior. Complete surgical resection has an oncologic benefit in localized disease and a potential palliative benefit for any functional tumor as well.

REFERENCES

1. Yao JC, Eisner MP, Leary C, et al. Population-based study of islet cell carcinoma. Ann Surg Oncol 2007;14(12):3492–500.
2. Rindi G, Wiedenmann B. Neuroendocrine neoplasms of the gut and pancreas: new insights. Nat Rev Endocrinol 2012;8(1):54–64.
3. Vortmeyer AO, Huang S, Lubensky I, et al. Non-islet origin of pancreatic islet cell tumors. J Clin Endocrinol Metab 2004;89(4):1934–8.
4. Yao JC, Shah MH, Ito T, et al. Everolimus for advanced pancreatic neuroendocrine tumors. N Engl J Med 2011;364(6):514–23.
5. Raymond E, Dahan L, Raoul JL, et al. Sunitinib malate for the treatment of pancreatic neuroendocrine tumors. N Engl J Med 2011;364(6):501–13.
6. Strosberg JR, Fine RL, Choi J, et al. First-line chemotherapy with capecitabine and temozolomide in patients with metastatic pancreatic endocrine carcinomas. Cancer 2011;117(2):268–75.
7. Strosberg JR, Cheema A, Weber JM, et al. Relapse-free survival in patients with nonmetastatic, surgically resected pancreatic neuroendocrine tumors: an analysis of the AJCC and ENETS staging classifications. Ann Surg 2012;256(2): 321–5.
8. Hellman P, Andersson M, Rastad J, et al. Surgical strategy for large or malignant endocrine pancreatic tumors. World J Surg 2000;24(11):1353–60.
9. Jensen RT, Berna MJ, Bingham DB, et al. Inherited pancreatic endocrine tumor syndromes: advances in molecular pathogenesis, diagnosis, management, and controversies. Cancer 2008;113(7 Suppl):1807–43.
10. Kulke MH, Anthony LB, Bushnell DL, et al. NANETS treatment guidelines: well-differentiated neuroendocrine tumors of the stomach and pancreas. Pancreas 2010;39(6):735–52.
11. Whipple AO, Frantz VK. Adenoma of islet cells with hyperinsulinism: a review. Ann Surg 1935;101(6):1299–335.
12. Hirshberg B, Livi A, Bartlett DL, et al. Forty-eight-hour fast: the diagnostic test for insulinoma. J Clin Endocrinol Metab 2000;85(9):3222–6.
13. Service FJ, Natt N, Thompson GB, et al. Noninsulinoma pancreatogenous hypoglycemia: a novel syndrome of hyperinsulinemic hypoglycemia in adults

independent of mutations in Kir6.2 and SUR1 genes. J Clin Endocrinol Metab 1999;84(5):1582–9.

14. Service GJ, Thompson GB, Service FJ, et al. Hyperinsulinemic hypoglycemia with nesidioblastosis after gastric-bypass surgery. N Engl J Med 2005;353(3): 249–54.

15. Clancy TE, Moore FD Jr, Zinner MJ. Post-gastric bypass hyperinsulinism with nesidioblastosis: subtotal or total pancreatectomy may be needed to prevent recurrent hypoglycemia. J Gastrointest Surg 2006;10(8):1116–9.

16. Friesen SR. Tumors of the endocrine pancreas. N Engl J Med 1982;306(10): 580–90.

17. Mehrabi A, Fischer L, Hafezi M, et al. A systematic review of localization, surgical treatment options, and outcome of insulinoma. Pancreas 2014;43(5):675–86.

18. Service FJ, Mcmahon MM, O'brien PC, et al. Functioning insulinoma–incidence, recurrence, and long-term survival of patients: a 60-year study. Mayo Clin Proc 1991;66(7):711–9.

19. Doppman JL, Chang R, Fraker DL, et al. Localization of insulinomas to regions of the pancreas by intra-arterial stimulation with calcium. Ann Intern Med 1995; 123(4):269–73.

20. King AD, Ko GT, Yeung VT, et al. Dual phase spiral CT in the detection of small insulinomas of the pancreas. Br J Radiol 1998;71(841):20–3.

21. Gouya H, Vignaux O, Augui J, et al. CT, endoscopic sonography, and a combined protocol for preoperative evaluation of pancreatic insulinomas. AJR Am J Roentgenol 2003;181(4):987–92.

22. Druce MR, Muthuppalaniappan VM, O'leary B, et al. Diagnosis and localisation of insulinoma: the value of modern magnetic resonance imaging in conjunction with calcium stimulation catheterisation. Eur J Endocrinol 2010;162(5):971–8.

23. Kisker O, Bartsch D, Weinel RJ, et al. The value of somatostatin-receptor scintigraphy in newly diagnosed endocrine gastroenteropancreatic tumors. J Am Coll Surg 1997;184(5):487–92.

24. Zollinger RM, Ellison EH. Primary peptic ulcerations of the jejunum associated with islet cell tumors of the pancreas. Ann Surg 1955;142(4):709–23 [discussion: 724–8].

25. Norton JA, Fraker DL, Alexander HR, et al. Surgery to cure the Zollinger-Ellison syndrome. N Engl J Med 1999;341(9):635–44.

26. Weber HC, Venzon DJ, Lin JT, et al. Determinants of metastatic rate and survival in patients with Zollinger-Ellison syndrome: a prospective long-term study. Gastroenterology 1995;108(6):1637–49.

27. Stabile BE, Passaro E Jr. Benign and malignant gastrinoma. Am J Surg 1985; 149(1):144–50.

28. Lamers CG, Van Tongeren JH. Comparative study of the value of the calcium, secretin, and meal stimulated increase in serum gastrin to the diagnosis of the Zollinger-Ellison syndrome. Gut 1977;18(2):128–35.

29. Stabile BE, Morrow DJ, Passaro E Jr. The gastrinoma triangle: operative implications. Am J Surg 1984;147(1):25–31.

30. Gibril F, Reynolds JC, Doppman JL, et al. Somatostatin receptor scintigraphy: its sensitivity compared with that of other imaging methods in detecting primary and metastatic gastrinomas. A prospective study. Ann Intern Med 1996;125(1):26–34.

31. Norton JA, Alexander HR, Fraker DL, et al. Does the use of routine duodenotomy (DUODX) affect rate of cure, development of liver metastases, or survival in patients with Zollinger-Ellison syndrome? Ann Surg 2004;239(5):617–25 [discussion: 626].

32. Norton JA, Kahn CR, Schiebinger R, et al. Amino acid deficiency and the skin rash associated with glucagonoma. Ann Intern Med 1979;91(2):213–5.
33. Vagefi PA, Razo O, Deshpande V, et al. Evolving patterns in the detection and outcomes of pancreatic neuroendocrine neoplasms: the Massachusetts General Hospital experience from 1977 to 2005. Arch Surg 2007;142(4):347–54.
34. Crippa S, Partelli S, Zamboni G, et al. Incidental diagnosis as prognostic factor in different tumor stages of nonfunctioning pancreatic endocrine tumors. Surgery 2014;155(1):145–53.
35. Ricke J, Klose KJ. Imaging procedures in neuroendocrine tumours. Digestion 2000;62(Suppl 1):39–44.
36. Rindi G, AR, Bosman FT, et al. Nomenclature and classification of neuroendocrine neoplasms of the digestive system. In: Bosman Tf CF, Hruban Rh, Theise Nd, editors. WHO classification of tumors of the digestive system, 13, 4th edition. Lyon (France): International Agency for Research on Cancer; 2010.
37. Klimstra DS, Modlin IR, Coppola D, et al. The pathologic classification of neuroendocrine tumors: a review of nomenclature, grading, and staging systems. Pancreas 2010;39(6):707–12.
38. Rindi G, Kloppel G, Alhman H, et al. TNM staging of foregut (neuro)endocrine tumors: a consensus proposal including a grading system. Virchows Arch 2006; 449(4):395–401.
39. Strosberg JR, Cheema A, Weber J, et al. Prognostic validity of a novel American Joint Committee on Cancer Staging classification for pancreatic neuroendocrine tumors. J Clin Oncol 2011;29(22):3044–9.
40. Hackert T, Hinz U, Fritz S, et al. Enucleation in pancreatic surgery: indications, technique, and outcome compared to standard pancreatic resections. Langenbecks Arch Surg 2011;396(8):1197–203.
41. Liu H, Peng C, Zhang S, et al. Strategy for the surgical management of insulinomas: analysis of 52 cases. Dig Surg 2007;24(6):463–70.
42. Iihara M, Kanbe M, Okamoto T, et al. Laparoscopic ultrasonography for resection of insulinomas. Surgery 2001;130(6):1086–91.
43. Fendrich V, Waldmann J, Bartsch DK, et al. Surgical management of pancreatic endocrine tumors. Nat Rev Clin Oncol 2009;6(7):419–28.
44. Hirshberg B, Libutti SK, Alexander HR, et al. Blind distal pancreatectomy for occult insulinoma, an inadvisable procedure. J Am Coll Surg 2002;194(6):761–4.
45. Morrow EH, Norton JA. Surgical management of Zollinger-Ellison syndrome; state of the art. Surg Clin North Am 2009;89(5):1091–103.
46. Bartsch DK, Waldmann J, Fendrich V, et al. Impact of lymphadenectomy on survival after surgery for sporadic gastrinoma. Br J Surg 2012;99(9):1234–40.
47. Macfarlane MP, Fraker DL, Alexander HR, et al. Prospective study of surgical resection of duodenal and pancreatic gastrinomas in multiple endocrine neoplasia type 1. Surgery 1995;118(6):973–9 [discussion: 979–80].
48. Tonelli F, Fratini G, Nesi G, et al. Pancreatectomy in multiple endocrine neoplasia type 1-related gastrinomas and pancreatic endocrine neoplasias. Ann Surg 2006;244(1):61–70.
49. Ellison EC, Johnson JA. The Zollinger-Ellison syndrome: a comprehensive review of historical, scientific, and clinical considerations. Curr Probl Surg 2009;46(1): 13–106.
50. O'toole D, Salazar R, Falconi M, et al. Rare functioning pancreatic endocrine tumors. Neuroendocrinology 2006;84(3):189–95.
51. Steinmuller T, Kianmanesh R, Falconi M, et al. Consensus guidelines for the management of patients with liver metastases from digestive (neuro)endocrine

tumors: foregut, midgut, hindgut, and unknown primary. Neuroendocrinology 2008;87(1):47–62.

52. Hill JS, Mcphee JT, Mcdade TP, et al. Pancreatic neuroendocrine tumors: the impact of surgical resection on survival. Cancer 2009;115(4):741–51.

53. Fischer L, Bergmann F, Schimmack S, et al. Outcome of surgery for pancreatic neuroendocrine neoplasms. Br J Surg 2014;101(11):1405–12.

54. Fischer L, Kleeff J, Esposito I, et al. Clinical outcome and long-term survival in 118 consecutive patients with neuroendocrine tumours of the pancreas. Br J Surg 2008;95(5):627–35.

55. Kleine M, Schrem H, Vondran FW, et al. Extended surgery for advanced pancreatic endocrine tumours. Br J Surg 2012;99(1):88–94.

56. Bettini R, Partelli S, Boninsegna L, et al. Tumor size correlates with malignancy in nonfunctioning pancreatic endocrine tumor. Surgery 2011;150(1):75–82.

57. Kuo EJ, Salem RR. Population-level analysis of pancreatic neuroendocrine tumors 2 cm or less in size. Ann Surg Oncol 2013;20(9):2815–21.

58. Zerbi A, Falconi M, Rindi G, et al. Clinicopathological features of pancreatic endocrine tumors: a prospective multicenter study in Italy of 297 sporadic cases. Am J Gastroenterol 2010;105(6):1421–9.

59. Gaujoux S, Partelli S, Maire F, et al. Observational study of natural history of small sporadic nonfunctioning pancreatic neuroendocrine tumors. J Clin Endocrinol Metab 2013;98(12):4784–9.

60. Lee LC, Grant CS, Salomao DR, et al. Small, nonfunctioning, asymptomatic pancreatic neuroendocrine tumors (PNETs): role for nonoperative management. Surgery 2012;152(6):965–74.

61. Libutti SK. Evolving paradigm for managing small nonfunctional incidentally discovered pancreatic neuroendocrine tumors. J Clin Endocrinol Metab 2013; 98(12):4670–2.

62. Haynes AB, Deshpande V, Ingkakul T, et al. Implications of incidentally discovered, nonfunctioning pancreatic endocrine tumors: short-term and long-term patient outcomes. Arch Surg 2011;146(5):534–8.

63. Cherenfant J, Stocker SJ, Gage MK, et al. Predicting aggressive behavior in nonfunctioning pancreatic neuroendocrine tumors. Surgery 2013;154(4):785–91 [discussion 791–3].

64. Hashim YM, Trinkaus KM, Linehan DC, et al. Regional lymphadenectomy is indicated in the surgical treatment of pancreatic neuroendocrine tumors (PNETs). Ann Surg 2014;259(2):197–203.

65. Falconi M, Mantovani W, Crippa S, et al. Pancreatic insufficiency after different resections for benign tumours. Br J Surg 2008;95(1):85–91.

66. Falconi M, Zerbi A, Crippa S, et al. Parenchyma-preserving resections for small nonfunctioning pancreatic endocrine tumors. Ann Surg Oncol 2010;17(6):1621–7.

67. Ferrone CR, Tang LH, Tomlinson J, et al. Determining prognosis in patients with pancreatic endocrine neoplasms: can the WHO classification system be simplified? J Clin Oncol 2007;25(35):5609–15.

68. Parekh JR, Wang SC, Bergsland EK, et al. Lymph node sampling rates and predictors of nodal metastasis in pancreatic neuroendocrine tumor resections: the UCSF experience with 149 patients. Pancreas 2012;41(6):840–4.

69. Bettini R, Boninsegna L, Mantovani W, et al. Prognostic factors at diagnosis and value of WHO classification in a mono-institutional series of 180 non-functioning pancreatic endocrine tumours. Ann Oncol 2008;19(5):903–8.

70. Tomassetti P, Campana D, Piscitelli L, et al. Endocrine pancreatic tumors: factors correlated with survival. Ann Oncol 2005;16(11):1806–10.
71. Bilimoria KY, Talamonti MS, Tomlinson JS, et al. Prognostic score predicting survival after resection of pancreatic neuroendocrine tumors: analysis of 3851 patients. Ann Surg 2008;247(3):490–500.
72. Ellison TA, Wolfgang CL, Shi C, et al. A single institution's 26-year experience with nonfunctional pancreatic neuroendocrine tumors: a validation of current staging systems and a new prognostic nomogram. Ann Surg 2014;259(2):204–12.
73. Kulke MH, Shah MH, Benson AB 3rd, et al. Neuroendocrine tumors, version 1.2015. J Natl Compr Canc Netw 2015;13(1):78–108.
74. Thomas-Marques L, Murat A, Delemer B, et al. Prospective endoscopic ultrasonographic evaluation of the frequency of nonfunctioning pancreaticoduodenal endocrine tumors in patients with multiple endocrine neoplasia type 1. Am J Gastroenterol 2006;101(2):266–73.
75. Kouvaraki MA, Shapiro SE, Cote GJ, et al. Management of pancreatic endocrine tumors in multiple endocrine neoplasia type 1. World J Surg 2006;30(5):643–53.
76. Triponez F, Goudet P, Dosseh D, et al. Is surgery beneficial for MEN1 patients with small (< or = 2 cm), nonfunctioning pancreaticoduodenal endocrine tumor? An analysis of 65 patients from the GTE. World J Surg 2006;30(5):654–62 [discussion 663–4].
77. D'souza SL, Elmunzer BJ, Scheiman JM. Long-term follow-up of asymptomatic pancreatic neuroendocrine tumors in multiple endocrine neoplasia type I syndrome. J Clin Gastroenterol 2014;48(5):458–61.
78. Fendrich V, Michl P, Habbe N, et al. Liver-specific therapies for metastases of neuroendocrine pancreatic tumors. World J Hepatol 2010;2(10):367–73.
79. Que FG, Nagorney DM, Batts KP, et al. Hepatic resection for metastatic neuroendocrine carcinomas. Am J Surg 1995;169(1):36–42 [discussion: 42–3].
80. Hodul P, Malafa M, Choi J, et al. The role of cytoreductive hepatic surgery as an adjunct to the management of metastatic neuroendocrine carcinomas. Cancer Control 2006;13(1):61–71.
81. Cusati D, Zhang L, Harmsen WS, et al. Metastatic nonfunctioning pancreatic neuroendocrine carcinoma to liver: surgical treatment and outcomes. J Am Coll Surg 2012;215(1):117–24 [discussion: 124–5].
82. Gaujoux S, Gonen M, Tang L, et al. Synchronous resection of primary and liver metastases for neuroendocrine tumors. Ann Surg Oncol 2012;19(13):4270–7.
83. Sarmiento JM, Heywood G, Rubin J, et al. Surgical treatment of neuroendocrine metastases to the liver: a plea for resection to increase survival. J Am Coll Surg 2003;197(1):29–37.
84. Glazer ES, Tseng JF, Al-Refaie W, et al. Long-term survival after surgical management of neuroendocrine hepatic metastases. HPB (Oxford) 2010;12(6):427–33.
85. Mayo SC, De Jong MC, Pulitano C, et al. Surgical management of hepatic neuroendocrine tumor metastasis: results from an international multi-institutional analysis. Ann Surg Oncol 2010;17(12):3129–36.
86. Zerbi A, Capitanio V, Boninsegna L, et al. Treatment of malignant pancreatic neuroendocrine neoplasms: middle-term (2-year) outcomes of a prospective observational multicentre study. HPB (Oxford) 2013;15(12):935–43.
87. Elias D, Lefevre JH, Duvillard P, et al. Hepatic metastases from neuroendocrine tumors with a "thin slice" pathological examination: they are many more than you think. Ann Surg 2010;251(2):307–10.
88. Bloomston M, Muscarella P, Shah MH, et al. Cytoreduction results in high perioperative mortality and decreased survival in patients undergoing pancreatectomy

for neuroendocrine tumors of the pancreas. J Gastrointest Surg 2006;10(10): 1361–70.

89. Kianmanesh R, Sauvanet A, Hentic O, et al. Two-step surgery for synchronous bilobar liver metastases from digestive endocrine tumors: a safe approach for radical resection. Ann Surg 2008;247(4):659–65.

Systemic Therapies for Advanced Pancreatic Neuroendocrine Tumors

Nitya Raj, MD*, Diane Reidy-Lagunes, MD, MS

KEYWORDS

- Neuroendocrine tumors • Pancreatic neuroendocrine tumors • Carcinoid tumors
- Octreotide • Lanreotide • Sunitinib • Everolimus

KEY POINTS

- Pancreatic neuroendocrine tumors (NETs) are genetically and clinically different than extrapancreatic NETs (ie, carcinoid tumors) and often respond to cytotoxic and targeted treatments.
- Asymptomatic patients with low-volume advanced pancreatic NETs often have indolent disease, and some can be followed expectantly. Careful evaluation of each individual patient with an initial interval of observation and assessment can help define who needs treatment sooner.
- Somatostatin analogues (octreotide and lanreotide) can decrease hormone production in functional tumors and can control neuroendocrine tumor growth; given their favorable toxicity profile, they are generally used as first-line treatment in unresectable patients.
- Sunitinib and everolimus are 2 targeted therapies approved for progressive pancreatic NETs and are generally reserved for use in tumors that have progressed on somatostatin analogue therapy.
- Pancreatic NETs can respond to cytotoxic chemotherapy; the most commonly used agents include alkylating, fluorouracil, and platinum drugs.

INTRODUCTION

Well-differentiated neuroendocrine tumors (NETs) are an uncommon and heterogeneous group of neoplasms that arise throughout the body, most commonly in the lung and gastrointestinal tract.[1] These tumors are subdivided into carcinoid tumors and pancreatic NETs (panNETs). Carcinoid tumors develop from the neuroendocrine

Disclosure Statement: Dr D. Reidy-Lagunes is on the advisory board for Novartis, Pfizer, and Ipsen. In addition, Dr D. Reidy-Lagunes does both research and consulting for Novartis. Dr N. Raj has nothing to disclose.
Gastrointestinal Oncology Service, Division of Solid Tumor Oncology, Department of Medicine, Memorial Sloan Kettering Cancer Center, 300 East 66th Street, 1039, New York, NY 10065, USA
* Corresponding author.
E-mail address: rajn@mskcc.org

tissues of the aerodigestive tract, and panNETs develop from the endocrine tissues of the pancreas (ie, islets of Langerhans). This group of well-differentiated NETs is both morphologically and clinically distinct from high-grade neuroendocrine carcinomas, tumors that are characterized by an extremely aggressive behavior and are treated along small cell lung cancer paradigms with platinum-based chemotherapy.[2] Epidemiologic data from the last 30 years have demonstrated that the incidence of NETs continues to increase, although there have been no significant changes in survival from this disease.[3,4]

panNETs are the second most common tumor of the pancreas and represent 1% to 2% of all pancreatic neoplasms.[5,6] Although most panNETs are slow growing, after the development of metastatic disease (most commonly in the liver), median survival ranges from 2 to 5 years; most patients with liver metastases will die of the disease.[7] About one-third of panNETs are functional tumors and produce clinical syndromes due to excessive hormone secretion; these functional panNETs are classified by the hormones they hypersecrete and include insulinoma (secrete insulin and cause hypoglycemia), gastrinoma (secrete gastrin and cause Zollinger-Ellison syndrome, which is characterized by severe peptic ulcer disease), glucagonoma (secrete glucagon and cause hyperglycemia), and vasoactive intestinal polypeptide (VIP) (VIPoma, secrete VIP and cause severe secretory diarrhea).[6,8–10] Nonfunctional panNETs are tumors that do not secrete hormones or the products they secrete do not cause a clinical syndrome, such as pancreatic polypeptide, chromogranin A, ghrelin, neurotensin, subunits of chorionic gonadotropin, and neuron-specific enolase.[10] Metastatic disease is a common presentation for most patients with panNETs, especially those with nonfunctioning tumors given the absence of clinical symptoms that would warrant earlier clinical evaluation.[7]

Asymptomatic patients diagnosed with advanced, metastatic panNETs are often monitored initially; however, with time, often their disease will progress and require treatment. The typical indications for therapy are pain and symptoms due to tumor bulk, symptoms from hormone secretion for functional tumors, high tumor burden, or progression of disease under observation.[8] Given the heterogeneous clinical presentations and complex spectrum of aggressiveness of panNETs, their treatment is challenging and requires multimodality management with surgeons, interventional radiologists, medical oncologists, endocrinologists, and gastroenterologists. This article focuses on the data and rationale supporting the use of systemic treatments for advanced, metastatic, well-differentiated panNETs.

PATHOLOGY

Since 2010, the classification of panNETs has been based on the revised criteria from the World Health Organization, which is defined by the cytologic grade and the proliferative index (as assessed by the Ki-67 and/or mitotic count).[11] In these revised criteria, tumors are broken down by differentiation status (well and poorly differentiated) and grade (grade 1, low; grade 2, intermediate; and grade 3, high). Although the family of well-differentiated tumors are classically of the grade 1 or grade 2 type and generally have a more indolent, less aggressive course, grade 3 or high-grade neuroendocrine carcinomas are typically poorly differentiated and classified as large or small cell carcinomas; these grade 3 neuroendocrine carcinomas are highly aggressive, akin to small cell lung cancers, and are associated with a poor prognosis.

To support this belief, many studies have looked at the relationship between tumor grade and survival; not surprisingly, tumor grade seems to be correlated with survival; in one retrospective analysis of 425 patients with panNETs, the 5-year survival rates for grade 1, grade 2, and grade 3 tumors were 75%, 62%, and 7%, respectively.[12] Unfortunately, this grading system is not universally incorporated into most of the clinical trials investigating panNETs and makes the interpretation of the published data somewhat challenging.

However, recent data also suggest that it may not be correct to consider all grade 3 gastroenteropancreatic (GEP)-NETs as a single entity. Specifically, it has been suggested that some well-differentiated grade 3 NETs may behave differently than poorly differentiated grade 3 NETs.[13] Furthermore, data on treatment outcomes suggest that NETs with a Ki-67 proliferation index in the lower end of the G3 range respond less robustly to chemotherapy agents, such as platinum drugs. In one study, it was shown that grade 3 GEP-NETs with a Ki-67 proliferation index less than 55% were less responsive to first-line platinum-based chemotherapy, though this subgroup achieved longer survival in comparison with grade 3 GEP-NETs with a Ki-67 proliferation index of 55% or greater (14 months vs 10 months).[14] Further corroborating these data, in an investigation of 45 patients specifically with grade 3 panNETs, studying survival and treatment response based on poorly or well-differentiated status, differences were appreciated both in survival and response by therapy type.[15] Specifically, the well-differentiated subgroup demonstrated improved overall survival (OS) in comparison with the poorly differentiated subgroup (52.0 months vs 10.1 months). Looking at responses to therapy, although both poorly and well-differentiated grade 3 panNETs responded to alkylating chemotherapy agents, poorly differentiated tumors had a higher response to platinum agents. Based on the findings of these studies, current research efforts are directed toward a better understanding of grade 3 NETs, both pancreatic and extrapancreatic, as they seem to be a more heterogeneous group than originally thought.

GENETICS
Inherited Pancreatic Neuroendocrine Tumors

Although panNETs often develop sporadically, inherited panNETs occur and are generally associated with 4 genetic disorders. These disorders include multiple endocrine neoplasia type 1 (MEN1), von Hippel Lindau (VHL) disease, neurofibromatosis 1 (NF1; von Recklinghausen disease), and tuberous sclerosis complex (TSC). All of these genetic disorders demonstrate autosomal dominant inheritance; additionally, the genes implicated in these disorders (MEN1, VHL, NF1, and TSC1/2) are all tumor suppressor genes and play a critical role in cellular development.[10] The most frequent occurrence of panNETs is in MEN1, followed by VHL, then NF1, and finally TSC.[10]

Nonfamilial (Sporadic) Pancreatic Neuroendocrine Tumors

More recently, effort has been made to better understand the genetic basis of nonfamilial panNETs through whole-exome sequencing; in this study, the exomic sequences of approximately 18,000 protein-coding genes in 10 nonfamilial panNETs were determined (small cell and large cell neuroendocrine carcinomas were excluded in order to ensure the set of tumors studied was clinically homogeneous).[16] The most commonly mutated genes in these 10 tumor samples were then screened in an additional 58 panNETs. In addition to observing an increased number of mutations in genes implicated in chromatin remodeling, mutations in the mammalian target of rapamycin (mTOR) pathway were also identified. Specifically, 44% of the tumors had somatic inactivating mutations in MEN1, the gene that encodes menin, which is a component of the histone methyltransferase complex. Forty-three percent of the tumors had mutations in genes encoding death-domain-associated protein (DAXX) and alpha thalassemia/mental retardation syndrome X-linked (ATRX), these proteins are subunits of a chromatin remodeling complex; no tumor had mutations in both DAXX and ATRX, which was expected given that these proteins function within the same pathway. Approximately 18% of the tumors had mutations along the mammalian target of rapamycin (mTOR) pathway; 7.3% of these mutations were in phosphatase and tensin homolog (PTEN), 8.8% in TSC2, and 1.4% in phosphatidylinositol-4, 5-bisphosphate 3-kinase, catalytic subunit alpha (PIK3CA).

In the aforementioned study, the patient population was composed of individuals pursuing surgical resection with curative intent, and those with metastatic disease. Looking specifically at survival in different subgroups, prolonged OS was appreciated in patients with mutations in MEN1, DAXX/ATRX, or the combination of both MEN1 and DAXX/ATRX. This survival benefit was most pronounced in those patients with the combination of mutations; in patients with mutations in both MEN1 and DAXX/ATRX, 100% survived for a minimum of 10 years; however, 60% of patients who lacked these mutations died within 5 years of diagnosis.

The aforementioned study has been critical to our understanding of the genomic basis of sporadic panNETs. The findings demonstrate that patients with mutations in chromatin remodeling genes may represent a more favorable panNET subgroup. In addition, this study also highlights the subgroup of patients with panNETs who may demonstrate a more favorable response to the mTOR inhibitor everolimus; further studies to test this hypothesis are ongoing.

SYSTEMIC TREATMENT OF ADVANCED PANCREATIC NEUROENDOCRINE TUMORS

The treatment of patients with advanced, metastatic panNETs, whether inherited or sporadic, is approached in a multidisciplinary manner and may include surgical resection, liver-directed therapies, and/or systemic treatments. In unresectable patients, the goals of these therapies are to palliate tumor-related symptoms and prolong the life span.

There are multiple systemic therapy options available for the treatment of metastatic panNETs. These systemic options include somatostatin analogue therapy, targeted agents, and cytotoxic chemotherapy.

Somatostatin Analogues

Somatostatin and its synthetic analogues (ie, octreotide and lanreotide) bind to G-protein couple receptors on the cell surface to exert their effects. There are 5 known subtypes of somatostatin receptors (SST1–SST5), and binding of somatostatin to these receptors can inhibit the release of hormones and secretory proteins and also stall tumor growth, offering cytostatic control.

More than 75% of panNETs express somatostatin receptors (most commonly SST2) on their surface and are octreotide avid on somatostatin analogue scintigraphy (ie, indium-111 pentetreotide [Octreoscan]).[17,18] In octreotide-positive disease, somatostatin analogues are often used as first line, as they are well tolerated, treat functional symptoms (in those tumors that are hormone secreting), and have been demonstrated to have an antiproliferative, cytostatic effect on the growth of tumors.

Somatostatin analogues and control of symptoms from hormone secretion

Therapy with octreotide and lanreotide has revolutionized the way we care for patients with hormone-producing, functional panNETs. As previously discussed, functional panNETs include insulinomas, gastrinomas, glucagonomas, and VIPomas. Somatostatin analogues seem to be highly useful in the treatment of functional symptoms from VIPomas and glucagonomas, with an improvement seem in secretory diarrhea in VIPomas and an improvement in necrolytic migratory erythema, a characteristic blistering skin rash, in glucagonomas.[19–21]

Although insulinomas and gastrinomas are the most common types of functional panNETs, somatostatin analogues seem to have a more limited role in controlling their hormone-related symptoms. In particular, when initiating somatostatin analogue therapy on insulinomas, close monitoring of glucose levels is required, as there can be transient worsening of hypoglycemia; hypoglycemia can occur as nearly half of insulinomas do not express SST2 and somatostatin analogue therapy can blunt a compensatory glucagon response.[8] In gastrinomas, rather than somatostatin analogues, proton pump inhibitors are the preferred treatment to blunt the effects of excessive gastric acid production.

Somatostatin analogues and control of tumor growth

In addition to treating hormone-related symptoms in functional tumors, octreotide and lanreotide have a role in controlling tumor growth. The earliest studies investigating a cytostatic role for somatostatin analogues included patients with many types of NETs, questioning the applicability to panNETs alone.[22,23] The only randomized data to support an antiproliferative role for octreotide in the treatment of NETs came from the phase III Placebo-Controlled, Double-Blind, Prospective, Randomized Study on the Effect of Octreotide LAR in the Control of Tumor Growth in Patients with Metastatic Neuroendocrine Midgut Tumors (PROMID) study, but this study only included midgut tumors and not pancreatic NETs.[24] In this study, 85 patients were randomized to either placebo or octreotide long-acting-release (LAR) 30 mg intramuscularly monthly until progression of disease or death. The primary end point was time to tumor progression (TTP), and the investigators observed a significant difference in TTP in the octreotide LAR and placebo groups (14.3 months vs 6 months, $P = .000072$). In clinical practice and by the National Comprehensive Cancer Network's guidelines, physicians were extrapolating the use of octreotide in midgut tumors to use in pancreatic NET; but no prospective randomized data exist.[25]

The Controlled Study of Lanreotide Antiproliferative Response in Neuroendocrine Tumors (CLARINET) study, however, confirmed the antiproliferative effect of somatostatin analogues in GEP-NETs. In this double-blind, placebo-controlled, multinational study in patients with low- or intermediate-grade, moderately or well-differentiated NETs (45% panNETs), 204 patients were randomized to receive an extended-release aqueous-gel formulation of lanreotide (Autogel) at a dose of 120 mg or placebo once every 28 days for 96 weeks; the primary end point was progression-free survival (PFS), defined as time to disease progression or death. The investigators observed that lanreotide was associated with significantly prolonged PFS in comparison with placebo (median not reached vs median of 18 months, $P<.001$). There were no significant differences between the two groups in quality of life (QOL) or OS. The most common adverse event was diarrhea, which was more prevalent in patients receiving lanreotide (26% in the lanreotide group and 9% in the placebo group). This study confirmed that in comparison with placebo, lanreotide is safely tolerated and significantly prolongs PFS in patients with metastatic NETs; based on these findings, lanreotide is approved by the Food and Drug Administration (FDA) to treat unresectable well-differentiated GEP-NETs. Of note, lanreotide is the only somatostatin analogue FDA approved for cytostatic tumor control in the treatment of NETs; however, octreotide is thought to have similar efficacy in controlling tumor growth.[26]

TARGETED THERAPIES

In recent years, targeted agents have been evaluated as therapy options for panNETs. All NETs are known to be highly vascular; for this reason, targeted angiogenic inhibitors have been heavily investigated as a treatment option in the spectrum of NETs.[27]

Specific biological agents that have been studied include those directed against vascular endothelial growth factor (VEGF) as well as those targeting mTOR. Sunitinib and everolimus are the only targeted therapies approved for progressive panNETs. Both single and combination therapies have been tested in clinical trials.

Sunitinib

Sunitinib is a small-molecule tyrosine kinase inhibitor that blocks many receptor tyrosine kinases, including VEGF receptor 1 to 3, platelet-derived growth factor receptor (PDGFR), mast/stem cell growth factor receptor (c-KIT), RET, and Fms-Related Tyrosine Kinase 3 (FLT-3).[9] A phase II multicenter study investigated the efficacy of sunitinib in both carcinoid and panNETs (107 treated patients; 41 carcinoid and 66 panNET).[28] Patients were treated with sunitinib 50 mg for 4 weeks followed by a 2-week break. The overall objective response rate in panNETs was 16.7% (11 of 66 patients), and 68% (45 of 66 patients) had stable disease; in panNETs, the median TTP was 7.7 months and 1-year OS was 81.1%. In comparison, only 2.4% of patients with carcinoid tumors achieved a confirmed partial response. The findings suggested that sunitinib has antitumor activity in panNETs; however, a lack of efficacy was seen in carcinoid tumors.

Based on the findings from this phase II study, a multinational, randomized double-blind placebo-controlled phase III trial was conducted of sunitinib in patients with advanced, well-differentiated panNETs.[29] In this study, 171 patients were randomly assigned to either sunitinib 37.5 mg/d or placebo; the study was discontinued early after observation of more serious adverse events and deaths in the placebo group as well as improved PFS in the sunitinib arm. Specifically, the median PFS was 11.4 months in the sunitinib group, compared with 5.5 months in the placebo group. The objective response rate was also improved with sunitinib in comparison with placebo (9.3% vs 0%). Sunitinib was most commonly associated with gastrointestinal side effects (diarrhea, nausea, vomiting) as well as asthenia and fatigue. These positive findings led to the FDA approval of sunitinib in progressive panNETs. In a more recent updated analysis of the survival data, at 2 years of additional follow-up, median OS was 33 months with sunitinib and 26.7 months with placebo ($P = .11$).[30]

Everolimus

Everolimus is an oral inhibitor of mTOR, a serine-threonine kinase that impacts cell proliferation, cell survival, and also controls angiogenic pathways via hypoxia-inducible factor-1a, VEGF, and by endothelial and smooth muscle cell proliferation.[31] In the phase II setting, everolimus demonstrated promising antitumor activity in both carcinoid tumors and panNETs.[32,33] Based on these findings, RAD001 in Advanced Neuroendocrine Tumors, Third Trial (RADIANT 3) Study Group, a randomized double-blind placebo-controlled study of 410 patients with low- or intermediate-grade, progressive, and advanced panNETs, was conducted.[34] In this study, patients were randomized to receive everolimus or placebo, and the investigators observed a significantly improved median PFS of 11.0 months with everolimus compared with 4.6 months with placebo. In the everolimus arm, the response rate was 5%, in comparison with 2% in the placebo arm. The most common adverse events were grade 1 or 2 and included stomatitis, rash, diarrhea, fatigue, and infections. More serious grade 3 or 4 events seen with everolimus included anemia (6%) and hyperglycemia (5%). Based on the RADIANT 3 study, everolimus received FDA approval in the treatment of panNETs. The findings of RADIANT 3 were concordant with those from whole-exome sequencing of panNETs, in which mutations along the mTOR pathway were observed with increased frequency, suggestive that this tumor type may respond to mTOR inhibition.[16]

CYTOTOXIC CHEMOTHERAPY

Through multiple studies, a role for chemotherapy (both single drug and combination drugs) has been demonstrated in the management of panNETs. Chemotherapy is most commonly used in the presence of a more aggressive clinical course and symptomatic, heavy tumor burden. In the treatment of panNETs, chemotherapy has been demonstrated to have both palliative and antitumor effects, though evidence regarding OS is conflicting. Chemotherapy agents that have been investigated and commonly used for the treatment of NETs include alkylating agents (streptozocin, temozolomide, dacarbazine) and platinum agents.

Alkylating Agents: Streptozocin

Three alkylating agents, streptozocin, temozolomide, and dacarbazine, have demonstrated activity in the management of panNETs. The earliest evidence for use of alkylating agents came from a case report in 1968 of a patient with a panNET who was suffering from recurrent hypoglycemia and received symptomatic relief as well as a decrease in hepatic tumor burden while on therapy with streptozocin.[35] Then, in 1971, through a phase II study, a 5-day intensive course of streptozocin was evaluated and demonstrated to be active against panNETs.[36]

A multicenter trial led by the Eastern Cooperative Oncology Group (ECOG) was conducted in which 105 patients with advanced panNETs were randomized to one of 3 treatment regimens: streptozocin plus 5-fluorouracil (5-FU), streptozocin plus doxorubicin, or chlorozotocin alone.[37] In terms of tumor regression, streptozocin plus doxorubicin was superior to streptozocin plus 5-FU (69% vs 45%, P = .05). It is important to recognize that, in this study, markers of response included radiographic tumor regression or alternatively improvements in tumor seen on physical examination and for patients without measurable tumor by imaging or examination; laboratory assays evaluating hormone production were used. Survival was short in both arms but favored the streptozocin arm (2.2 vs 1.4 years, P = .004).

In further investigation, however, these findings from the ECOG trial could not be confirmed. In a retrospective review of 16 patients with advanced panNETs treated at a single institution with streptozocin and doxorubicin, only 1 of 16 (6%) achieved an objective response by standard computed tomography response criteria; 9 of 16 (56%) had stable disease and 6 of 16 (38%) had progression of disease as their best response during treatment.[38] The investigators of this study were unable to confirm the high objective response rate previously appreciated, possibly because of the nonmodern response criteria (physical examination, laboratory biochemical parameters) used in the ECOG trial.

A retrospective study was subsequently conducted to investigate outcomes in 84 patients with metastatic panNETs treated with streptozocin, 5-FU, and doxorubicin; response evaluation criteria in solid tumors (RECIST) were used to evaluate response.[39] In this study, the response rate to chemotherapy was 39%; the median duration of response was 9.3 months, and the 2-year PFS and OS rates were 41% and 74%, respectively.

Alkylating Agents: Dacarbazine

Dacarbazine (DTIC) is a nonclassic synthetic alkylating agent and has been investigated as a treatment option for panNETs.[40,41] Early investigations of DTIC, first in carcinoid tumors, suggested a benefit in terms of tumor shrinkage in about half of treatment patients, along with an improvement in QOL; the most commonly appreciated side effect was nausea, with no major organ toxicities noted.[42,43] Based on these early data, a phase II study of DTIC in patients with advanced panNETs was conducted by ECOG (E6282).[41] In this study, 50 patients with documented clinical or radiographic disease progression received DTIC every 4 weeks. In this patient cohort, the response rate was 34%, with chemotherapy-naïve patients deriving the greatest benefit; the median OS was 19.3 months. Notable lethal toxicities were septic shock in one patient and myocardial infarction in one patient. The most common grade 4 toxicity was hematological (in 5 patients), and 13% of patients experienced grade 3 vomiting. Based on the results of this study, DTIC was thought to have activity in previously untreated, progressive, panNETs; but given the potential toxicities, as with streptozocin, widespread use of DTIC for panNET treatment has been limited.

Alkylating Agents: Temozolomide

Temozolomide is an oral alkylating agent developed to be a less toxic alternative to DTIC.[44] The earliest data for a rationale for temozolomide in the therapy for pan-NETs came from a phase II trial in which 29 patients with metastatic NETs (including carcinoid tumors, pheochromocytoma, and panNETs) received a combination of temozolomide and thalidomide.[45] In this study, temozolomide was given in a dose-intense regimen (150 mg/m^2 for 7 days, every other week). A 40% biochemical response rate (chromogranin A) and a 25% radiologic response rate were appreciated with the combination of temozolomide and thalidomide; when breaking the radiologic response rate down by tumor type, it was 45% in panNETs, 33% in pheochromocytomas, and 7% in carcinoid tumors. The median duration of response was 13.5 months, with 1-year and 2-year survival of 79% and 61% respectively. The most severe toxicity was grade 3 to 4 lymphopenia, seen in 69% of patients; the dose-intense regimen of temozolomide used in this study likely contributed to the high rates of lymphopenia observed. Of note, a separate single phase II study of thalidomide in 18 patients with NETs (5 with panNETs) showed no antitumor activity with thalidomide, with no patients achieving a complete or partial response.[46] Taking these two studies together, temozolomide may have been the active drug in the combination study, and temozolomide seems to offer the greatest benefit in panNETs compared with other types of NETs.

The panNET treatment with monotherapy temozolomide was subsequently evaluated. In a retrospective analysis of 36 patients with metastatic NETs (12 patients with panNETs) treated with single-agent temozolomide (dosed at 200 mg/m^2 for 5 days, every 4 weeks), the medial overall time to progression was 7 months, with objective response appreciated in 14% of patients and stable disease in 53% of patients by RECIST criteria.[47] The most common side effects were hematologic, with 14% of patients experiencing grade 3/4 thrombocytopenia. This small series suggested a role for single-agent temozolomide in panNETs.

Through small retrospective studies, the combination of capecitabine and temozolomide for panNET treatment has also been investigated. A retrospective review was undertaken of 18 patients with metastatic NETs to the liver (7 with panNETs), all who had progression on octreotide LAR and were then treated on a pilot study of capecitabine and temozolomide.[48] Using RECIST, 1 patient (5.6%) had a complete response, 10 patients (55.5%) had a partial response, and 4 patients (22.2%) had stable disease; the median PFS was 14 months, with median OS from the diagnosis of liver metastases was 83 months. The most recent study to evaluate the combination of capecitabine and temozolomide was conducted retrospectively on 30 patients with metastatic panNETs who had not received any prior systemic therapy.[49] Patients were treated with combination capecitabine and temozolomide; 21 of 30 (70%)

patients demonstrated an objective radiographic response, with a median PFS of 18 months and 2-year OS of 92%. Notable toxicities included grade 4 hematologic abnormalities in 2 patients. This study provided further support that these two oral drugs, used in combination, offer a high and durable response in metastatic panNETs. However, careful monitoring of blood counts is essential with the administration of temozolomide, given the potential hematologic toxicity. An ongoing ECOG study is randomizing patients to temozolomide single agent versus capecitabine plus temozolomide and is poised to ask the question of benefit of single versus combination therapy.

Platinum Agents

Platinum chemotherapy drugs have also been evaluated as a treatment option for panNETs; however, the benefit may be more limited to patients with higher-grade tumors. In a phase II trial of cisplatin and etoposide in 45 patients with metastatic NETs, the tumor response was restricted to the patients with higher-grade, more aggressive tumors; among 18 patients classified with anaplastic neuroendocrine carcinomas, there were 9 partial responses and 3 complete responses. In comparison, among the 27 patients with well-differentiated carcinoid tumors or panNETs, there were only 2 partial responses observed, both in carcinoid tumors.[2]

In a separate study, the combination of cisplatin, 5-FU, and streptozocin was investigated in 79 patients with metastatic or locally advanced NETs (47 patients with panNETs). Among panNETs, the overall response rate was 38%; this study, however, also included patients with high-grade, poorly differentiated tumors, which tend to be more chemosensitive, and it is unknown if most responders were of higher grade.[50]

ADDITIONAL EXPERIMENTAL SYSTEMIC TREATMENTS
Peptide Receptor Radiation Therapy

Peptide receptor radiation therapy (PRRT), therapy that targets and treats NETs with radiolabeled somatostatin analogues, is based on the understanding that NETs highly expresses somatostatin receptors on their surface. In PRRT, a somatostatin analogue is linked to a therapeutic beta-emitting radioisotope, with the goal of the radiation emitted from the radiolabeled peptide binding to the surface of a tumor cell to both kill the tumor cell as well as neighboring cells, as the path length of beta particles extends across many cells.[51]

Several studies have demonstrated a role for PRRT in the treatment of advanced, metastatic NETs. Multiple radioisotopes have been investigated, including yttrium-90 (^{90}Y), indium-111, and lutetium-177 (^{177}Lu); these radioisotopes are linked to a somatostatin analogue to exert their therapeutic effects.

Yttrium-90–DOTATOC

A phase II study of ^{90}Y-DOTA-d-Phe(1)-Tyr(3)-octreotide (DOTATOC) included 39 patients with progressive NETs (of gastrointestinal and lung origin) who received 4 intravenous injections at 6-week intervals. The investigators observed an objective response rate of 38%, and 5% of patients (2 of 39 patients) had complete remissions, 18% of patients (7 of 39 patients) had partial remissions, and 69% of patients (27 of 39 patients) had stable disease. There was a similar reduction in clinical symptoms, including diarrhea, flushing, wheezing, and pellagra. The most severe grade 3 or 4 toxicities were hematologic.[51]

Building on this phase II data, the Multicenter Analysis of a Universal Receptor Imaging and Treatment Initiative, a European Study (MAURITIUS) trial was conducted.[52] In

MAURITIUS, 154 patients were treated with ^{90}Y-DOTA-lanreotide; stable disease was observed in 63 patients (41%), and tumor regression was seen in 22 patients (14%). In contrast to the aforementioned studies, the investigators did not appreciate any severe hematologic toxicity.

Lutetium-177–DOTATATE

^{177}Lu-DOTATATE has also been studied, with results demonstrating a benefit in terms of reduction in tumor size as well as QOL.

In the largest study of ^{177}Lu-DOTATATE, 504 patients with advanced NETs were treated with 4 treatment cycles, with treatment intervals of 6 to 10 weeks.[53] Among 310 evaluable patients, the investigators appreciated complete tumor remission in 2% of patients and partial tumor remission in 28% of patients. Median TTP was 40 months; from the start of treatment, the median OS was 46 months (128 months from diagnosis). Using historical controls, a survival benefit of 40 to 72 months from diagnosis was observed. In terms of adverse events, 3 patients did develop myelodysplastic syndrome and temporary liver toxicity was seen in 2 patients.

Other Experimental Targeted Treatments

Bevacizumab-containing regimens

Bevacizumab is a humanized monoclonal antibody that binds to soluble VEGF and inhibits tumor growth by preventing endothelial cell proliferation.[54] Most of the studies of bevacizumab in NETs have investigated a role for bevacizumab in patients with advanced carcinoid tumors.[55,56] However, subsequently, a role for bevacizumab has been studied in panNETs. In a phase II study of bevacizumab plus temozolomide in patients with advanced NETs, 34 patients (44% with panNETs, 56% with carcinoid) received bevacizumab 5 mg/kg on day 1 and 15 of a 28-day cycle and temozolomide 150 mg/m^2 on days 1 through 7 and days 15 through 21.[57] The investigators observed an overall radiographic response of 15% (5 of 34); however, when broken down by subgroup, the response rate was 33% in panNETs (5 of 15) and 0% (0 of 19) in carcinoid tumors. The median PFS was 11 months (14.3 months for panNETs and 7.3 months for carcinoid tumors), and the median OS was 33.3 months (41.7 months for panNETs and 18.8 months for carcinoid tumors).

The combination of 5-FU, oxaliplatin, and bevacizumab was also studied in panNETs. In one study, there was a 33% response rate in 6 patients with progressive panNETs who received short-term infusional 5-FU, leucovorin, oxaliplatin, and bevacizumab.[58] In another study, 40 patients (20 panNETs) were treated with capecitabine, oxaliplatin, and bevacizumab; of 31 evaluable patients, 7 patients (23%) were observed to have partial responses; 6 of these 7 patients (85.7%) had panNETs.[59] A phase II study has also been conducted in patients with panNETs investigating the combination of the mTOR inhibitor temsirolimus and bevacizumab; in this study of 58 patients (56 evaluable), confirmed response rate (RR) was 41% (23 of 56), median PFS was 13.2 months, and median OS was 34 months.[60] The findings from this study suggested possible activity for the combination of mTOR and VEGF pathway inhibitors.

Based on the findings of the aforementioned study, there has been continued investigation of the combination of mTOR and VEGF inhibition. CALGB 80701 (NCT01229943) was a randomized phase II trial of octreotide LAR, bevacizumab, and everolimus versus octreotide LAR and everolimus in 150 patients with metastatic panNETs; data analysis was just recently reported at the American Society of Clinical Oncology 2015 convention.[61] The study met its primary end point. PFS was

16.7 months in the combination arm versus 14 months in the single-agent everolimus arm. Response rates were higher in the combination arm (31% vs 12%). It is a paradigm shift to see targeted therapies cause such a high response rate. However, toxicity was significantly greater; 84% of patients on the combination bevacizumab/everolimus arm experienced serious grade 3 to 4 events. The toxicity, therefore, calls combination therapy into question.

A phase II study of single-agent bevacizumab for progressive moderately or well-differentiated panNETs was also recently reported.[62] In this study of 22 patients, partial response rates were 9% (2 of 22). In a heavily treated patient population, the median PFS was 13.6 months. Notably, 36% of patients did experience grade 3 hypertension. The findings from this study were thought to be promising, given that patients were required to have disease progression by RECIST within 7 months of study enrollment and patients overall experienced minimal systemic toxicity. Further investigation is warranted.

SUMMARY AND FUTURE DIRECTIONS

As discussed in this article, there are multiple types of systemic therapy options to manage and treat panNETs, including somatostatin analogue therapy, targeted therapy, and chemotherapy. Surgery remains the mainstay of treatment of patients with limited and localized disease and offers the potential for cure. However, as discussed, most patients with panNETs present with advanced disease; goals of therapy in the metastatic setting are directed toward control of symptoms (both due to tumor bulk and hormone hypersecretion in functional tumors), halting growth of disease, and prolonging life spans, all while preserving QOL.

For grade 1 and grade 2 metastatic panNETs, in the absence of symptoms and with low tumor volume, a trial of observation is generally encouraged to better understand the pace of disease growth. In the setting of disease progression, somatostatin analogues are typically started as first-line therapy; these analogues are also sometimes administered on patient presentation to control hormone-related symptoms from functional tumors.

Subsequently, the order of treatment varies and is individualized to each patient. Multimodality therapy is essential for the management of panNETs; over time, patients will receive several types of therapy, potentially including surgical debulking, liver-directed therapies, as well as systemic treatments to control their disease. As has been discussed, chemotherapy is generally reserved for use in the presence of rapid tumor growth or heavy disease burden. Targeted agents are another option to consider, which improve PFS, although response rates are generally less than 10%.

After decades of stagnation, in the past 5 years, an improved understanding of this rare disease has led to more treatment options. As noted, the appropriate selection and sequencing of treatment approaches for patients with advanced pancreatic NETs is unknown and currently depends on clinical judgment. The hope is that increased understanding of the disease will lead to a more personalized individualized treatment of patients. In addition, it is hoped that tumor mutational analysis will identify biomarkers that can serve as predictors of response and/or resistance to the different agents.

When designing clinical trials in the future, it will be essential that these trials separate panNETs from NETs originating in other locations; from the knowledge to date, panNETs seem to respond differently to the available systemic therapies and need to be studied in isolation. Randomized trials are also clearly needed to test the role of combination therapies to assess toxicity and confirm their efficacy compared with our currently available agents.

REFERENCES

1. Kunz PL, Reidy-Lagunes D, Anthony LB, et al. Consensus guidelines for the management and treatment of neuroendocrine tumors. Pancreas 2013;42(4):557–77.
2. Moertel CG, Kvols LK, O'Connell MJ, et al. Treatment of neuroendocrine carcinomas with combined etoposide and cisplatin - evidence of major therapeutic activity in the anaplastic variants of these neoplasms. Cancer 1991;68(2): 227–32.
3. Modlin IM, Oberg K, Chung DC, et al. Gastroenteropancreatic neuroendocrine tumours. Lancet Oncol 2008;9(1):61–72.
4. Modlin IM, Lye KD, Kidd M. A 5-decade analysis of 13,715 carcinoid tumors. Cancer 2003;97(4):934–59.
5. Dumlu EG, Karakoc D, Ozdemir A. Nonfunctional pancreatic neuroendocrine tumors: advances in diagnosis, management and controversies. Int Surg 2015; 100(6):1089–97.
6. Metz DC, Jensen RT. Gastrointestinal neuroendocrine tumors: pancreatic endocrine tumors. Gastroenterology 2008;135(5):1469–92.
7. Yao JC, Hassan M, Phan A, et al. One hundred years after "carcinoid": epidemiology of and prognostic factors for neuroendocrine tumors in 35,825 cases in the United States. J Clin Oncol 2008;26(18):3063–72.
8. Reidy-Lagunes DL. Systemic therapy for advanced pancreatic neuroendocrine tumors: an update. J Natl Compr Canc Netw 2012;10(6):777–83.
9. Castellano D, Grande E, Valle J, et al. Expert consensus for the management of advanced or metastatic pancreatic neuroendocrine and carcinoid tumors. Cancer Chemother Pharmacol 2015;75(6):1099–114.
10. Jensen RT, Berna MJ, Bingham DB, et al. Inherited pancreatic endocrine tumor syndromes: advances in molecular pathogenesis, diagnosis, management, and controversies. Cancer 2008;113(7 Suppl):1807–43.
11. The International Agency for Research on Cancer. In: Bosman FT, Carneiro F, Hruban RH, et al, editors. WHO classification of tumours of the digestive system. 4th edition. Lyon (France): International Agency for Research on Cancer; 2010. p. 417.
12. Strosberg JR, Cheema A, Weber J, et al. Prognostic validity of a novel American Joint Committee on Cancer Staging classification for pancreatic neuroendocrine tumors. J Clin Oncol 2011;29(22):3044–9.
13. Basturk O, Yang Z, Tang LH, et al. The high-grade (WHO G3) pancreatic neuroendocrine tumor category is morphologically and biologically heterogeneous and includes both well differentiated and poorly differentiated neoplasms. Am J Surg Pathol 2015;39(5):683–90.
14. Sorbye H, Welin S, Langer SW, et al. Predictive and prognostic factors for treatment and survival in 305 patients with advanced gastrointestinal neuroendocrine carcinoma (WHO G3): The NORDIC NEC study. Ann Oncol 2013;24(1):152–60.
15. Raj NP, et al. Treatment response and outcomes of grade 3 (G3) pancreatic neuroendocrine carcinomas (HGNEC) based on pathologic differentiation [Meeting Abstracts]. J Clin Oncol 2015;33(suppl) [abstract: e15185].
16. Jiao Y, Shi C, Edil BH, et al. DAXX/ATRX, MEN1, and mTOR pathway genes are frequently altered in pancreatic neuroendocrine tumors. Science 2011;331(6021): 1199–203.
17. Reubi JC, Waser B. Concomitant expression of several peptide receptors in neuroendocrine tumours: molecular basis for in vivo multireceptor tumour targeting. Eur J Nucl Med Mol Imaging 2003;30(5):781–93.

18. Oberg KE, Reubi JC, Kwekkeboom DJ, et al. Role of somatostatins in gastroen-teropancreatic neuroendocrine tumor development and therapy. Gastroenterology 2010;139(3):742–53, 753.e1.

19. Kraenzlin ME, Ch'ng JL, Wood SM, et al. Long-term treatment of a VIPoma with somatostatin analogue resulting in remission of symptoms and possible shrinkage of metastases. Gastroenterology 1985;88(1 Pt 1):185–7.

20. Nikou GC, Toubanakis C, Nikolaou P, et al. VIPomas: an update in diagnosis and management in a series of 11 patients. Hepatogastroenterology 2005;52(64):1259–65.

21. Frankton S, Bloom SR. Gastrointestinal endocrine tumours. Glucagonomas. Baillieres Clin Gastroenterol 1996;10(4):697–705.

22. Saltz L, Trochanowski B, Buckley M, et al. Octreotide as an antineoplastic agent in the treatment of functional and nonfunctional neuroendocrine tumors. Cancer 1993;72(1):244–8.

23. Arnold R, Neuhaus C, Benning R, et al. Somatostatin analog sandostatin and inhibition of tumor growth in patients with metastatic endocrine gastroenteropancreatic tumors. World J Surg 1993;17(4):511–9.

24. Rinke A, Müller HH, Schade-Brittinger C, et al. Placebo-controlled, double-blind, prospective, randomized study on the effect of octreotide LAR in the control of tumor growth in patients with metastatic neuroendocrine midgut tumors: a report from the PROMID Study Group. J Clin Oncol 2009;27(28):4656–63.

25. Clark OH, Benson AB 3rd, Berlin JD, et al. NCCN clinical practice guidelines in oncology: neuroendocrine tumors. J Natl Compr Canc Netw 2009;7(7):712–47.

26. Caplin ME, Pavel M, Ruszniewski P. Lanreotide in metastatic enteropancreatic neuroendocrine tumors. N Engl J Med 2014;371(3):224–33.

27. Turner HE, Harris AL, Melmed S, et al. Angiogenesis in endocrine tumors. Endocr Rev 2003;24(5):600–32.

28. Kulke MH, Lenz HJ, Meropol NJ, et al. Activity of sunitinib in patients with advanced neuroendocrine tumors. J Clin Oncol 2008;26(20):3403–10.

29. Raymond E, Dahan L, Raoul JL, et al. Sunitinib malate for the treatment of pancreatic neuroendocrine tumors. N Engl J Med 2011;364(6):501–13.

30. Vinik A, Van Cutsem E, Niccoli P, et al. Updated results from a phase III trial of sunitinib versus placebo in patients with progressive, unresectable, well-differentiated pancreatic neuroendocrine tumor (NET) [Meeting Abstracts]. J Clin Oncol 2012; 30(suppl) [abstract: 4118].

31. O'Donnell A, Faivre S, Burris HA 3rd, et al. Phase I pharmacokinetic and pharmacodynamic study of the oral mammalian target of rapamycin inhibitor everolimus in patients with advanced solid tumors. J Clin Oncol 2008;26(10):1588–95.

32. Yao JC, Phan AT, Chang DZ, et al. Efficacy of RAD001 (everolimus) and octreotide LAR in advanced low- to intermediate-grade neuroendocrine tumors: results of a phase II study. J Clin Oncol 2008;26(26):4311–8.

33. Yao JC, Lombard-Bohas C, Baudin E, et al. Daily oral everolimus activity in patients with metastatic pancreatic neuroendocrine tumors after failure of cytotoxic chemotherapy: a phase II trial. J Clin Oncol 2010;28(1):69–76.

34. Yao JC, Shah MH, Ito T, et al. Everolimus for advanced pancreatic neuroendocrine tumors. N Engl J Med 2011;364(6):514–23.

35. Murray-Lyon IM, Eddleston AL, Williams R, et al. Treatment of multiple-hormone-producing malignant islet-cell tumour with streptozotocin. Lancet 1968;2(7574): 895–8.

36. Moertel CG, Reitemeier RJ, Schutt AJ, et al. Phase II study of strepozotocin (NSC-85998) in the treatment of advanced gastrointestinal cancer. Cancer Chemother Rep 1971;55(3):303–7.

37. Moertel CG, Lefkopoulo M, Lipsitz S, et al. Streptozocin-doxorubicin, streptozocin-fluorouracil or chlorozotocin in the treatment of advanced islet-cell carcinoma. N Engl J Med 1992;326(8):519–23.
38. Cheng PN, Saltz LB. Failure to confirm major objective antitumor activity for streptozocin and doxorubicin in the treatment of patients with advanced islet cell carcinoma. Cancer 1999;86(6):944–8.
39. Kouvaraki MA, Ajani JA, Hoff P, et al. Fluorouracil, doxorubicin, and streptozocin in the treatment of patients with locally advanced and metastatic pancreatic endocrine carcinomas. J Clin Oncol 2004;22(23):4762–71.
40. Loo TL, Housholder GE, Gerulath AH, et al. Mechanism of action and pharmacology studies with DTIC (NSC-45388). Cancer Treat Rep 1976;60(2):149–52.
41. Ramanathan RK, Cnaan A, Hahn RG, et al. Phase II trial of dacarbazine (DTIC) in advanced pancreatic islet cell carcinoma. Study of the Eastern Cooperative Oncology Group-E6282. Ann Oncol 2001;12(8):1139–43.
42. Altimari AF, Badrinath K, Reisel HJ, et al. DTIC therapy in patients with malignant intra-abdominal neuroendocrine tumors. Surgery 1987;102(6):1009–17.
43. Kessinger A, Foley JF, Lemon HM. Use of DTIC in the malignant carcinoid syndrome. Cancer Treat Rep 1977;61(1):101–2.
44. Stevens MF, Hickman JA, Langdon SP, et al. Antitumor activity and pharmacokinetics in mice of 8-carbamoyl-3-methyl-imidazo[5,1-d]-1,2,3,5-tetrazin-4(3H)-one (CCRG 81045; M & B 39831), a novel drug with potential as an alternative to dacarbazine. Cancer Res 1987;47(22):5846–52.
45. Kulke MH, Stuart K, Enzinger PC, et al. Phase II study of temozolomide and thalidomide in patients with metastatic neuroendocrine tumors. J Clin Oncol 2006;24(3):401–6.
46. Varker KA, Campbell J, Shah MH. Phase II study of thalidomide in patients with metastatic carcinoid and islet cell tumors. Cancer Chemother Pharmacol 2008; 61(4):661–8.
47. Ekeblad S, Sundin A, Janson ET, et al. Temozolomide as monotherapy is effective in treatment of advanced malignant neuroendocrine tumors. Clin Cancer Res 2007;13(10):2986–91.
48. Fine RL, Gulati AP, Krantz BA, et al. Capecitabine and temozolomide (CAPTEM) for metastatic, well-differentiated neuroendocrine cancers: the Pancreas Center at Columbia University experience. Cancer Chemother Pharmacol 2013;71(3): 663–70.
49. Strosberg JR, Fine RL, Choi J, et al. First-line chemotherapy with capecitabine and temozolomide in patients with metastatic pancreatic endocrine carcinomas. Cancer 2011;117(2):268–75.
50. Turner NC, Strauss SJ, Sarker D, et al. Chemotherapy with 5-fluorouracil, cisplatin and streptozocin for neuroendocrine tumours. Br J Cancer 2010;102(7):1106–12.
51. Waldherr C, Pless M, Maecke HR, et al. Tumor response and clinical benefit in neuroendocrine tumors after 7.4 GBq (90)Y-DOTATOC. J Nucl Med 2002;43(5): 610–6.
52. Virgolini I, Britton K, Buscombe J, et al. In- and Y-DOTA-lanreotide: results and implications of the MAURITIUS trial. Semin Nucl Med 2002;32(2):148–55.
53. Kwekkeboom DJ, de Herder WW, Kam BL, et al. Treatment with the radiolabeled somatostatin analog [177 Lu-DOTA 0,Tyr3] octreotate: toxicity, efficacy, and survival. J Clin Oncol 2008;26(13):2124–30.
54. Ranieri G, Patruno R, Ruggieri E, et al. Vascular endothelial growth factor (VEGF) as a target of bevacizumab in cancer: from the biology to the clinic. Curr Med Chem 2006;13(16):1845–57.

55. Yao JC, Phan A, Hoff PM, et al. Targeting vascular endothelial growth factor in advanced carcinoid tumor: a random assignment phase II study of depot octreotide with bevacizumab and pegylated interferon alpha-2b. J Clin Oncol 2008; 26(8):1316–23.
56. Kulke MH, Chan JA, Meyerhardt JA, et al. A prospective phase II study of 2-methoxyestradiol administered in combination with bevacizumab in patients with metastatic carcinoid tumors. Cancer Chemother Pharmacol 2011;68(2): 293–300.
57. Chan JA, Stuart K, Earle CC, et al. Prospective study of bevacizumab plus temozolomide in patients with advanced neuroendocrine tumors. J Clin Oncol 2012; 30(24):2963–8.
58. Venook AP, Ko AH, Tempero MA, et al. Phase II trial of FOLFOX plus bevacizumab in advanced, progressive neuroendocrine tumors [Meeting Abstracts]. J Clin Oncol 2008;26(15_suppl 15545). Available at: http://meeting.ascopubs.org/cgi/content/short/26/15_suppl/15545.
59. Kunz PL, Kuo T, Zahn JM, et al. A phase II study of capecitabine, oxaliplatin, and bevacizumab for metastatic or unresectable neuroendocrine tumors [Meeting Abstracts]. J Clin Oncol 2010;28(15_suppl 4104). Available at: http://meeting.ascopubs.org/cgi/content/abstract/28/15_suppl/4104.
60. Hobday TJ, Qin R, Reidy-Lagunes D, et al. Multicenter phase II trial of temsirolimus and bevacizumab in pancreatic neuroendocrine tumors. J Clin Oncol 2015; 33(14):1551–6.
61. Kulke MH, Niedzwiecki D, Foster NR, et al. Randomized phase II study of everolimus (E) versus everolimus plus bevacizumab (E+B) in patients (Pts) with locally advanced or metastatic pancreatic neuroendocrine tumors (pNET), CALGB 80701 (Alliance) [Meeting Abstracts]. J Clin Oncol 2015;33(suppl) [abstract: 4005].
62. Hobday TJ, Yin J, Pettinger A, et al. Multicenter prospective phase II trial of bevacizumab (bev) for progressive pancreatic neuroendocrine tumor (PNET) [Meeting Abstracts]. J Clin Oncol 2015;33(suppl) [abstract: 4096].

Pheochromocytoma and Paraganglioma

Genetics, Diagnosis, and Treatment

Lauren Fishbein, MD, PhD, MTR

KEYWORDS

- Pheochromocytoma • Paraganglioma • Genetics • Treatment • Malignant
- Metastatic

KEY POINTS

- Pheochromocytomas and paragangliomas (PCCs/PGLs), both benign and malignant, have high morbidity and mortality, especially when not properly diagnosed or treated.
- Blood pressure management, usually with the alpha-blocker phenoxybenzamine, is critical perioperatively for all patients and surrounding treatments for those with metastatic disease.
- Surgery is the only cure for PCC/PGL, but limited biochemical and tumor control of metastatic disease occurs with treatments, including ^{131}I-MIBG, chemotherapy, and radiation.
- Up to 40% of patients with PCC/PGL have germline mutations in susceptibility genes; therefore, all patients should be considered for clinical genetic testing.
- Future work is needed to identify predictors of metastatic potential and novel targets for therapy.

INTRODUCTION

Neuroendocrine tumors arising from the adrenal medulla and extra-adrenal ganglia are called pheochromocytomas and paragangliomas (PCCs/PGLs), respectively. PCCs/PGLs are rare tumors with an incidence of 2 to 8 per million.[1] PCCs/PGLs occur in 0.2% to 0.6% of hypertensive patients and account for up to 5% of adrenal incidentalomas.[2] Most PCCs/PGLs are benign yet associated with high morbidity and mortality secondary to hypersecretion of catecholamines and metanephrines leading to hypertension, cardiovascular disease and even death. Approximately a quarter of PCCs/PGLs are malignant, defined by the World Health Organization as the presence

Disclosure Statement: The author has nothing to disclose.
Division of Endocrinology, Diabetes and Metabolism, Department of Medicine, Perelman School of Medicine, University of Pennsylvania, 351 BRB II/III, 421 Curie Boulevard, Philadelphia, PA 19104, USA
E-mail address: lauren.fishbein@ucdenver.edu

Hematol Oncol Clin N Am 30 (2016) 135–150
http://dx.doi.org/10.1016/j.hoc.2015.09.006

of distant metastases.[1] Diagnosing PCCs/PGLs can be challenging, and treatments for metastatic disease are most often not curative. This review discusses the inherited genetics, diagnosis, and treatment of PCCs/PGLs.

GENETICS

Up to 40% of patients with PCCs/PGLs have a germline mutation in a known susceptibility gene,[3–5] more than any other solid tumor type. **Table 1** describes the susceptibility genes and the associated syndromes. The risk of PCC/PGL with each syndrome is discussed in the following sections.

Classic Tumor Syndromes

Neurofibromatosis type 1 (NF1) is an autosomal dominant syndrome found in 1 in 3000 individuals caused by mutations in the *NF1* gene. The diagnosis of NF1 is made when patients meet at least 2 of the clinical criteria (see **Table 1**).[6] PCCs, although not in the diagnostic criteria, occur at a higher frequency than in the general population. Approximately 5% of patients develop unilateral or bilateral PCC, and 12% of those are metastatic.[6] The mean age at diagnosis of PCC is 42, similar to sporadic PCC. Guidelines suggest screening for PCC in patients with NF1 who have hypertension.[6]

Multiple endocrine neoplasia type 2 (MEN2) is an autosomal dominant syndrome found in 1 in 30,000 individuals caused by activating mutations in the *RET* proto-oncogene. There are 3 subgroups of MEN2 described in **Table 1**. MEN2A accounts for more than 90% of cases, whereas MEN2B and the rare familial medullary thyroid cancer subtype account for the rest.[7] Fifty percent of patients with MEN2 develop PCC and half have bilateral disease. There are strong genotype phenotype correlations; therefore, screening recommendations for PCC vary depending on the mutation.[7] Patients with MEN2A with *RET* codon 630 or 634 mutations and patients with MEN2B (most with *RET* codon 918 mutations) should begin screening for PCC at age 8. Patients with all other MEN2A mutations should begin screening for PCC at age 20. The mean age at diagnosis of PCC is between 30 and 40 years old, and the malignancy rate is less than 5%.[7]

von Hippel Lindau disease (vHL) is an autosomal dominant syndrome affecting 1 in 36,000 births per year and caused by mutations in the *VHL* gene. vHL is defined by several benign and malignant tumors described in **Table 1**.[8] Unilateral or bilateral PCC occurs in 10% to 20% of patients, with rare reports of extra-adrenal or head and neck PGL (HNPGL).[8] Similar to MEN2, there are strong genotype phenotype correlations.[9,10] Patients with truncating mutations or exonic deletions in the VHL protein have a lower penetrance for PCC but a high penetrance for renal cell carcinoma. On the other hand, patients with missense mutations in VHL more frequently develop PCC when mutations are on the surface of the protein rather than the core.[11] Screening for PCC in patients with vHL should begin at age 5 for families with high-risk mutations. The mean age at diagnosis of PCC is 30 years old, and approximately 5% develop metastatic disease.[8]

Hereditary Paraganglioma Syndromes

Autosomal dominant mutations in succinate dehydrogenase (SDH), complex II of the mitochondrial respiratory chain, cause the hereditary paraganglioma syndromes. Mutations can occur in any of the subunit genes (*SDHA, SDHB, SDHC, SDHD*) or cofactor (*SDHAF2* also called *SDH5*) (see **Table 1**). SDHB is the most commonly mutated subunit leading to PCC/PGL. Mutation carriers develop extra-adrenal PGL

Table 1
Pheochromocytoma and paraganglioma susceptibility genes and the associated syndromes

Gene	Protein	Function	Syndrome (Inheritance Pattern)	Metastatic PCC/PGL
Classic tumor syndromes				
NF1	Neurofibromin	GTPase, which inactivates RAS to control the MAPK signaling pathway	Neurofibromatosis type 1 (AD) • Cutaneous neurofibromas (2 or more) • Plexiform neurofibromas • Café-au-lait spots (6 or more ≥1.5 cm in postpubertal patients and ≥ 0.5 cm in prepubertal patients) • Lisch nodules (benign iris hamartoma) • Inguinal or axillary freckling • Long bone dysplasia • Optic gliomas • First-degree relative with NF1 Not part of diagnostic criteria, but associated • PCC (possibly bilateral) • Malignant peripheral nerve sheath tumors • Chronic myelogenous leukemia	12%
RET	RET	Membrane tyrosine kinase receptor signals through PI3K	Multiple endocrine neoplasia type 2A (AD) • Medullary thyroid cancer • PCC (possibly bilateral) • Hyperparathyroidism Multiple endocrine neoplasia type 2B (AD) • Medullary thyroid cancer • PCC (possibly bilateral) • Marfanoid habitus • Mucocutaneous neuromas • Gastrointestinal ganglioneuromas Familial medullary thyroid cancer (AD) • Medullary thyroid cancer	<5%

(continued on next page)

Table 1
(continued)

Gene	Protein	Function	Syndrome (Inheritance Pattern)	Metastatic PCC/PGL
VHL	von Hippel Lindau protein	Ubiquitin ligase 3E activity which inactivates hypoxia inducible factors to control transcription of genes involved in angiogenesis	von Hippel Lindau disease (AD) • Hemangioblastomas of the central nervous system (including retina) • Endolymphatic sac tumors • Epididymal cystadenomas • PCC (possibly bilateral) • Renal cell carcinomas (clear cell) • Renal cysts • Pancreatic neuroendocrine tumors • Pancreatic cysts	5%
Succinate dehydrogenase complex genes		Complex II of the mitochondria respiratory chain that transfers electrons to the terminal acceptor ubiquinone and also converts succinate to fumarate in the TCA cycle		
SDHA	Succinate dehydrogenase subunit A	Catalytic subunit	Hereditary Paraganglioma Syndrome (AD) • PCC/PGL • GI stromal tumors	Low
SDHB	Succinate dehydrogenase subunit B	Catalytic subunit	Hereditary paraganglioma syndrome (AD) • EAPGL • PCC and HNPGL possible • Renal cell carcinoma (clear cell) • GI stromal tumors • Pituitary adenomas rare	23%
SDHC	Succinate dehydrogenase subunit C	Anchoring subunit	Hereditary Paraganglioma Syndrome (AD) • HNPGL • EAPGL possible (often thoracic) • PCC rare • Renal cell carcinoma (clear cell) rare • GI stromal tumors • Pituitary adenomas rare	Low

Gene	Name	Function	Clinical	Malignancy
SDHD	Succinate dehydrogenase subunit D	Anchoring subunit	Hereditary paraganglioma syndrome (AD, paternal inheritance) • Multifocal HNPGL • PCC and EAPGL possible • Renal cell carcinoma (clear cell) • GI stromal tumors • Pituitary adenoma rare	<5%
SDHAF2 (*SDH5*)	Succinate dehydrogenase cofactor AF2	Cofactor for complex II leading to flavination of SDHA	Hereditary paraganglioma syndrome (AD, paternal inheritance) • Multifocal HNPGL	Low
Additional susceptibility genes				
TMEM127	Transmembrane protein 127	Transmembrane protein in the endosome involved in the mTOR pathway	(AD) • PCC • EAPGL and HNPGL possible • Renal cell carcinoma rare	Low
MAX	MYC-associated protein X	Transcription factor heterodimerizes with MYC to control cellular proliferation, differentiation and apoptosis	(AD) • PCC (bilateral)	Intermediate
EPAS1	Hypoxia inducible factor 2A	Activates transcription of angiogenesis genes	Polycythemia paraganglioma syndrome (AD, often somatic mosaicism) • Polycythemia • PCC/PGL • Somatostatinoma	NK
FH	Fumarate hydratase	TCA cycle enzyme which converts fumarate to malate	Hereditary leiomyomatosis and renal cell carcinoma (AD) • Cutaneous and uterine leiomyomas • Renal cell carcinoma (type 2 papillary) • PCC/PGL rare	Possibly high
MDH2	Malate dehydrogenase	TCA cycle enzyme which converts malate to oxaloacetate	(AD) • PCC/PGL	NK

Abbreviations: AD, autosomal dominant; EAPGL, extra-adrenal paraganglioma; GI, gastrointestinal; HNPGL, head and neck paraganglioma; MAPK, mitogen-activated protein kinase; NK, not known; PCC, pheochromocytoma; PGL, paraganglioma; TCA, tricarboxylic acid cycle.

but can also have PCC and HNPGL. The mean age at initial diagnosis of PCC/PGL is 32 years.[12] *SDHB* mutation carriers with PCC/PGL have the highest risk of developing metastases at 23% based on a meta-analysis and systematic review.[13] Long-term surveillance studies of mutation carrier families are needed to determine the true rate of malignancy and penetrance of disease.

SDHD is the next most commonly mutated subunit leading to PCC/PGL. Interestingly, only paternally inherited *SDHD* mutations cause disease phenotype, with extremely rare exception.[14,15] *SDHD* mutation carriers develop multiple HNPGL but can have PCC and extra-adrenal PGL. The mean age at diagnosis of initial PCC/PGL is 33 years.[12] The risk of malignancy is lower than 5%.[13]

Mutations in the remaining SDH subunits occur much less frequently and also are associated with specific phenotypes. Eighty-one percent of the *SDHC*-associated tumors are HNPGL, 10% are thoracic PGL, and the remaining tumors are abdominal PGL and PCC.[16] The mean age at first PCC/PGL is 38 years, and the risk of malignancy is very low.[12] Only a few reported families with PCC/PGL have mutations in *SDHA* or *SDHAF2*.[17,18] Similar to *SDHD* mutations, *SDHAF2* mutations have a parent-of-origin effect with paternal transmission of disease, and affected patients develop only HNPGL.[18]

There are no guidelines on when to begin screening or what screening to do in asymptomatic *SDHx* mutation carriers. PCCs/PGLs have been reported in children as young as 5 years old. The full spectrum of clinical syndromes associated with *SDHx* mutations is still being defined but includes a risk of gastrointestinal stromal tumors, renal cell carcinoma, and pituitary adenomas (see **Table 1**).[19] Therefore, most experts recommend annual biochemical screening for PCC/PGL starting between age 5 and 10 and full-body MRI screening for all associated tumor types every 2 to 5 years until more information is known.

Additional Susceptibility Genes

Other susceptibility genes have been implicated in PCC/PGL at low frequency (less than 2% of cases) including *MAX (Myc-associated protein X)* and *TMEM127 (Transmembrane protein 127)*, both of which are usually associated with PCC (see **Table 1**).[20,21] Rare patients with PCC/PGL, with or without polycythemia and somatostatinomas, have somatic mosaicism for *EPAS1* mutations, encoding a mutant hypoxia-inducible factor 2α.[22–24] There are case reports of other susceptibility genes in the tricarboxylic acid cycle (TCA) cycle. A few families with germline *fumarate hydratase, FH,* mutations and one family with germline *malate dehydrogenase, MDH2,* mutations have been found to have PCC/PGL.[25–27] Clearly, dysregulation of the TCA cycle (by *SDHx, FH, MDH2* mutations) predisposes to PCC/PGL, and it will not be surprising in the future to find rare families with PCC/PGL who have mutations in other TCA cycle enzymes.

In sporadic PCC/PGL, there are low rates of somatic mutations in the classic susceptibility genes, such as *NF1, VHL* and *RET*, but surprisingly, not in *SDHx* genes.[28,29] Up to 10% of sporadic tumors have somatic mutations in *HRAS*.[30] Recently, approximately 13% of PCCs/PGLs were found to have somatic mutations in *ATRX*, a chromatin-remodeling gene also mutated in pancreatic neuroendocrine tumors, and these mutations were associated with clinically aggressive PCC/PGL.[31]

Given the high rate of inherited mutations associated with PCC/PGL, the Endocrine Society guidelines recommend referring all patients with PCC/PGL for consideration of clinical genetic testing.[32] The clinical phenotype, as discussed previously, can guide the order of gene testing, as can the biochemical profile (**Table 2**).[33,34] As panel

Table 2 Biochemical profile can be associated with inherited mutation	
Biochemical Profile	**Possible Gene Mutation**
Noradrenergic	*SDHx* or *VHL* or sporadic (no mutation identified)
Adrenergic	*RET* or *NF1*
Dopaminergic	*SDHx* (often *SDHB*)
Methoxytyramine[a]	*SDHx* (or seen in metastatic disease even without a known mutation)

[a] Not routinely tested for in the United States.

gene testing is becoming more cost effective, it is replacing single-gene testing in most centers.

SYMPTOMS AND DIAGNOSIS

Patients with PCC/PGL often present with the classic triad of diaphoresis, headache, and palpitations and have hypertension, but the clinical presentation associated with catecholamine/metanephrine excess can vary (**Box 1**). The number of asymptomatic patients is higher than previously appreciated.[35]

Both 24-hour urine-fractionated and plasma-free metanephrines have more than 90% sensitivity for PCC/PGL. Plasma metanephrines are the first-line screening test given the ease of collection and higher specificity compared with 24-hour urine tests (ranging from 79% to 98% versus 69% to 95%, respectively).[32] Plasma and urine catecholamines have frequent false-positive results, as minimal stimulation can raise epinephrine levels; therefore, these tests are not routinely part of the initial screening except in *SDHx* mutation carriers, as they may have dopamine-only secreting tumors.[34] Many medications interfere with the testing of plasma metanephrines leading to false-positive results including acetaminophen, selective serotonin reuptake inhibitors, tricyclic antidepressants, monoamine oxidase inhibitors, and certain beta-adrenergic and alpha-adrenergic blockers.[36] These medications should be stopped for 10 to 14 days before testing if possible. If the medications

Box 1 Common symptoms and signs associated with pheochromocytoma/paraganglioma
Headache
Diaphoresis
Palpitations
Tachycardia
Hypertension (persistent, episodic, or relative to baseline)
Syncope
Anxiety
Tremor
New-onset hyperglycemia (or worsening of controlled diabetes mellitus)
Weight changes
No symptoms

cannot be stopped and there are metanephrine elevations, it is appropriate to move on to imaging studies.

Once biochemical hypersecretion is confirmed, cross-sectional imaging studies will help localize the tumor. Computed tomography (CT) or magnetic resonance imaging (MRI) of the abdomen/pelvis are the best initial test because approximately 75% of tumors will be in the adrenal glands. For patients with known susceptibility gene mutations, imaging other locations may be necessary based on associated phenotype (as discussed in the genetics section). Parasympathetic PGLs, including HNPGL, are rarely secretory, and if suspected, imaging should be done regardless of biochemical results. Furthermore, if patients with known HNPGL have elevated metanephrines, imaging studies should be done to rule out an additional primary PCC/PGL in another location. ^{123}I- metaiodobenzylguanidine (MIBG) imaging is most useful to identify metastatic disease in preparation for possible ^{131}I-MIBG treatment or if cross-sectional imaging does not reveal the tumor.[32] ^{123}I-MIBG is not as useful for first-line imaging because up to 50% of normal adrenal glands have increased symmetric or asymmetric physiologic uptake leading to false-positive results.[37] The Endocrine Society guidelines recommend the use of 18F-fluoro-deoxyglucose PET scanning with CT imaging over ^{123}I-MIBG imaging to diagnose patients with metastatic disease, especially for those with known *SDHB* inherited mutations, as the sensitivity of PET imaging is 74% to 100%.[32]

PERIOPERATIVE MANAGEMENT

Surgery is the mainstay of treatment for PCCs/PGLs. Catecholamine excess can cause significant morbidity and mortality in the perioperative setting with initial mortality rates as high as 30% to 45%; however, the current surgical techniques and medical management have significantly decreased the mortality rate to 0% to 2.9%.[38] Comparable outcomes are seen with laparoscopic surgery for PCC compared with open procedures.[39] Adrenal cortical-sparing surgery should be considered for patients with increased risk of bilateral PCC and low risk of malignancy, such as patients with vHL and MEN2. If adrenal cortical function can be preserved, patients avoid the long-term dependence on corticosteroids.

Patients with benign or malignant PCC/PGL must be treated with medical blockade before any surgery or procedure to avoid a hypertensive crisis. Most centers use alpha-adrenergic receptor blockers, although there are no published prospective randomized trials to suggest the best regimen. **Table 3** lists the common medication regimens. Several retrospective single-drug studies show good outcomes with alpha-blockade,[40,41] but very few studies compare multiple regimens. The largest retrospective multiregimen study compared practices at the Mayo Clinic using phenoxybenzamine (n = 50) with that of the Cleveland Clinic using doxazosin (n = 37), often combined with calcium channel blockers.[42] Both sites used beta-blockers if tachycardia occurred with the alpha-blockade. Results showed phenoxybenzamine was associated with increased postoperative hypotension but a shorter duration of severe intraoperative hypertension compared with doxazosin. There were no differences in surgical outcomes or length of hospital stay. Another retrospective study compared several alpha-blockade regimens in 39 patients from a single center (phenoxybenzamine, n = 21; doxazosin, n = 17; prazosin, n = 11).[43] There were no differences in intraoperative hypertension, postoperative blood pressure, or volume-replacement needs between regimens.

Given the limited data, guidelines recommend phenoxybenzamine as first-line treatment with an alternative regimen of doxazocin plus or minus a calcium channel blocker.[32] Metyrosine, which blocks catecholamine production, is not usually

Table 3
Perioperative blockade regimens to begin 10 to 14 days before surgery

Category	Drug	Dosing	Common Side Effects
Nonselective alpha-blocker	Phenoxybenzamine	10 mg given 2–3 times per day (up to 60 mg daily)	Orthostatic hypotension, nasal congestion, tachycardia
	Phentolamine	Intravenous 2.5–5 mg boluses	
Selective alpha-1 blockers	Doxazosin	2–4 mg given 2–3 times per day	Orthostatic hypotension, dizziness, tachycardia
	Prazosin	1–2 mg given 2 times per day	
	Terazosin	1–4 mg given once daily	
Dihydropyridine calcium channel blockers	Nicardipine Amlodipine	30 mg 2 times per day 5–10 mg once daily	Headache, edema
Tyrosine hydroxylase inhibitor	Metyrosine	250–500 mg titrated up to 4 times per day	Severe fatigue, extrapyramidal neurologic side effects, nausea
Selective beta-1 blocker only after full alpha-blockade	Metoprolol	25–100 mg given 2 times per day	Fatigue, dizziness, asthma exacerbation
Nonselective beta-blocker only after full alpha-blockade	Propranolol	20–40 mg given 2–3 times per day	Fatigue, dizziness, asthma exacerbation

recommended because it is expensive and has significant side effects (see **Table 3**); but it may be useful in high-risk patients with cardiovascular disease to minimize perioperative hemodynamic swings. Preoperative blood pressure under 130/80 mm Hg and heart rate less than 80 bpm are ideal. Development of orthostatic hypotension and tachycardia are expected side effects of effective blockade and should not necessarily prompt a dose reduction. Instead, supportive therapy should be given with hydration and high salt intake, as well as initiation of beta-blockers to control tachycardia. Beta-blockers should not be used until a patient is fully alpha-blocked to prevent the theoretic unopposed alpha-adrenergic stimulation leading to severe vasoconstriction and hypertensive crisis. Plasma metanephrines should be monitored 4 to 8 weeks postoperatively to ensure successful removal of all tumor tissue and then at least annually for life given the potential for multiple primary tumors, recurrence and the long latency for metastatic disease.

METASTATIC PHEOCHROMOCYTOMAS AND PARAGANGLIOMAS

A quarter of PCCs/PGLs are malignant ($\sim$10% of PCCs and $\sim$20% of PGLs), defined by distant metastases, commonly in the liver, lung, bone, and lymph nodes, which can be seen at diagnosis of the primary tumor or develop even 20 years later.[44] Patients with metastatic PCC/PGL have a 50% 5-year overall survival.[44] Approximately half of patients with metastatic PCC/PGL have inherited *SDHB* mutations,[4] and many have no known mutation. In addition, there are clinically aggressive tumors, without metastases but with extensive local invasion into adjacent tissue, which cannot be easily surgically cured and share the burden of catecholamine hypersecretion.

Predicting malignant potential is difficult. Tumors larger than 4 to 5 cm, secreting methoxytyramine or associated with germline *SDHB* mutations carry an increased risk of malignancy.[33,44] In 2002, the Pheochromocytoma of the Adrenal Gland Scaled Score (PASS), a pathologic scoring system, was published to predict malignant potential (**Table 4**).[45] A retrospective analysis of 100 PCCs found that tumors with a PASS less than 4 were always clinically benign, whereas tumors with a PASS of 4 or more had the potential to become metastatic. Unfortunately, given high interobserver and intraobserver variability,[46] most centers do not use the PASS.

A second pathologic score was developed called the GAPP (Grading system for Adrenal Pheochromocytoma and Paraganglioma), which includes not only histologic features but also biochemical secretion and Ki67 index (see **Table 4**).[47] The scoring system more closely resembles that for gastroenteropancreatic neuroendocrine tumors by classifying tumors as well differentiated (score: 0–2), moderately differentiated (score: 3–6), and poorly differentiated (score: 7–10). In a cohort of 163 PCCs/PGLs, the GAPP distinguished between malignant and benign PCCs/PGLs with a

Table 4
Comparison of features in the PASS and GAPP pathologic scoring systems for predicting malignancy in PCC/PGL

PASS Features (Points)	GAPP Features (Points)
Histologic pattern • Large nests or diffuse growth (2)	Histologic pattern • Zellballen (0) • Large or irregular nests (1) • Pseudorosettes (1)
Cellularity • High (2)	Cellularity • Low <150 cells/U (0) • Moderate 15–200 cells/U (1) • High >250 cells/U (2)
Necrosis • Present (2)	Necrosis • Absent (1) • Present (2)
Invasion • Vascular invasion (1) • Capsular invasion (1)	Invasion (vascular or capsular) • Absent (0) • Present (1)
Mitosis • Mitotic figures (more than 3/10 high-powered fields) (2) • Atypical mitoses (2)	Ki67 proliferation index • <1% (0) • 1%–3% (1) • >3% (2)
Other features • Extension to adipose tissue (2) • Cell spindling (2) • Cellular monotony (2) • Nuclear pleomorphism (1) • Nuclear hyperchromasia (1)	Catecholamine type • Epinephrine elevated with or without norepinephrine (0) • Norepinephrine and/or dopamine but without epinephrine (1) • Nonsecreting (0)
Maximum Score = 20	Maximum Score = 10

Abbreviations: GAPP, Grading system for Adrenal Pheochromocytoma and Paraganglioma; PASS, Pheochromocytoma of the Adrenal Gland Scaled Score; PCC, pheochromocytoma; PGL, paraganglioma.

Data from Thompson LD. Pheochromocytoma of the Adrenal gland Scaled Score (PASS) to separate benign from malignant neoplasms: a clinicopathologic and immunophenotypic study of 100 cases. Am J Surg Pathol 2002;26:551–66; and Kimura N, Takayanagi R, Takizawa N, et al. Pathological grading for predicting metastasis in phaeochromocytoma and paraganglioma. Endocr Relat Cancer 2014;21:405–14.

mean score of 5.33 ± 0.43 and 2.08 ± 0.17, respectively.[47] The GAPP may be useful to predict malignancy, but it must be validated by independent investigators before it can be implemented into clinical care.

Treatments for Metastatic Pheochromocytomas and Paragangliomas

Unless full surgical resection is possible, metastatic disease cannot be cured; however, treatments with chemotherapy, ^{131}I-MIBG, and/or radiation can offer disease control. Given the often indolent nature of disease, therapies usually are reserved for patients with clear progression or severe symptoms. There are no studies to direct the timing or order of treatments. Alpha-blockade is required during any treatment to prevent hypertensive crisis from catecholamine release during tumor cell lysis.

Chemotherapy

Cyclophosphamide, vincristine, and dacarbazine (CVD) chemotherapy is the standard regimen for treating metastatic PCC/PGL despite no prospective clinical trials. A systematic review and meta-analysis was done to evaluate the effects of CVD chemotherapy in patients with metastatic PCC/PGL.[48] Four studies met inclusion criteria for a combined total of 50 patients. Results showed a complete or partial tumor response rate in 4% and 37% of patients, respectively, and a complete or partial biochemical response rate of 14% and 40% of patients, respectively. Of note, 14% of patients had stable disease. Tumor responses usually occurred after 2 to 4 cycles of CVD therapy, and the median duration of response for the 2 studies that reported it was 20 months and 40 months. The most common toxicities were myelosuppression, peripheral neuropathy and gastrointestinal toxicity, which were sometimes severe but usually transient.[48]

One group of investigators evaluated the response to temozolomide in patients with metastatic PCC/PGL.[49] Tumors with epigenetic silencing by methylation of the *MGMT (O(6)-methylguanine-DNA methyltransferase)* promoter lack the enzyme needed to repair DNA alkylating damage caused by temozolomide, and, hence, are more sensitive to temozolomide-based therapies. Therefore, the investigators hypothesized that *SDHB*-associated PCCs/PGLs, which have global hypermethylation,[3] may respond better to treatment with temozolomide. They replaced dacarbazine in the CVD regimen with temozolomide (CTD chemotherapy) and reported retrospective data for 15 patients with metastatic PCC/PGL, 10 of whom had *SDHB* mutations. Median progression-free survival was longer in *SDHB* mutation carriers (19.7 months) compared with non-mutation carriers (2.9 months) ($P = .007$).[49] MGMT expression was measured in only 10 of 15 samples but was deficient in 5 *SDHB*-associated tumors, 4 of which had response to treatment.[49] This study was very small and not all patients had sufficient material to correlate MGMT expression with outcomes; however, it is one of the first in PCC/PGL to link genomic data with treatment regimens for personalized care. Future prospective studies need to be done to confirm and support these findings.

[123]I-Metaiodobenzylguanidine

Sixty percent of PCCs/PGLs are MIBG avid, and therefore, are susceptible to systemic ^{131}I-MIBG therapy.[50] MIBG is transported into cells by the norepinephrine transporter and causes cell death by emitting ionizing radiation from the decaying ^{131}I radionuclide. A systematic review and meta-analysis was done to examine the effect of ^{131}I-MIBG treatment on tumor volume in patients with metastatic PCC/PGL.[51] Seven studies met the inclusion criteria for a combined total of 243 patients of varying ages who may or may not have had previous therapies and received ^{131}I-MIBG through numerous protocols and dose regimens. The results showed a complete or partial tumor response in 3% and 27% of patients, respectively, and a complete or partial hormonal response in 11% and 40% of patients, respectively. Of note, 52% of patients had stable disease,[51] but given the often indolent nature of metastatic PCC/PGL, it is unclear if this is due to treatment effects or the natural history of disease. Two studies within the cohort reported mean progression-free survival times of 23.1 and 28.5 months. Hematologic toxicity with severe grade 3 to 4 neutropenia and thrombocytopenia were the most commonly reported side effects in 87% and 83% of patients, respectively.[51] Since the meta-analysis was done, a multicenter cohort of 48 patients with metastatic PCC/PGL was reported and showed similar results.[52] More work is being done to understand the best dosing regimen, to create different formulations of MIBG with higher purity and specificity, and to use MIBG in combination with chemotherapy or radiation.

In addition to standard radiation precautions and myelosuppression associated with all systemic radiation treatments, there are other important considerations with the use of ^{131}I-MIBG. Free iodine from the treatment will accumulate in the thyroid gland; therefore, patients require potassium iodide before and after treatment to prevent a thyroiditis and subsequent hypothyroidism. Thyroid stimulating hormone (TSH) levels should be monitored periodically before and after treatment. Despite appropriate blockade, hypothyroidism can occur in 11% to 32% of patients.[53] ^{131}I-MIBG should be avoided in patients with renal failure because it is excreted through the kidney,[54] although of note, the meta-analysis did not report renal toxicity.[51] Many medications interfere with MIBG uptake, but patients can remain on alpha-blockade, which is particularly important in this disease.[54]

Targeted Therapies

Several small studies have looked at targeted therapies for metastatic PCC/PGL. Results using the mammalian target of rapamycin (mTOR) inhibitor everolimus have been disappointing in this disease.[55] Sunitinib, a receptor tyrosine kinase inhibitor, was evaluated in a retrospective report of 17 patients with metastatic PCC/PGL. There was a partial response (n = 3) or stable disease (n = 4) in 47% of patients.[56] The median progression-free survival was only 4.1 months. Grade 4 hypertension was the most significant adverse event. There are ongoing prospective clinical trials in Europe and the United States with various tyrosine kinase inhibitors, which will provide better information on the efficacy and safety of these targeted therapies.

External Beam Radiotherapy

External beam radiotherapy (EBRT) in the management of metastatic PCC/PGL has been controversial. Malignant PCCs/PGLs were believed to be resistant to radiation, but recent work suggests that EBRT can affect long-term local control in most cases. The largest retrospective cohort examined EBRT in 24 patients with metastatic PCC/PGL with a 3-dimensional conformal EBRT to a mean dose of 31.8 Gy or fractionated stereotactic radiosurgery to 21.9 Gy.[57] Symptomatic control or stable disease by imaging was seen in 81% and 87% of the lesions, respectively. The next largest reported series was a retrospective review of 17 patients with non–head and neck malignant PCC/PGL treated with various EBRT regimens to a median dose of 40 Gy.[58] Seventy-six percent of patients had local control (attributable to disease stabilization and/or symptom control). EBRT appears to offer symptomatic control in patients with limited burden of metastases. Because metastatic PCC/PGL can be an indolent disease, prospective studies are needed to determine if EBRT truly contributes to disease stability in terms of tumor growth.

SUMMARY

PCCs/PGLs are rare but unique tumors. Up to 40% of patients have germline mutations in known susceptibility genes. Knowledge of the germline mutation has implications in the treatment, screening, and surveillance of patients and their family members; therefore, all patients with PCC/PGL should be referred for clinical genetic testing. Surgery is the mainstay of treatment, and patients require appropriate perioperative blockade. For patients with metastatic PCC/PGL, treatment options can provide symptomatic relief but only limited control of disease progression. Hopefully, the recent expansion of knowledge about both germline and somatic genetics will lead to better predictors of malignant potential and better targets for therapy.

REFERENCES

1. DeLellis RA, Lloyd RV, Heitz PU, et al. World Health Organization Classification of Tumours. Pathology and genetics of tumours of endocrine organs. Lyon (France): IARC Press; 2004.
2. Kasperlik-Zaluska AA, Roslonowska E, Slowinska-Srzednicka J, et al. 1,111 patients with adrenal incidentalomas observed at a single endocrinological center: incidence of chromaffin tumors. Ann N Y Acad Sci 2006;1073:38–46.
3. Favier J, Amar L, Gimenez-Roqueplo AP. Paraganglioma and phaeochromocytoma: from genetics to personalized medicine. Nat Rev Endocrinol 2015;11: 101–11.
4. Fishbein L, Merrill S, Fraker DL, et al. Inherited mutations in pheochromocytoma and paraganglioma: why all patients should be offered genetic testing. Ann Surg Oncol 2013;20:1444–50.
5. Mannelli M, Castellano M, Schiavi F, et al. Clinically guided genetic screening in a large cohort of Italian patients with pheochromocytomas and/or functional or nonfunctional paragangliomas. J Clin Endocrinol Metab 2009;94:1541–7.
6. Williams VC, Lucas J, Babcock MA, et al. Neurofibromatosis type 1 revisited. Pediatrics 2009;123:124–33.
7. Wells SA Jr, Asa SL, Dralle H, et al. Revised American Thyroid Association guidelines for the management of medullary thyroid carcinoma: the American Thyroid Association Guidelines Task Force on medullary thyroid carcinoma. Thyroid 2015; 25(6):567–610.
8. Maher ER, Neumann HP, Richard S. von Hippel-Lindau disease: a clinical and scientific review. Eur J Hum Genet 2011;19:617–23.
9. Maher ER, Webster AR, Richards FM, et al. Phenotypic expression in von Hippel-Lindau disease: correlations with germline VHL gene mutations. J Med Genet 1996;33:328–32.
10. Zbar B, Kishida T, Chen F, et al. Germline mutations in the Von Hippel-Lindau disease (VHL) gene in families from North America, Europe, and Japan. Hum Mutat 1996;8:348–57.
11. Ong KR, Woodward ER, Killick P, et al. Genotype-phenotype correlations in von Hippel-Lindau disease. Hum Mutat 2007;28:143–9.
12. Pasini B, Stratakis CA. SDH mutations in tumorigenesis and inherited endocrine tumours: lesson from the phaeochromocytoma-paraganglioma syndromes. J Intern Med 2009;266:19–42.
13. van Hulsteijn LT, Dekkers OM, Hes FJ, et al. Risk of malignant paraganglioma in SDHB-mutation and SDHD-mutation carriers: a systematic review and meta-analysis. J Med Genet 2012;49:768–76.

14. Bayley JP, Oldenburg RA, Nuk J, et al. Paraganglioma and pheochromocytoma upon maternal transmission of SDHD mutations. BMC Med Genet 2014;15:111.
15. Yeap PM, Tobias ES, Mavraki E, et al. Molecular analysis of pheochromocytoma after maternal transmission of SDHD mutation elucidates mechanism of parent-of-origin effect. J Clin Endocrinol Metab 2011;96:E2009–13.
16. Else T, Marvin ML, Everett JN, et al. The clinical phenotype of SDHC-associated hereditary paraganglioma syndrome (PGL3). J Clin Endocrinol Metab 2014;99: E1482–6.
17. Burnichon N, Briere JJ, Libe R, et al. SDHA is a tumor suppressor gene causing paraganglioma. Hum Mol Genet 2010;19:3011–20.
18. Kunst HP, Rutten MH, de Monnink JP, et al. SDHAF2 (PGL2-SDH5) and hereditary head and neck paraganglioma. Clin Cancer Res 2011;17:247–54.
19. Evenepoel L, Papathomas TG, Krol N, et al. Toward an improved definition of the genetic and tumor spectrum associated with SDH germ-line mutations. Genet Med 2015;17(8):610–20.
20. Comino-Mendez I, Gracia-Aznarez FJ, Schiavi F, et al. Exome sequencing identifies MAX mutations as a cause of hereditary pheochromocytoma. Nat Genet 2011;43:663–7.
21. Jiang S, Dahia PL. Minireview: the busy road to pheochromocytomas and paragangliomas has a new member, TMEM127. Endocrinology 2011;152:2133–40.
22. Buffet A, Smati S, Mansuy L, et al. Mosaicism in HIF2A-related polycythemia-paraganglioma syndrome. J Clin Endocrinol Metab 2014;99:E369–73.
23. Comino-Mendez I, de Cubas AA, Bernal C, et al. Tumoral EPAS1 (HIF2A) mutations explain sporadic pheochromocytoma and paraganglioma in the absence of erythrocytosis. Hum Mol Genet 2013;22:2169–76.
24. Zhuang Z, Yang C, Lorenzo F, et al. Somatic HIF2A gain-of-function mutations in paraganglioma with polycythemia. N Engl J Med 2012;367:922–30.
25. Cascon A, Comino-Mendez I, Curras-Freixes M, et al. Whole-exome sequencing identifies MDH2 as a new familial paraganglioma gene. J Natl Cancer Inst 2015;107 [pii:djv053].
26. Castro-Vega LJ, Buffet A, De Cubas AA, et al. Germline mutations in FH confer predisposition to malignant pheochromocytomas and paragangliomas. Hum Mol Genet 2014;23:2440–6.
27. Clark GR, Sciacovelli M, Gaude E, et al. Germline FH mutations presenting with pheochromocytoma. J Clin Endocrinol Metab 2014;99:E2046–50.
28. Burnichon N, Vescovo L, Amar L, et al. Integrative genomic analysis reveals somatic mutations in pheochromocytoma and paraganglioma. Hum Mol Genet 2011;20(20):3974–85.
29. Welander J, Larsson C, Backdahl M, et al. Integrative genomics reveals frequent somatic NF1 mutations in sporadic pheochromocytomas. Hum Mol Genet 2012; 21:5406–16.
30. Oudijk L, de Krijger RR, Rapa I, et al. H-RAS mutations are restricted to sporadic pheochromocytomas lacking specific clinical or pathological features: data from a multi-institutional series. J Clin Endocrinol Metab 2014;99:E1376–80.
31. Fishbein L, Khare S, Wubbenhorst B, et al. Whole-exome sequencing identifies somatic ATRX mutations in pheochromocytomas and paragangliomas. Nat Commun 2015;6:6140.
32. Lenders JW, Duh QY, Eisenhofer G, et al. Pheochromocytoma and paraganglioma: an Endocrine Society clinical practice guideline. J Clin Endocrinol Metab 2014;99:1915–42.

33. Eisenhofer G, Lenders JW, Siegert G, et al. Plasma methoxytyramine: a novel biomarker of metastatic pheochromocytoma and paraganglioma in relation to established risk factors of tumour size, location and SDHB mutation status. Eur J Cancer 2012;48:1739–49.
34. Eisenhofer G, Lenders JW, Timmers H, et al. Measurements of plasma methoxytyramine, normetanephrine, and metanephrine as discriminators of different hereditary forms of pheochromocytoma. Clin Chem 2011;57:411–20.
35. Cohen DL, Fraker D, Townsend RR. Lack of symptoms in patients with histologic evidence of pheochromocytoma: a diagnostic challenge. Ann N Y Acad Sci 2006; 1073:47–51.
36. Neary NM, King KS, Pacak K. Drugs and pheochromocytoma–don't be fooled by every elevated metanephrine. N Engl J Med 2011;364:2268–70.
37. Mozley PD, Kim CK, Mohsin J, et al. The efficacy of iodine-123-MIBG as a screening test for pheochromocytoma. J Nucl Med 1994;35:1138–44.
38. Bruynzeel H, Feelders RA, Groenland TH, et al. Risk factors for hemodynamic instability during surgery for pheochromocytoma. J Clin Endocrinol Metab 2010;95:678–85.
39. Agarwal G, Sadacharan D, Aggarwal V, et al. Surgical management of organ-contained unilateral pheochromocytoma: comparative outcomes of laparoscopic and conventional open surgical procedures in a large single-institution series. Langenbecks Arch Surg 2012;397:1109–16.
40. Conzo G, Musella M, Corcione F, et al. Role of preoperative adrenergic blockade with doxazosin on hemodynamic control during the surgical treatment of pheochromocytoma: a retrospective study of 48 cases. Am Surg 2013;79: 1196–202.
41. Prys-Roberts C, Farndon JR. Efficacy and safety of doxazosin for perioperative management of patients with pheochromocytoma. World J Surg 2002;26: 1037–42.
42. Weingarten TN, Cata JP, O'Hara JF, et al. Comparison of two preoperative medical management strategies for laparoscopic resection of pheochromocytoma. Urology 2010;76:508.e6–11.
43. Kocak S, Aydintug S, Canakci N. Alpha blockade in preoperative preparation of patients with pheochromocytomas. Int Surg 2002;87:191–4.
44. Ayala-Ramirez M, Feng L, Johnson MM, et al. Clinical risk factors for malignancy and overall survival in patients with pheochromocytomas and sympathetic paragangliomas: primary tumor size and primary tumor location as prognostic indicators. J Clin Endocrinol Metab 2011;96:717–25.
45. Thompson LD. Pheochromocytoma of the Adrenal gland Scaled Score (PASS) to separate benign from malignant neoplasms: a clinicopathologic and immunophenotypic study of 100 cases. Am J Surg Pathol 2002;26:551–66.
46. Wu D, Tischler AS, Lloyd RV, et al. Observer variation in the application of the Pheochromocytoma of the Adrenal Gland Scaled Score. Am J Surg Pathol 2009;33:599–608.
47. Kimura N, Takayanagi R, Takizawa N, et al. Pathological grading for predicting metastasis in phaeochromocytoma and paraganglioma. Endocr Relat Cancer 2014;21:405–14.
48. Niemeijer ND, Alblas G, van Hulsteijn LT, et al. Chemotherapy with cyclophosphamide, vincristine and dacarbazine for malignant paraganglioma and pheochromocytoma: systematic review and meta-analysis. Clin Endocrinol (Oxf) 2014; 81:642–51.

49. Hadoux J, Favier J, Scoazec JY, et al. SDHB mutations are associated with response to temozolomide in patients with metastatic pheochromocytoma or paraganglioma. Int J Cancer 2014;135:2711–20.

50. Timmers HJ, Chen CC, Carrasquillo JA, et al. Comparison of 18F-fluoro-L-DOPA, 18F-fluoro-deoxyglucose, and 18F-fluorodopamine PET and 123I-MIBG scintigraphy in the localization of pheochromocytoma and paraganglioma. J Clin Endocrinol Metab 2009;94:4757–67.

51. van Hulsteijn LT, Niemeijer ND, Dekkers OM, et al. (131)I-MIBG therapy for malignant paraganglioma and phaeochromocytoma: systematic review and meta-analysis. Clin Endocrinol (Oxf) 2014;80:487–501.

52. Yoshinaga K, Oriuchi N, Wakabayashi H, et al. Effects and safety of 131I-metaiodobenzylguanidine (MIBG) radiotherapy in malignant neuroendocrine tumors: results from a multicenter observational registry. Endocr J 2014;61:1171–80.

53. Carrasquillo JA, Pandit-Taskar N, Chen CC. Radionuclide therapy of adrenal tumors. J Surg Oncol 2012;106:632–42.

54. Giammarile F, Chiti A, Lassmann M, et al. EANM procedure guidelines for 131I-meta-iodobenzylguanidine (131I-mIBG) therapy. Eur J Nucl Med Mol Imaging 2008;35:1039–47.

55. Oh DY, Kim TW, Park YS, et al. Phase 2 study of everolimus monotherapy in patients with nonfunctioning neuroendocrine tumors or pheochromocytomas/paragangliomas. Cancer 2012;118:6162–70.

56. Ayala-Ramirez M, Chougnet CN, Habra MA, et al. Treatment with sunitinib for patients with progressive metastatic pheochromocytomas and sympathetic paragangliomas. J Clin Endocrinol Metab 2012;97:4040–50.

57. Vogel J, Atanacio AS, Prodanov T, et al. External beam radiation therapy in treatment of malignant pheochromocytoma and paraganglioma. Front Oncol 2014;4:166.

58. Fishbein L, Bonner L, Torigian DA, et al. External beam radiation therapy (EBRT) for patients with malignant pheochromocytoma and non-head and -neck paraganglioma: combination with 131I-MIBG. Horm Metab Res 2012;44:405–10.

Poorly Differentiated Neuroendocrine Tumors

Jennifer R. Eads, MD

KEYWORDS

- Poorly differentiated • High-grade • G3 • Neuroendocrine tumor
- Neuroendocrine carcinoma

KEY POINTS

- Poorly differentiated neuroendocrine carcinomas (NECs) are a rare disease entity that is not well understood and for which there is a poor prognosis.
- Clinical trial data to guide therapy are extremely limited and treatment recommendations have been based on data derived from small cell lung cancer.
- Pathologic and clinical data are emerging that suggest that poorly differentiated NECs are likely a distinct disease that differs from small cell lung cancer.
- Patients with localized disease are typically treated with surgery followed by chemotherapy with or without radiation therapy.
- Patients with advanced disease are treated with a platinum and etoposide chemotherapeutic regimen, although a temozolomide-based regimen may be more appropriate for some patients.

INTRODUCTION

Poorly differentiated neuroendocrine carcinomas (NECs) are rare cancers with likely fewer than 1000 cases diagnosed annually based on best estimates.[1,2] Owing to its rarity, it has been greatly understudied and very little is known about the tumor biology, molecular characteristics, and optimal treatment strategy for patients with this disease. Historically, poorly differentiated NECs have been considered as nearly equivalent to small cell lung cancer given the histologic similarities observed between the 2 diseases. As such, many of the treatment recommendations for poorly differentiated NECs are based on the small cell lung cancer literature and there are sparse clinical data specific to poorly differentiated NECs available to guide therapy. During the

Disclosures: Research support—Novartis; Consulting—Portola
Division of Hematology and Oncology, University Hospitals Seidman Cancer Center, Case Western Reserve University, Case Comprehensive Cancer, 11100 Euclid Avenue, Lakeside 1200, Cleveland, OH 44106, USA
E-mail address: jennifer.eads@uhhospitals.org

Hematol Oncol Clin N Am 30 (2016) 151–162
http://dx.doi.org/10.1016/j.hoc.2015.09.007
0889-8588/16/$ – see front matter

past decade, both pathologic and clinical data have started to emerge suggesting that poorly differentiated NECs are likely distinct from small cell lung cancer. In this article, we focus on poorly differentiated NECs of the gastrointestinal tract and review the pathologic and clinical nuances associated with this rare disease as well as both historical and developing treatment strategies used in the management of poorly differentiated NECs.

EPIDEMIOLOGY AND PROGNOSIS

Neuroendocrine tumors are rare, with approximately 8000 new cases diagnosed annually.[2] The incidence of these tumors seems to be increasing, with most recent reports showing an annual incidence of 5.25 to 5.86 per 100,000 population.[1,3] Tumors of the poorly differentiated subtype most often arise within the gastrointestinal tract with the most common primary sites being the esophagus (30%–53%) and the large bowel (20%–39%) with the stomach, gallbladder, pancreas, small bowel, ampulla of Vater, bile ducts, and liver also being affected primary sites of disease.[4,5] Of all gastrointestinal neuroendocrine tumors, poorly differentiated NECs account for only approximately 11% of cases.[1] More than one-half of patients (57%–66%) present with metastatic disease at the time of their diagnosis[4,6,7] and without treatment, typically succumb to their disease within weeks.[8,9] Unfortunately, even with treatment, the median overall survival for patients with metastatic disease is only 5 months,[7] although patients with non–small cell histology are reported to have improved 5-year survival rates as compared with patients with small cell histology (32% vs 6%).[10] Patients with localized disease have a better prognosis, but most often their disease is still fatal. Administration of some form of treatment including surgery, chemotherapy and/or radiation therapy does prolong survival but 2-year survival is 23%[11] and reports of median overall survival range from 8 to 20 months.[11–13]

PATIENT PRESENTATION AND DIAGNOSIS
Clinical Presentation

Unlike patients with well-differentiated neuroendocrine tumors who typically present with a relatively indolent disease process and who have a good chance of cure with full surgical resection, patients with poorly differentiated NECs may seem to be acutely ill and have a more rapidly evolving disease course. Tumor markers (such as serum chromogranin A and urinary 5-hydroxyindoleacetic acid levels) are typically not helpful[7] and there are no identified tumor markers that are useful in either diagnosing or following poorly differentiated NECs. As with any malignancy, a tissue biopsy is critical for identifying that the tumor is of neuroendocrine origin and then for further classifying it as well or poorly differentiated.

Pathology

The most recent classification of neuroendocrine tumors by the World Health Organization characterizes poorly differentiated NECs as grade 3 (G3) tumors[14] (**Table 1**).

The terminology associated with this disease is complicated and these tumors may be reported as many synonymous entities, including poorly differentiated carcinomas, high-grade neuroendocrine tumors, high-grade NECs, G3 neuroendocrine tumors, G3 NECs, and well-differentiated neuroendocrine tumors with a high proliferative rate. A G3 NEC is defined as having a Ki-67 proliferative index of greater than 20% or a mitotic rate of greater than 20 per 10 high-powered fields.[14] Histologically these tumors are categorized as small cell, large cell, or mixed NECs, where small cell carcinomas are thought to be distinctive pathologically from the large cell and mixed NEC

Table 1
WHO histologic classification of neuroendocrine tumors

Differentiation	Grade	Mitotic Count (per 10 hpf)	Ki-67 Proliferative Index	WHO Classification
Well differentiated	1	<2	≤2	Neuroendocrine tumor, grade 1
Moderately differentiated	2	2–20	3–20	Neuroendocrine tumor, grade 2
Poorly differentiated	3	>20	>20	Neuroendocrine carcinoma, grade 3 (small cell or large cell)

Abbreviations: hpf, high-power field; WHO, World Health Organization.
From Bosman FT, Carneiro F, Hruban RH, et al. WHO classification of tumors of the digestive system. 4th edition. Geneva (Switzerland): WHO Press; 2010; with permission.

subtypes.[15,16] In an assessment of Ki-67 in lung primaries, the Ki-67 exhibited by tumors with small cell histology is significantly higher than among tumors with large cell histology.[17] Two retrospective studies have demonstrated disease heterogeneity among the G3 subgroup from a clinical perspective where patients having tumors with a Ki-67 of less than 60% and less than 55% exhibited a lack of response to treatment with standard front-line therapy for poorly differentiated NECs and instead demonstrated responses to chemotherapeutic regimens more commonly active in well-differentiated tumors.[16,18] The broad spectrum of Ki-67 values included within the G3 category (>20%–100%), coupled with observed pathologic differences and clinical data suggesting that subgroups within the G3 population may respond differently to different treatment regimens raises the question as to whether this group of tumors is more heterogeneous than is accounted for in the current classification system and if a modification of this system is indicated.

Staging

Management of poorly differentiated NECs is guided by small cell lung cancer recommendations; as such, G3 NECs may be staged as either limited stage versus extensive stage (**Table 2**) or the TNM staging system may be used.[19,20]

Table 2
Staging of G3 neuroendocrine carcinomas

Stage	Definition
Limited stage	AJCC (7th edition) stage I-III (T any, N any, M0) that can be safely treated with definitive radiation doses. Excludes T3-4 owing to multiple lung nodules that are too extensive or have tumor/nodal volume that is, too large to be encompassed in a tolerable radiation plan.
Extensive stage	AJCC (7th edition) stage IV (T any, N any, M 1a/b), or T3-4 owing to multiple lung nodules that are too extensive or have tumor/nodal volume that is, too large to be encompassed in a tolerable radiation plan.

Abbreviation: AJCC, American Joint Committee on Cancer.
Data from Edge SB, Byrd DR, Compton CC, et al, editors. AJCC Cancer staging manual. 7th edition. New York: Springer; 2009. p. 1–748; and National comprehensive cancer network (NCCN) Clinical practice guidelines in oncology, neuroendocrine tumors version 1.2015. 2015. Available at: http://www.nccn.org. Accessed May 20, 2015.

Imaging

Aside from tissue histology, the most useful diagnostic tools for neuroendocrine tumors may be in the form of imaging. Routine staging scans at diagnosis include a computed tomography scan of the chest, abdomen, and pelvis and are additionally used for following tumor size to assess for response to therapy. The presence of brain metastases in small cell lung cancer is common, thereby deeming imaging of the central nervous system standard. However, brain metastases in high-grade NECs are not as common and therefore no standard imaging of the central nervous system is recommended.[21] Nuclear imaging with octreotide scans and ^{18}F-fluorodeoxyglucose (FDG)-PET scans are very useful in the diagnosis of neuroendocrine tumors.[22,23] These functional imaging studies provide information pertaining to tumor activity. Octreotide scans are more often positive in tumors with high levels of somatostatin receptor expression (most commonly seen in well-differentiated tumors as opposed to low expression in poorly differentiated NECs),[24] whereas FDG-PET scans are most often positive for tumors with underlying high metabolic activity, as is seen more often in poorly differentiated tumors.[25] Additionally, it has been demonstrated that a significant correlation exists between FDG-PET positivity and both Ki-67 and World Health Organization tumor grade.[26] Particularly when the Ki-67 is greater than 15%, the sensitivity of FDG-PET is greater than 92%.[27] As such, these imaging modalities may be useful in distinguishing low- versus high-grade tumors.

MANAGEMENT OF LOCALIZED DISEASE

The role for surgical resection, chemotherapy, and radiation therapy in the management of localized disease is controversial, because many patients have a rapid time to recurrence despite undergoing what would be considered a curative cancer operation. Most recurrences occur at distant sites suggesting that occult metastatic disease is likely present even at the time of diagnosis.[10,28] To date, no prospective trial assessing the optimal approach to the management of localized disease has been conducted. As a result, it is unclear what contribution each of these treatment modalities makes to patient outcomes.

Surgical Resection

Small case series and retrospective studies have demonstrated a role for surgery in patients with localized poorly differentiated gastrointestinal NECs. In rare cases, surgical resection has resulted in long-term survival, with patients showing no evidence of disease recurrence for as long as 5 to 7 years after surgery.[29,30] In a retrospective study including 14 evaluable patients with small cell carcinoma in various locations throughout the gastrointestinal tract and who had undergone surgical resection for limited disease, 7 (50%) had a period of prolonged disease control. In some cases, chemotherapy and/or radiation therapy was also administered.[4] In a larger retrospective review of 126 patients with high-grade NECs of the colon and rectum, no survival advantage was conferred with resection of either a localized or a metastatic tumor.[28] In a large, retrospective evaluation of 1367 patients with colorectal NEC from the Survey of Epidemiology and End Results database, patients with non–small cell NECs demonstrated an improved median overall survival of 21 months if treated with surgery versus only 6 months without surgery (P<.0001). Patients with small cell histology did not demonstrate a survival benefit (median overall survival of 18 months with surgery vs 14 months without surgery; P = .95).[12] Data regarding a multimodal approach in these patients, such as receipt of chemotherapy and/or radiation therapy, was not available.

Neoadjuvant and Adjuvant Chemotherapy

The administration of chemotherapy seems to improve outcomes when combined with surgery. In a review of 199 patients with small cell carcinoma of the esophagus, 93 of whom (46.7%) had limited stage disease, administration of systemic chemotherapy in addition to surgery resulted in a significantly improved overall survival of 20 months with combination therapy versus 5 months with surgery alone.[11] Most often, 4 to 6 cycles of adjuvant chemotherapy with either cisplatin or carboplatin and etoposide are administered in combination with radiation therapy[31–33] and this treatment strategy has been endorsed by both the National Comprehensive Cancer Network and the North American Neuroendocrine Tumor Society.[20,34,35]

Radiation Therapy

The use of radiation therapy is limited typically to localized or unresectable disease. There are no clinical trials specifically addressing the role of radiation in localized poorly differentiated NECs, but chemoradiation therapy is known to be beneficial in patients with limited stage small cell lung cancer. Ideally, radiation is administered concurrently with systemic platinum and etoposide chemotherapy because this combination has demonstrated a superior survival advantage as compared with chemotherapy followed by radiation, albeit with greater toxicity. Survival outcomes in a phase III study of 231 patients with limited stage small cell lung cancer showed a median overall survival of 19.7 months with sequential administration versus 27.2 months with concurrent administration.[36] In cases of localized disease where patients have either not undergone surgical resection or have had surgery but then developed a localized disease recurrence, either radiation alone or chemoradiation has demonstrated long-term survival outcomes of up to greater than 5 years in some cases.[13,37–39]

MANAGEMENT OF ADVANCED DISEASE
First-Line Chemotherapeutic Options

Very limited clinical trial data are available regarding front-line therapy for patients with poorly differentiated NECs, particularly as defined by the current classification system. Similar to localized disease, owing to the long-standing association of poorly differentiated NECs with small cell lung cancer, current treatment recommendations are extrapolated from the small cell lung cancer literature, which is reflected as well in the National Comprehensive Cancer Network guidelines.[20] Standard therapy involves administration of a platinum agent (cisplatin or carboplatin) and etoposide. Multiple randomized phase III clinical trials in small cell lung cancer patients have demonstrated excellent response rates of up to 85% (**Table 3**) as well as complete responses and cure in very limited instances. Other regimens, including cisplatin/irinotecan and carboplatin/gemcitabine have been compared with cisplatin/etoposide therapy.[41–44] Although an initial study of 154 patients demonstrated an improved overall survival benefit of 12.8 versus 9.4 months with the use of cisplatin and irinotecan, a larger follow-up study of 661 patients reported no difference in median overall survival (9.1 months with cisplatin/etoposide vs 9.9 months with cisplatin/irinotecan; $P = .71$). Based on these results, platinum/etoposide has remained the standard front-line treatment in small cell lung cancer and, hence, poorly differentiated NECs.

Among poorly differentiated NECs, primarily retrospective data are available with reports of median overall survival ranging from 5.8 to 19 months with cisplatin and etoposide treatment (see **Table 3**). The Moertel study, which reported a 19-month overall survival, used outdated response criteria as well as an outdated classification system where patients with "anaplastic" NECs were included.[45] In the only other reported

Table 3
Select front-line chemotherapy trials in small cell lung cancer and poorly differentiated neuroendocrine carcinomas

Drug/Study	No. of Patients	Response Rate	Median Overall Survival
Small cell lung cancer			
Ihde, 1994 (phase III)[40]			
Standard dose cisplatin/etoposide	71	72%–83%[a]	10.7 mo
High-dose cisplatin/etoposide	44	86% P = NS	11.4 mo P = .68
Noda, 2002 (phase III)[41]			
Cisplatin/etoposide	77	67.5%	9.4 mo
Cisplatin/irinotecan	77	84.4% P = .02	12.8 mo P = .002
Hanna, 2006 (phase III)[42]			
Cisplatin/etoposide	110	43.6%	10.2 mo
Cisplatin/irinotecan	221	48% P = NS	9.3 mo P = .74
Lara, 2009 (phase III)[43]			
Cisplatin/etoposide	327	60%	9.1 mo
Cisplatin/irinotecan	324	57% P = .56	9.9 mo P = .71
Lee, 2009 (phase III)[44]			
Cisplatin/etoposide	120	62.7%	8.1 mo
Carboplatin/gemcitabine	121	63.3% P = .92	8.0 mo P = .96
High-grade neuroendocrine carcinomas			
Moertel, 1991 (phase II)[45]			
Cisplatin/etoposide	18	67%	19 mo
Mitry, 1999 (retrospective)[46]			
Cisplatin/etoposide	41	42%	15 mo
Hainsworth, 2006 (phase II)[47]			
Paclitaxel/carboplatin/etoposide[b]	78	53%	14.5 mo
Iwasa, 2010 (retrospective)[48]			
Cisplatin/etoposide[c]	21	14%	5.8 mo
Sorbye 2012 (retrospective)[16]			
Cisplatin/etoposide	129	31%	12 mos
Carboplatin/etoposide	67	30%	11 mo
Carboplatin/etoposide/vincristine	28	44%	10 mo
Yamaguchi T, 2014 (retrospective)[49]			
Cisplatin/etoposide	46	28%	7.3 mo
Cisplatin/irinotecan	160	50%	13 mo P = .389
Okuma, 2014 (retrospective)[50]			
Cisplatin/irinotecan[d]	12	50%	12.6 mo

[a] Of the 71 patients in this arm, 25 were not randomized to this arm but rather placed in this arm owing to high concern for administration of high dose cisplatin/etoposide.
[b] Included primary sites outside of the gastrointestinal system.
[c] Primary tumor sites included poorly differentiated neuroendocrine carcinomas arising from the hepatobiliary tract and pancreas.
[d] Includes only high-grade neuroendocrine carcinomas of the esophagus.
Data from Refs.[16,40–50]

Table 4
Select second-line and beyond chemotherapy trials in small cell lung cancer and poorly differentiated neuroendocrine carcinomas

Drug/Study	No. Patients (S/R)[a]	Response Rate (S/R)	Median Overall Survival (S/R)
Small cell lung cancer			
Hoang, 2003 (phase II)[51]			
Gemcitabine	15/12	0%/0%	8.8/4.2 mo
Masters, 2003 (phase II)[52]			
Gemcitabine	26/20	16.7%/5.6%	7.3/6.9 mo
Ohyanagi, 2008 (phase II)[53]			
Gemcitabine/irinotecan	20/10	45%/20%	14.4/7.4 mo
Mori, 2006 (phase II)[54]			
Carboplatin/paclitaxel	18/11	83%/45%	7.9/5.3 mo
Dongiovanni, 2006 (phase II)[55]			
Gemcitabine/paclitaxel	21/10	29%/20%	8.2/2.4 wk
Schuette, 2005 (phase II)[56]			
Gemcitabine/irinotecan	20/15	17%	5.8 months
Pallis, 2009 (phase II)[57]			
Gemcitabine/irinotecan	38	23.7%	6.8 mo
Irinotecan	31	0% $P = .004$	4.6 mo $P = NS$
Rocha-Lima, 2007 (phase II)[58]			
Gemcitabine/irinotecan	35/36	31%/11%	7.1/3.5 mo
Evans, 1985 (phase II)[59]			
Cisplatin/etoposide	54	52%	6 mo
Yamamoto, 2006 (phase II)[60]			
Paclitaxel	11/10	27.3%/20%	5.8 mo
Ramalingam, 2010 (phase II)[61]			
Irinotecan/paclitaxel	28/14	25%/14%	7.6/5.5 mo
Pietanza, 2012 (phase II)[62]			
Temozolomide	48/16	23%/13%	6/5.6 mo
High-grade neuroendocrine carcinomas			
Bajetta, 2007 (phase II)[63]			
Capecitabine/oxaliplatin	13	23%	5 mo
Hadoux, 2015 (retrospective)[64]			
5-fluorouracil/oxaliplatin	20[b]	29%	9.9 mo
Olsen, 2012 (retrospective)[65]			
Temozolomide	28	0%	3.5 mo
Welin, 2011 (retrospective)[18]			
Temozolomide ± capecitabine ± bevacizumab	25	33%	22 mo
Hentic, 2012 (retrospective)[66]			
5-Fluorouracil/irinotecan	19	31%	18 mo

[a] (S/R) indicates sensitive/refractory, where patients with sensitive disease developed disease recurrence in greater than 3 months and refractory patients developed disease recurrence in less than 3 months after initial therapy. If only 1 value was provided, assessment was based on entire population.
[b] Only 12 patients were known to have gastrointestinal neuroendocrine carcinomas.
Data from Refs.[18,51–66]

phase II study, paclitaxel was added to carboplatin and etoposide.[47] Although the median overall survival of 14.5 months is on the higher ended of all reported ranges, this regimen had increased toxicity and included patients with primary lesions located outside of the gastrointestinal tract. Given the limitations of these prospective studies combined with otherwise only retrospective data, future prospective studies in this population are needed to gain a better understanding of the optimal front-line treatment for these patients.

Chemotherapeutic Options for Second-Line Therapy and Beyond

Clinical data for treatment in the second-line setting are also quite limited and are similarly extrapolated from small cell lung cancer studies. Multiple chemotherapeutic regimens have been evaluated in the second-line setting for small cell lung cancer with a smaller number of studies (primarily retrospective) available for poorly differentiated NECs (**Table 4**).

Based on results of the small cell lung cancer studies, there is no dominant regimen that is used standardly in the second-line treatment of poorly differentiated NEC. Emerging data do suggest, however, that a temozolomide-based regimen may be of greatest benefit, particularly in patients with a Ki-67 of less than 55% to 60%, although this has not been evaluated prospectively. In a retrospective study of 25 patients receiving temozolomide with or without capecitabine with or without bevacizumab, patients with a Ki-67 of less than 60%, features consistent with a well-differentiated neuroendocrine tumor (positive immunohistochemistry for chromogranin A, positive octreotide scans) and lack of a treatment response to platinum based therapy in the front-line setting had a better response to temozolomide-based therapy.[18] Response rate in this study was 33%, but the reported median overall survival of 22 months is the most impressive survival benefit reported for any study in either poorly differentiated NEC or small cell lung cancer. In a follow-up retrospective study of 305 patients with poorly differentiated NEC, patients with a Ki-67 of 20% to 54% showed a poorer response to platinum-based therapy as compared with patients in the higher Ki-67 range at 15% and 42%, respectively. Survival was improved in the low Ki-67 group, however, despite lack of response to front-line platinum-based therapy; the 30-month survival in the Ki-67 20% to 54% group versus the 55% to 100% group were 23% and 7%, respectively.[16]

SUMMARY

Poorly differentiated NECs of the gastrointestinal tract are rare tumors that have not been well studied and for which limited data are available to guide treatment. They are managed similarly to small cell lung cancer; however, recent pathologic and clinical data suggest that these tumors are a distinct disease entity and that even under the current classification system, the poorly differentiated NEC population is likely composed of a heterogeneous group of tumors. For patients with localized disease, surgical resection is reasonable, particularly for patients with non–small cell histology and in most cases, this should be followed by a course of adjuvant cisplatin/carboplatin and etoposide chemotherapy with or without radiation therapy. For advanced disease, front-line treatment with platinum and etoposide chemotherapy is the current treatment standard although patients with a Ki-67 in the lower range (<55%–60%) may be less responsive to this treatment and may benefit more from a temozolomide-based regimen. No clear regimen has emerged as the next best line of therapy upon disease progression. Given the paucity of data available in all clinical scenarios, further studies in both the localized and advanced disease settings are greatly needed.

REFERENCES

1. Yao JC, Hassan M, Phan A, et al. One hundred years after "carcinoid": epidemiology of and prognostic factors for neuroendocrine tumors in 35,825 cases in the United States. J Clin Oncol 2008;26:3063–72.
2. Available at: http://www.cancer.net/cancer-types/neuroendocrine-tumor/statistics. Accessed May 15, 2015.
3. Hallet J, How Lim Law C, Cukier M, et al. Exploring the rising incidence of neuroendocrine tumors: a population-based analysis of epidemiology, metastatic presentation and outcomes. Cancer 2015;121:589–97.
4. Brenner B, Shah MA, Gonen M, et al. Small-cell carcinoma of the gastrointestinal tract: a retrospective study of 64 cases. Br J Cancer 2004;90:1720–6.
5. Brenner B, Tang LH, Klimstra DS, et al. Small-cell carcinomas of the gastrointestinal tract: a review. J Clin Oncol 2004;22:2730–9.
6. Bernick PE, Klimstra DS, Shia J, et al. Neuroendocrine carcinomas of the colon and rectum. Dis Colon Rectum 2004;47:163–9.
7. Sorbye H, Strosberg J, Baudin E, et al. Gastroenteropancreatic high-grade neuroendocrine carcinoma. Cancer 2014;120:2814–23.
8. Redman BG, Pazdur R. Colonic small cell undifferentiated carcinoma: a distinct pathological diagnosis with therapeutic implications. Am J Gastroenterol 1987; 82:382–5.
9. Bunn PA Jr, Lichter A, Makuch RW, et al. Chemotherapy alone or chemotherapy with chest radiation therapy in limited stage small cell lung cancer: a prospective, randomized trial. Ann Intern Med 1987;106:655–62.
10. Korse CM, Taal BG, van Velthuysen ML, et al. Incidence and survival of neuroendocrine tumours in The Netherlands according to histological grade: experience of 2 decades of cancer registry. Eur J Cancer 2013;49:1975–83.
11. Casas F, Ferrer F, Farrus B, et al. Primary small cell carcinoma of the esophagus: a review of the literature with emphasis on therapy and prognosis. Cancer 1997; 80:1366–72.
12. Shafqat H, Ali S, Salhab M, et al. Survival of patients with neuroendocrine carcinoma of the colon and rectum: a population-based analysis. Dis Colon Rectum 2015;58:294–303.
13. Casas F, Farrus B, Daniels M, et al. Six-year followup of primary small cell carcinoma of the esophagus showing a complete response: a case report. Jpn J Clin Oncol 1996;26:180–4.
14. Bosman FT, Carneiro F, Hruban RH, et al. WHO classification of tumors of the digestive system. 4th edition. Geneva (Switzerland): WHO Press; 2010.
15. Shia J, Tang LH, Weiser MR, et al. Is nonsmall cell type high-grade neuroendocrine carcinoma of the tubular gastrointestinal tract a distinct disease entity? Am J Surg Pathol 2008;32:719–31.
16. Sorbye H, Welin S, Langer SW, et al. Predictive and prognostic factors for treatment and survival in 305 patients with advanced gastrointestinal neuroendocrine carcinoma (WHO G3): the NORDIC NEC study. Ann Oncol 2013;24: 152–60.
17. Skov BG, Holm B, Erreboe A, et al. ERCC1 and Ki67 in small cell lung carcinoma and other neuroendocrine tumors of the lung: distribution and impact on survival. J Thorac Oncol 2010;5:453–9.
18. Welin S, Sorbye H, Sebjornsen S, et al. Chemotherapy in poorly differentiated endocrine carcinoma after progression on first-line chemotherapy. Cancer 2011;117:4617–22.

19. Edge SB, Byrd DR, Compton CC, et al, editors. AJCC cancer staging manual. 7th edition. New York: Springer; 2009. p. 1–718.

20. National Comprehensive Cancer Network (NCCN). Clinical Practice Guidelines in Oncology, Neuroendocrine Tumors Version 1.2015. 2015. Available at: http://www.nccn.org. Accessed May 20, 2015.

21. Cicin I, Karagol H, Uzunoglu S, et al. Extrapulmonary small-cell carcinoma compared with small-cell lung carcinoma. A retrospective single-center study. Cancer 2007;110:1068–75.

22. Koopmans KP, Neels ON, Kema IP, et al. Molecular imaging in neuroendocrine tumours: molecular uptake mechanisms and clinical results. Crit Rev Oncol Hematol 2009;71:199–213.

23. Raderer M, Kurtaran A, Leimer M, et al. Value of peptide receptor scintigraphy using 123I-vasoactive intestinal peptide and 111In-DTPA-D-Phe1-octreotide in 194 carcinoid patients: Vienna University experience, 1993-1998. J Clin Oncol 2000;18:1331–6.

24. Ezziddin S, Logvinski T, Yong-Hing C, et al. Factors predicting tracer uptake in somatostatin receptor and MIBG scintigraphy of metastatic gastroenteropancreatic neuroendocrine tumors. J Nucl Med 2006;47:223–33.

25. Pasquali C, Rubello D, Sperti C, et al. Neuroendocrine tumor imaging: can ^{18}F-fluorodeoxyglucose positron emission tomography detect tumors with poor prognosis and aggressive behavior? World J Surg 1998;22:588–92.

26. Garin E, Le Jeune F, Devillers A, et al. Predictive value of ^{18}F-FDG PET and somatostatin receptor scintigraphy in patients with metastatic endocrine tumors. J Nucl Med 2009;50(6):858–64.

27. Binderup T, Knigge U, Loft A, et al. Functional imaging of neuroendocrine tumors: a head-to-head comparison of somatostatin receptor scintigraphy, 123I-MIGB scintigraphy, and 18F-FDG PET. J Nucl Med 2010;51:704–12.

28. Smith JD, Reidy DL, Goodman KA, et al. A retrospective review of 126 high-grade neuroendocrine carcinomas of the colon and rectum. Ann Surg Oncol 2014;21:2956–62.

29. Yachida S, Matsushita K, Usuki H, et al. Long-term survival after resection for small cell carcinoma of the esophagus. Ann Thorac Surg 2001;72:596–7.

30. Nishimaki T, Suzuki T, Nakagawa S, et al. Tumor spread and outcome of treatment in primary esophageal small cell carcinoma. J Surg Oncol 1997;64:130–4.

31. Turrisi AT 3rd, Kim K, Bulm R, et al. Twice-daily compared with once-daily thoracic radiotherapy in limited small-cell lung cancer treated concurrently with cisplatin and etoposide. N Engl J Med 1999;340:265–71.

32. Saito H, Takeda Y, Ichinose Y, et al. Phase II study of etoposide and cisplatin with concurrent twice-daily thoracic radiotherapy followed by irinotecan and cisplatin in patients with limited-disease small-cell lung cancer: West Japan Thoracic Oncology Group 9902. J Clin Oncol 2006;24:5247–52.

33. Skarlos DV, Samantas E, Briassoulis E, et al. Randomized comparison of early versus late hyperfractionated thoracic irradiation concurrently with chemotherapy in limited disease small-cell lung cancer: a randomized phase II study of the Hellenic Cooperative Oncology Group (HeCOG). Ann Oncol 2001;12:1231–8.

34. Kunz PL, Reidy-Lagunes D, Anthony LB, et al. Consensus guidelines for the management and treatment of neuroendocrine tumors. Pancreas 2013;42:557–77.

35. Strosberg JR, Coppola D, Klimstra DS, et al. The NANETS consensus guidelines for the diagnosis and management of poorly differentiated (high-grade) extrapulmonary neuroendocrine carcinomas. Pancreas 2010;39:799–800.

36. Takada M, Fukuoka M, Kawahara M, et al. Phase III study of concurrent versus sequential thoracic radiotherapy in combination with cisplatin and etoposide for limited-stage small-cell lung cancer: results of the Japan Clinical Oncology Group Study 9104. J Clin Oncol 2002;20:3054–60.
37. Ku GY, Minsky BD, Rusch VW, et al. Small-cell carcinoma of the esophagus and gastroesophageal junction: review of the Memorial Sloan-Kettering experience. Ann Oncol 2008;19:533–7.
38. Huncharek M, Muscat J. Small cell carcinoma of the esophagus: the Massachusetts General Hospital experience, 1978-1993. Chest 1995;13:179–81.
39. Medgyesy CD, Wolff RA, Putnam JB, et al. Small cell carcinoma of the esophagus: the University of Texas MD Anderson Cancer Center experience and literature review. Cancer 2000;88:262–7.
40. Ihde DC, Mulshine JL, Kramer BS, et al. Prospective randomized comparison of high-dose and standard-dose etoposide and cisplatin chemotherapy in patients with extensive-stage small-cell lung cancer. J Clin Oncol 1994;12:2022–34.
41. Noda K, Nishiwaki Y, Kawahara M, et al. Irinotecan plus cisplatin compared with etoposide plus cisplatin for extensive small-cell lung cancer. N Engl J Med 2002; 346:85–91.
42. Hanna N, Bunn PA Jr, Langer C, et al. Randomized phase III trial comparing irinotecan/cisplatin with etoposide/cisplatin in patients with previously untreated extensive-stage disease small-cell lung cancer. J Clin Oncol 2006; 24:2038–43.
43. Lara PN Jr, Natale R, Crowley J, et al. Phase III trial of irinotecan/cisplatin compared with etoposide/cisplatin in extensive-stage small-cell lung cancer: clinical and pharmacogenomics results from SWOG S0124. J Clin Oncol 2009;27: 2530–5.
44. Lee SM, James LE, Qian W, et al. Comparison of gemcitabine and carboplatin versus cisplatin and etoposide for patients with poor-prognosis small cell lung cancer. Thorax 2009;64:75–80.
45. Moertel CG, Kvols LK, O'Connell MJ, et al. Treatment of neuroendocrine carcinomas with combined etoposide and cisplatin, evidence of major therapeutic activity in the anaplastic variants of these neoplasms. Cancer 1991;68:227–32.
46. Mitry E, Baudin E, Ducreux M, et al. Treatment of poorly differentiated neuroendocrine tumours with etoposide and cisplatin. Br J Cancer 1999;81:1351–5.
47. Hainsworth JD, Spigel DR, Litchy S, et al. Phase II trial of paclitaxel, carboplatin and etoposide in advanced poorly differentiated neuroendocrine carcinoma: a Minnie Pearl Cancer Research Network study. J Clin Oncol 2006;24:3548–54.
48. Iwasa S, Morizane C, Okusaka T, et al. Cisplatin and etoposide as first-line chemotherapy for poorly differentiated neuroendocrine carcinoma of the hepatobiliary tract and pancreas. Jpn J Clin Oncol 2010;40:313–8.
49. Yamaguchi T, Machida N, Morizane C, et al. Multicenter retrospective analysis of systemic chemotherapy for advanced neuroendocrine carcinoma of the digestive system. Cancer Sci 2014;105:1176–81.
50. Okuma HS, Iwasa S, Shoji H, et al. Irinotecan plus cisplatin in patients with extensive-disease poorly differentiated neuroendocrine carcinoma of the esophagus. Anticancer Res 2014;34:5037–41.
51. Hoang T, Kim K, Jaslowski A, et al. Phase II study of second-line gemcitabine in sensitive or refractory small cell lung cancer. Lung Cancer 2003;42:97–102.
52. Masters GA, Declerck L, Blanke C, et al. Phase II trial of gemcitabine in refractory or relapsed small-cell lung cancer: Eastern Cooperative Oncology Group Trial 1597. J Clin Oncol 2003;21:1550–5.

53. Ohyanagi F, Horiike A, Okano Y, et al. Phase II trial of gemcitabine and irinotecan in previously treated patients with small-cell lung cancer. Cancer Chemother Pharmacol 2008;61:503–8.
54. Mori K, Kamiyama Y, Kondo T, et al. Pilot phase II study of weekly chemotherapy with paclitaxel and carboplatin for refractory or relapsed small-cell lung cancer. Cancer Chemother Pharmacol 2006;58:86–90.
55. Dongiovanni V, Buffoni L, Berruti A, et al. Second-line chemotherapy with weekly paclitaxel and gemcitabine in patients with small-cell lung cancer pretreated with platinum and etoposide: a single institution phase II trial. Cancer Chemother Pharmacol 2006;58:203–9.
56. Schuette W, Nagel S, Juergens S, et al. Phase II trial of gemcitabine/irinotecan in refractory or relapsed small-cell lung cancer. Clin Lung Cancer 2005;7:133–7.
57. Pallis AG, Agelidou A, Agelaki S, et al. A multicenter randomized phase II study of the irinotecan/gemcitabine doublet versus irinotecan monotherapy in previously treated patients with extensive stage small-cell lung cancer. Lung Cancer 2009;65:187–91.
58. Rocha-Lima CM, Herndon JE, Lee ME, et al. Phase II trial of irinotecan/gemcitabine as second-line therapy for relapsed and refractory small-cell lung cancer: Cancer and Leukemia Group B Study 39902. Ann Oncol 2007;18:331–7.
59. Evans WK, Osoba D, Feld R, et al. Etoposide (VP-16) and cisplatin: an effective treatment for relapse in small-cell lung cancer. J Clin Oncol 1985;3:65–71.
60. Yamamoto N, Tsurutani J, Yoshimura N, et al. Phase II study of weekly paclitaxel for relapsed and refractory small cell lung cancer. Anticancer Res 2006;26:777–82.
61. Ramalingam SS, Foster J, Gooding W, et al. Phase 2 study of irinotecan and paclitaxel in patients with recurrent or refractory small cell lung cancer. Cancer 2010;116:1344–9.
62. Pietanza MC, Kadota K, Huberman K, et al. Phase II trial of temozolomide in patients with relapsed sensitive or refractory small cell lung cancer, with assessment of methylguanine-DNA methyltransferase as a potential biomarker. Clin Cancer Res 2012;18:1138–45.
63. Bajetta E, Catena L, Procopio G, et al. Are capecitabine and oxaliplatin (XELOX) suitable treatments for progressing low-grade and high-grade neuroendocrine tumours? Cancer Chemother Pharmacol 2007;59:637–42.
64. Hadoux J, Malka D, Planchard D, et al. Post-first-line FOLFOX chemotherapy for grade 3 neuroendocrine carcinoma. Endocr Relat Cancer 2015;22:289–98.
65. Olsen IH, Sorensen JB, Federspiel B, et al. Temozolomide as second or third line treatment of patients with neuroendocrine carcinomas. ScientificWorldJournal 2012;2012:170496.
66. Hentic O, Hammel P, Couvelard A, et al. FOLFIRI regimen: an effective second-line chemotherapy after failure of etoposide-platinum combination in patients with neuroendocrine carcinomas grade 3. Endoc Relat Cancer 2012;19:751–7.

Role of Somatostatin Analogues in the Treatment of Neuroendocrine Tumors

 CrossMark

Sujata Narayanan, MD, Pamela L. Kunz, MD*

KEYWORDS

- Neuroendocrine tumors • Somatostatin analogues • Somatostatin receptors
- Carcinoid syndrome • Peptide receptor radionuclide therapy

KEY POINTS

- Functional neuroendocrine tumors (NETs) cause various clinical symptoms depending on the activity of the hormone secreted.
- Carcinoid syndrome, the classic example of a functional NET, is caused by serotonin over-production and leads to flushing, diarrhea, edema, telangiectasia, bronchospasm, and hypotension.
- Somatostatin receptors (SSTRs) are expressed in NETs, with SSTR-2 expression being predominant in gastroenteropancreatic NETs.
- Somatostatin analogues (SSAs) control clinical symptoms arising from hormone excess in SSTR-expressing NETs.
- Recently published data from have established the antiproliferative effects of SSAs and their role in control of tumor growth.

INTRODUCTION

Neuroendocrine tumors (NETs) are epithelial neoplasms with neuroendocrine differentiation that arise in various anatomic locations throughout the body. The annual incidence of NETs in the United States is about 3.65 per 100, 000 and recent analyses have indicated a rise in the incidence of carcinoid tumors in the United States and elsewhere,[1–4] owing in part to improvements in diagnostics and increased awareness.[2,5–7]

Disclosure statement: Dr P.L. Kunz receives research funding from Genentech, Merck, Lexicon, Advanced Accelerator Applications and Oxigene. She serves as an advisor for Ipsen, Lexicon and Novartis and also received the research funding from Esanex. Dr S. Narayanan has no relationships to disclose.
Medicine/Oncology, Stanford University School of Medicine, 875 Blake Wilbur Drive, Stanford, CA 94305-5826, USA
* Corresponding author.
E-mail address: pkunz@stanford.edu

The clinical presentation of carcinoid tumors can be variable, depending on their anatomic site of origin. Whereas patients with indolent disease can remain asymptomatic for years, some patients may present with symptoms related to tumor bulk or from secretion of various peptides or amines from these tumors. Such secretory tumors, also called "functional tumors," cause various clinical symptoms depending on the activity of the hormone secreted. The minority of NETs are truly functional; approximately 10% of patients with small bowel NETs and 40% of patients with pancreatic NETs meet this definition. Carcinoid syndrome, caused by serotonin overproduction, is the classic example of a functional NET and is associated with symptoms such as flushing, diarrhea, edema, telangiectasia, bronchospasm, and hypotension. These symptoms occur when the secretory products from the NETs bypass metabolism in the liver and enter the systemic circulation directly. This usually occurs in the presence of liver metastases, bulky retroperitoneal disease, or primary sites of disease outside the gastrointestinal tract.[8,9] Hindgut tumors (ie, transverse, descending, and sigmoid colon; rectum; and genitourinary) are rarely functional and almost never associated with classic carcinoid syndrome. **Table 1** lists examples of various clinical syndromes arising from hormone secretion in gastroenteropancreatic (ETs).[10]

The management of NETs is multidisciplinary. For patients with unresectable and metastatic disease the intent is 2-fold: controlling tumor growth and alleviating symptoms arising from peptide hormone secretion. The treatment options for tumor control include observation (stable disease and mild tumor burden), systemic therapy with somatostatin (SST) analogues (SSAs), molecularly targeted agents and cytotoxic chemotherapies, cytoreductive surgery, and regional therapies (hepatic arterial embolization and ablative procedures). SSAs are the mainstay for control of hormone secretion. Recently, SSAs have also been recognized as antiproliferative agents in well-differentiated metastatic disease. This article reviews the application and role of SSAs in the treatment of well-differentiated NETs.

SOMATOSTATIN AND SOMATOSTATIN RECEPTOR PHYSIOLOGY

SST is a peptide hormone that was initially discovered as an inhibitor of growth hormone release in the hypothalamus of rats.[11] Subsequent studies found that SST was secreted by paracrine cells scattered throughout the gastrointestinal tract,[12] and also found in various locations in the nervous system. The physiologic effects of SST are largely inhibitory, and it has been known to reduce gastrointestinal motility and gallbladder contraction; inhibit secretion of most gastrointestinal hormones, including insulin, glucagon, and gastrin; reduce blood flow in the gastrointestinal tract; and inhibit growth hormone release from the pituitary and neurotransmission in the brain.[11,13]

SST mediates its primarily inhibitory effects by binding to at least 5 high-affinity G-protein-coupled membrane receptors (SSTR1–5).[14,15] The antiproliferative actions of SST result from cell cycle arrest and/or apoptosis downstream from tumor SSTR activation, and SSTR-induced inhibition of tumor angiogenesis and the production of factors that support tumor growth.[16–20] The SSTRs share about 40% to 60% homology, but mediate different biological actions upon activation.[12] All 5 SSTRs have been identified throughout the central nervous system, the gastrointestinal tract, and endocrine and exocrine glands, as well as on inflammatory and immune cells. Tumors arising from SST target tissues, such as the pancreas and small intestine, express a high density of SSTRs.[15,21,22] The expression of SSTR2 has been noted to be predominant in most gastroenteropancreatic NETs.[21] Well-differentiated tumors express SSTRs more often, and at higher density, than do poorly differentiated tumors.[15]

Table 1
Examples of clinical syndromes associated with functioning neuroendocrine tumors

Syndrome	Secreted Hormone(s)	Symptom(s)
Intestinal neuroendocrine tumors		
Carcinoid syndrome	5-hydroxytryptamine (5-HT) Prostaglandin Substance P Gastrin Vasoactive intestinal polypeptide Prostaglandin Serotonin Bradykinin Kallikrein Histamine	Abdominal pain Secretory diarrhea Flushing Heart disease Telangiectasias (face) Bronchospasm Arthropathy Hypotension Pellagra
Pancreatic neuroendocrine tumors		
Calcitoninoma	Calcitonin	Diarrhea, facial flushing
CRHoma	Corticotropin release hormone	Cushing's syndrome
Gastrinoma	Gastrin	Zollinger Ellison syndrome (peptic ulcers)
GHRHoma	Growth hormone releasing hormone	Acromegaly
Glucagonoma	Glucagon	Necrolytic migratory erythema Cheilitis Diabetes mellitus Anemia Weight loss Diarrhea Venous thrombosis Neuropsychiatric symptoms
Insulinoma	Insulin	Hypoglycemia
PPoma	Pancreatic polypeptide	Considered nonfunctioning
Somatostatinoma	Somatostatin	Diabetes mellitus Cholelithiasis Diarrhea with steatorrhea
VIPoma	Vasoactive intestinal polypeptide	Watery diarrhea Hypokalemia Hypochlorhydria Dehydration Weight loss Flushing Hypercalcemia Hyperglycemia

Syndromes listed in alphabetical order.
Data from Oberg K, Knigge U, Kwekkeboom D, et al; ESMO Guidelines Working Group. Neuroendocrine gastro-entero-pancreatic tumors: ESMO clinical practice guidelines for diagnosis, treatment and follow-up. Ann Oncol 2012;23(Suppl 7):vii124–30.

CLINICAL APPLICATION OF SOMATOSTATIN AND SYNTHETIC ANALOGUES

The inhibitory effects of SST were initially recognized in the 1970s.[23,24] However, given its short half-life requiring a cumbersome continuous infusion and rebound hypersecretion of hormones, its routine clinical application was limited. Given the limitations of native SST, synthetic analogues were developed from the early 1980s to present time and these include octreotide, lanreotide, and pasireotide. These peptides are more resistant to degradation and their half-lives and hence their biological activities are substantially longer than native SST (1.5–2 h vs 1–2 min).[25] They vary in their affinity toward different SSTR subtypes,[12,26] and bind mainly to SSTR2, and much less to SSTR5. The newly developed SSA pasireotide is a new 'universal' or 'pan-receptor' SSA, having a high affinity for SSTR 1, 2, 3, and 5 subtypes.[27] Although initially approved for the treatment of acromegaly, the clinical application of SSAs now extends to multiple indications, such as the treatment of secretory diarrhea, gastrointestinal bleeding, inhibition of tumor growth, treatment of functional NET, and for the imaging of NETs.

SOMATOSTATIN ANALOGUES IN THE TREATMENT OF NEUROENDOCRINE TUMORS

In patients with NETs, indications for the use of an SSA include the treatment of symptoms arising from clinical syndromes caused by hormone excess, and for control of tumor growth. The SSAs are also used perioperatively for the prevention of carcinoid crisis.[25]

Controlling Symptoms Arising From Hormone Excess

SSAs can control hypersecretion in NETs that express SST receptors. These include functional NETs such as glucagonomas, VIPomas, gastrinomas, and metastatic insulinomas. Octreotide was the first SSA developed for this clinical indication, and has a half-life of 2 hours and high affinity toward SSTR 2 and 5. This short-acting formulation of octreotide requires administration by continuous infusion or as a subcutaneous injection 2 to 3 times per day, and is not associated with the side effect of rebound hormonal hypersecretion. Octreotide long-acting release (LAR), a longer acting formulation, was developed in the 1990s to provide more sustained drug levels and is administered at 20 to 30 mg as a monthly intramuscular (IM) injection. Studies comparing the shorter acting and longer acting forms of octreotide have demonstrated equal efficacy in terms of symptom control, with symptomatic response rates of 60% to 72% across groups.[28] For adequate symptom control during the initial administration of octreotide LAR, coverage with short acting octreotide for the initial 2 to 3 weeks is recommended until steady-state levels of octreotide LAR are achieved.

Lanreotide is another SSA with similar SSTR binding affinity as octreotide. Lanreotide has 2 formulations that are currently available, lanreotide sustained release (LA), given as an IM injection every 2 weeks and lanreotide prolonged release (Somatuline Autogel), given as a deep subcutaneous injections every 4 weeks. Lanreotide is approved both in Europe and the United States for the treatment of acromegaly. In a number of small prospective and retrospective studies, lanreotide has led to improvement of symptoms associated with carcinoid syndrome.[29–31] Short-acting octreotide and lanreotide LA have also demonstrated equal efficacy in controlling carcinoid syndrome.[32] Additionally, in a recent phase III study (A Double-blind, Randomized Placebo-controlled Clinical Trial Investigating the Efficacy and Safety of Somatuline Depot (Lanreotide) Injection in the Treatment of Carcinoid Syndrome [ELECT]) of lanreotide versus placebo in SSA-naïve patients or those responsive to conventional doses of octreotide, lanreotide reduced the need for short-acting octreotide (49% vs 34%, absolute difference 15%; $P = .02$).[33] A large cross-sectional observation study evaluated patient-reported satisfaction with lanreotide use for carcinoid syndrome, and found that patients achieved good and sustained control of symptoms arising from carcinoid syndrome.[34]

Pasireotide was developed as an agent with a broader SSTR profile similar to that of natural SST. It binds with high affinity to SSTR subtypes SSTR 1, 2, 3, and 5 and displays a 30- to 40-fold higher affinity for SSTR1 and SSTR5 than octreotide or lanreotide.[27] Given its greater binding affinity, it has been hypothesized that it may have a greater inhibitory effect than octreotide on hormones secreted by carcinoid tumors.[35] A multicenter, randomized, blinded phase III study of pasireotide LAR versus octreotide LAR in patients with symptomatic metastatic NET demonstrated equal efficacy of both these drugs in controlling symptoms of hormone secretion.[36] The safety profile was similar with the exception of hyperglycemia, which was higher in the pasireotide arm (11% vs 0%).

Dosing of Somatostatin Analogues for Hormone-Related Symptoms

When SSAs are used for symptom control, it is recommended to start short-acting SSA immediately in an effort to provide immediate symptom relief and then overlap with long-acting SSA until steady-state levels are reached (approximately 2 weeks). The suggested starting dose of octreotide acetate ranges from 100 to 600 µg/d in 2 to 4 divided doses; test doses are not required routinely. Doses are initiated usually at the lower dose range and can be individually titrated to control symptoms; some patients may require significantly higher doses ($\leq$1.5 mg/d). The recommended dose of octreotide LAR is 20 to 30 mg by deep IM injection repeated every 4 weeks. Correct IM injection can be challenging. One report noted that only 52% of injections were delivered successfully and correct IM injection was associated with improved control of flushing among patients with carcinoid syndrome.[37] Some patients also require "rescue" doses of short-acting octreotide for control of breakthrough symptoms even after initiation of the long-acting formulation; this commonly occurs in the days preceding a scheduled octreotide injection. Dose and frequency of both short- and long-acting SSAs may be increased further for symptoms control as needed.[38] The duration of treatment with SSAs is usually lifelong, unless there is loss of symptom control or occurrence of unmanageable side effects. The risk of tachyphylaxis after long-term use of SSAs has been postulated, although the mechanism of tachyphylaxis is poorly understood and rigorous prospective data are lacking.

The dosing of SSAs in elderly patients with carcinoid syndrome requires special mention, particularly given that the majority of NET patients are diagnosed in their 70s.[2] In a recent study of the Surveillance, Epidemiology, and End Results–Medicare databases,[39] Yao and colleagues showed that only 50% of elderly patients with US Food and Drug Administration–approved indications (carcinoid syndrome or metastatic disease) started Octreotide LAR within 6 months of diagnosis. Octreotide LAR use was lowest among patients aged 80 years and older. Also, the use of octreotide LAR within 6 months of diagnosis of carcinoid syndrome was associated with better survival for patients with metastatic disease. This study suggests that SSA use in elderly patients with functional NETs may be underused and should be evaluated in future studies.

Control of Tumor Growth

SSAs have also demonstrated antiproliferative properties in NETs with varying effect depending on primary site and SSTR subtype. For example, SSTRs 2 and 5 have been shown to mediate the antimitotic activity leading to cell cycle arrest.[40] SSAs may also exert an indirect antiproliferative effect by inhibiting the release of growth factors and various trophic hormones such as growth hormone, insulin-like growth factor-1, insulin, gastrin, and epidermal growth factor, both from the neoplastic cell and from the surrounding tumor matrix.[41] SSAs have also been postulated to reduce the vascularization of the neoplastic tissue in experimental models via inhibition of vascular endothelial growth factor.[42]

The first clinical trial to demonstrate the antiproliferative effect of SSAs in NETs was the PROMID (Placebo controlled, double-blind, prospective, Randomized study on the effect of Octreotide LAR in the control of tumor growth in patients with metastatic neuroendocrine midgut tumors) study.[43] In this phase III randomized, double-blind, placebo-controlled, multiinstitutional German study 85 patients with well-differentiated metastatic midgut NETs were randomized to receive 30 mg octreotide LAR monthly via IM injection versus placebo. In 85 enrolled patients, octreotide significantly improved time to progression when compared with placebo (14.3 vs 6 months in the placebo arm; hazard ratio, 0.34; 95% CI, 0.20–0.59; $P = .000072$); median overall survival (OS) could not be calculated at the time of initial analysis. The study also found that functionally active and inactive tumors responded similarly and the most favorable effect was observed in patients with low hepatic tumor volume and resected primary tumors. Updated OS data were presented in 2013; median OS was not reached in the octreotide LAR arm versus 84 months in the placebo arm (hazard ratio, 0.85; 95% CI, 0.46–1.56; $P = .59$). Although this study did not formally impact the US Food and Drug Administration label for octreotide LAR, octreotide was adopted widely for controlling tumor growth in patients with metastatic midgut NETs.

The CLARINET (Controlled study of Lanreotide Antiproliferative Response In NeuroEndocrine Tumors) study was a phase III randomized, double-blind, placebo-controlled, multinational study of lanreotide in patients with advanced, well-differentiated or moderately differentiated, nonfunctioning, SST receptor–positive NETs of grade 1 or 2 (with a Ki-67 antigen of <10%). Patients were randomized to receive lanreotide 120 mg via a deep subcutaneous injection every 28 days versus placebo. In 205 enrolled patients, lanreotide significantly improved progression-free survival when compared with placebo (median not reached vs 18.0 months; hazard ratio, 0.47; 95% CI, 0.30–0.73, $P<.001$); there was no difference in median OS. In an open-label extension study, 88 patients from the CLARINET core study continued on lanreotide (41 from the lanreotide arm and 47 from the placebo arm.) Of the subset of patients who had progressive disease while on placebo in the core study, median time to further progression was 14 months.[44]

The PROMID and CLARINET studies demonstrate the antiproliferative effect of SSAs in the treatment of NETs. However, there are key differences between these studies worth highlighting (**Table 2**). Most notably, PROMID included patients with small bowel NETs, grade 1 tumors, low hepatic tumor volume, and a relative short interval from diagnosis. CLARINET included a broader patient population with a predominance of pancreas and small bowel primary sites, both grade 1 and 2 tumors (Ki67 <10%), greater hepatic tumor volume, a majority of patients with stable disease during a 3 to 6 months before the study observation period, and a longer median time from diagnosis. CLARINET contributes new information to the field because it demonstrates activity of SSAs in pancreas, hindgut, and unknown primary NETs with higher grade and higher hepatic tumor volume. This study raises an important question, as to whether we should be using SSAs in patients with stable disease. Notably, the 18-month median progression-free survival in the placebo arm is encouraging and may provide evidence that active surveillance in select patients is reasonable. The CLARINET study has not demonstrated an OS difference, which could be attributed to crossover, need for longer follow-up, and perhaps a more indolent disease as evidenced by a longer time from diagnosis as compared with PROMID. Other completed and ongoing clinical trials evaluating SSAs for control of tumor growth in NETs are summarized in **Tables 3** and **4**.

Table 2 Key differences between the PROMID and CLARINET trials		
Characteristic	PROMID	CLARINET
n	85	204
Primary site	Midgut only	Pancreas (45%) Midgut (35%) Hindgut (7%) Unknown primary/other (13%)
Tumor grade	1 (Ki67 ≤2%)	1 and 2 (Ki67 <10%)
Hepatic tumor volume	0%–10% volume (75%) 10%–25% volume (6%) >25% volume (19%)	≤25% volume (67%) >25% volume (33%)
Tumor progression at baseline	Unknown	4%
Time from diagnosis	Octreotide: 7.5 mo Placebo: 3.3 mo	Lanreotide: 13.2 mo Placebo: 16.5 mo
Tumor response assessment tool	WHO	RECIST

Abbreviations: CLARINET, Controlled study of Lanreotide Antiproliferative Response In NeuroEndocrine Tumors; PROMID, Placebo controlled, double-blind, prospective, Randomized study on the effect of Octreotide LAR in the control of tumor growth in patients with metastatic neuroendocrine midgut tumors; RECIST, Response Evaluation Criteria in Solid Tumors; WHO, World Health Organization.

Data from Rinke A, Muller HH, Schade-Brittinger C, et al. Placebo-controlled, double-blind, prospective, randomized study on the effect of octreotide LAR in the control of tumor growth in patients with metastatic neuroendocrine midgut tumors: a report from the PROMID Study Group. J Clin Oncol 2009;27(28):4656–63; and Caplin M, Ruszniewski P, Pavel M, et al. Progression-free survival (PFS) with lanreotide autogel/depot (LAN) in enteropancreatic NETs patients: the CLARINET extension study. J Clin Oncol 2014;32(Suppl 5s):[abstract: 4107].

Dosing for Control of Tumor Growth

The standard SSA doses used for tumor control are octreotide LAR 20 to 30 mg via IM injection monthly and lanreotide 120 mg via a deep subcutaneous injection every 4 weeks, respectively. In contrast with dosing for hormone control, a 2-week overlap with short-acting octreotide is not required. The use of above-standard doses of SSAs for tumor control is controversial because high-quality data are lacking.

The Use of Somatostatin Analogues for Carcinoid Crisis

Carcinoid crisis is thought to be a syndrome of sudden onset severe carcinoid syndrome and vasomotor collapse; however, the physiology is poorly understood. It is also not clear which NET patients are at risk for carcinoid crisis, and may include patients with classic carcinoid syndrome and those with nonfunctional tumors. It has historically been recommended that patients with functional NETs receive prophylactic periprocedural intravenous octreotide to prevent carcinoid crisis. In a recently reported a single-institution retrospective experience of 97 patients with carcinoid tumors undergoing surgery, octreotide LAR and bolus octreotide were insufficient in preventing intraoperative complications.[45] Future definitive studies are needed to better understand carcinoid crisis and develop preventive strategies.

Side Effects of Somatostatin Analogue Therapy

The most commonly encountered side effects SSAs include nausea, abdominal cramps, diarrhea, steatorrhea, flatulence, hyperglycemia, and cholelithiasis/biliary sludging. Most of these symptoms are dose dependent, and resolve within the first

Table 3
Select completed randomized clinical trials with somatostatin analogues

Phase	Therapy	n	Patients	TTP or PFS		RR (%)
				Months	HR/P	
Single agent studies						
II (PROMID)[43]	Octreotide vs Placebo	85	Midgut	14.3 vs 6.0[a]	0.34 P<.001	2
III (CLARINET)[44]	Lanreotide vs Placebo	204	Pancreas, midgut, hindgut, unknown	NR vs 18.0[a]	0.47 P<.001	NA
Combination studies						
III (RADIANT-2)[57]	Everolimus + octreotide vs Placebo + octreotide	429	NETs with carcinoid syndrome	16.4 11.3	0.77 P=.026	2 2
II (COOPERATE-2)[58]	Everolimus vs Everolimus + pasireotide	160	pNET	16.6 16.8	0.99 P=.488	5 16
III (SWOG 0518)[59]	IFN + octreotide vs Bevacizumab + octreotide	427	High risk NET, nonpancreatic	16.6 15.4	0.93 P=.55	12 4
II (CALGB 80701)[a,60]	Everolimus + bevacizumab + octreotide vs Everolimus + octreotide	160	pNET	16.7 14.0	0.80 P=.12	31 12

Abbreviations: CALGB, Randomized Phase II Study of Everolimus Alone Versus Everolimus Plus Bevacizumab in Patients With Locally Advanced or Metastatic Pancreatic Neuroendocrine Tumors; CLARINET, Controlled study of Lanreotide Antiproliferative Response In NeuroEndocrine Tumors; COOPERATE-2, A trial looking at everolimus and pasireotide for neuroendocrine tumours of the pancreas; HR, hazard ratio; IFN, interferon; NA, not applicable; NET, neuroendocrine tumor; NR, not reported; PFS, progression-free survival; pNETs, pancreatic neuroendocrine tumors; PROMID, Placebo controlled, double-blind, prospective, Randomized study on the effect of Octreotide LAR in the control of tumor growth in patients with metastatic neuroendocrine midgut tumors; RADIANT-2, RAD001 in Advanced Neuroendocrine Tumors, second trial; SWOG 0518, Phase III Prospective Randomized Comparison of Depot Octreotide plus Interferon Alpha versus Depot Octreotide plus Bevacizumab; TTP, time to progression.
[a] Statistically significant difference.
Data from Refs.[43,44,57–60]

Table 4
Select ongoing randomized clinical trials with somatostatin analogues

Phase	Therapy	N	Patients	Primary Endpoint	NCT	Status
III (LUNA)	Pasireotide vs everolimus vs both	120	Lung/thymus	PFS (9 mo)	01563354	Active, not recruiting
III (NETTER-1)	177Lu-DOTA0-Tyr3-octreotate vs high-dose octreotide	280	Midgut	PFS	01578239	International, recruiting
II/III (REMINET)	Lanreotide vs placebo after SD/CR on chemotherapy or biotherapy	118	Duodenopancreatic NET	PFS (6 mo)	02288377	France, recruiting
III (CASTOR)	177Lu-octreotate vs IFN	60	GI NET	PFS	01860742	Belgium, not yet recruiting
II	177Lu-octreotate and capecitabine/temozolomide (CAPTEM) vs (i) CAPTEM alone (pNETs) (ii) vs 177Lu-octreotate alone (midgut)	165	pNETs and midgut	PFS (12 mo for pNETs and 24 mo for midgut)	02358356	Australia and Asia, not yet recruiting

Abbreviations: CASTOR, Randomized Phase III of PRRT Versus Interferon; GI, gastrointestinal; IFN, interferon; LUNA, 3-arm Trial to Evaluate Pasireotide LAR/Everolimus Alone/in Combination in Patients With Lung/Thymus NET; NETTER-1, 177Lu-DOTA0-Tyr3-Octreotate to Octreotide LAR in Patients With Inoperable, Progressive, Somatostatin Receptor Positive Midgut Carcinoid Tumours; PFS, progression-free survival; pNETs, pancreatic neuroendocrine tumors; REMINET, Lanreotide as Maintenance Therapy in Patients With Non-Resectable Duodeno-Pancreatic Neuroendocrine Tumors.
Data from Refs.[61–65]

few weeks of treatment. Cholelithilasis and/or gallbladder sludge occurs secondary to the inhibition of gallbladder contraction and emptying and can develop in approximately 50% of patients on SSAs. Although this side effect is also dose dependent, only 1% of patients develop acute symptoms requiring cholecystectomy.[25] It has been recommended that cholecystectomy be performed prophylactically in NET patients on or considering SSA therapy. Local discomfort may also be experienced for all methods of administration (subcutaneous, deep subcutaneous, IM injection). SSAs should be used with caution in patients with insulinomas because they have the potential to worsen hypoglycemia by suppressing glucagon secretion.

MONITORING PATIENTS ON SOMATOSTATIN ANALOGUE THERAPY

Routine clinical evaluation, including history and physical examination, and laboratory evaluation of tumor markers is recommended for patients on treatment with SSAs, usually every 3 months. Patients may exhibit symptomatic response to treatment with a decrease in the intensity and duration of their hormonally mediated symptoms (such as diarrhea, cramping, flushing, and hypoglycemia) and also experience improvement in their performance status and quality of life. Biochemical responses can be measured by evaluating specific tumor markers, such as plasma chromogranin and 24-hour urine 5-hydroxy indole acetic acid in patients with gastrointestinal NETs, and measurement of the predominant peptide in patients with pancreatic NETs. A biochemical response is generally defined as a 50% or greater decrease in serum or urine tumor markers. However, the clinical implication of biochemical responses is controversial, and significant early reduction in the tumor markers may indicate a more durable response to octreotide.[46] Data demonstrating benefit of plasma octreotide monitoring is lacking; therefore, routine use is not recommended.

Objective responses to therapy with SSAs are evaluated with imaging (computed tomography, MRI, or ultrasonography). SST receptor scintigraphy, or octreoscan, is usually used for the initial localization of primary and metastatic SST positive tumors, but they are not used routinely for monitoring response to treatment. ^{68}Ga-DOTATATE PET/computed tomography scans, a new-generation SST receptor scintigraphy, are available in Europe but considered investigational in the United States. These scans are considered more sensitive than octreoscans and may replace octreoscans in the future.[47,48]

APPLICATION OF RADIOLABELED SOMATOSTATIN ANALOGUES IN NEUROENDOCRINE TUMORS THERAPEUTICS

Peptide receptor radionuclide therapy (PRRT) with radiolabeled SSAs is a relatively new and promising treatment modality for patients with inoperable or metastatic NET tumors. This treatment is based on the same principle used in SST receptor scintigraphy, such as [111]indium octreoscans and the newer ^{68}Ga DOTA PET scans. The radiolabeled SSAs bind to SST receptors and get internalized into the tumor cells, and can be used for diagnostic and therapeutic purposes (termed theranostics). By targeting SST receptors in NET tumors with radiolabeled SSAs, a tumoricidal radiation dose is delivered, thus causing a localized antitumor effect.[49]

SST peptides with higher receptor affinity are conjugated with radio–metal labeling chelators. DOTA is a chelator capable of encapsulating hard metals such as gallium, yttrium, or lutetium. The first generation of PRRT studies in the 1990s used [111]In a [gamma] emitter. Although they showed encouraging responses with regard to symptom relief, tumor shrinkage, and patient survival, they were also associated with significant bone marrow toxicity, including myelodysplastic syndrome and leukemia. The second generation of PRRT used ^{90}Y-DOTA Tyr^3-octreotide that has been evaluated in several phase I and II studies.[50–54] ^{90}Y is a pure [beta] emitter with a relatively long tissue penetration range (12 mm), which enables it to easily penetrate larger lesions. These studies reported a modest response rates ranging from 25% to 30%. However, it was noted that renal toxicity was often a dose-limiting side effect of this treatment, and the administration of ^{90}Y PRRT required amino acid infusion for nephroprotection. Since 2000, [^{177}Lu-DOTA^0,Tyr^3]octreotate has been used for PRRT. ^{177}Lu is a medium-energy [beta]-emitter with an approximate half-life of 6.7 days and with the maximal tissue penetration of 2 mm.

In 2008, Kwekkeboom and colleagues[55] reported a retrospective analysis of 500 patients treated with [^{177}Lu-DOTA^0,Tyr^3]octreotate up to a cumulative dose of 750 to 800 mCi (27.8–29.6 GBq), usually in 4 treatment cycles, with treatment intervals of 6 to 10 weeks. Complete and partial tumor remissions occurred in 2% and 28% of the patients, respectively, and minor tumor response (decrease in size >25% and <50%) occurred in 16%. Median time to progression was 40 months; median OS from start of treatment was 46 months. Acute toxicities included nausea and vomiting; subacute toxicities included grade 3 to 4 hematologic toxicity (occurred in 9.5% of patients 4–8 weeks after 3.6% of administrations) and alopecia (62%). Serious delayed toxicities occurred in 9 patients, including renal insufficiency (2 patients), liver toxicity (3 patients), and myelodysplastic syndrome (4 patients).

Although PRRT has been used for treatment of metastatic SSTR-positive NETs in Europe since the 1990s, it is not approved by the US Food and Drug Administration given the lack of randomized data. The first phase III, randomized, multinational clinical trial of PRRT is now underway. The NETTER-1 (177Lu-DOTA0-Tyr3-Octreotate to Octreotide LAR in Patients With Inoperable, Progressive, Somatostatin Receptor Positive Midgut Carcinoid Tumours) study will compare 177Lu-DOTA0-Tyr3-octreotate with high-dose octreotide LAR (60 mg monthly) in patients with inoperable, SST receptor-positive metastatic midgut NETs who have experienced progressive disease on standard doses (20–30 mg every 3 to 4 weeks) of octreotide LAR (NCT01578239). The accrual goal is 280 patients and the primary endpoint is progression-free survival. Additionally, novel radiolabeled SST antagonists are being developed for both imaging and treatment.[56] Other future studies also include a phase II study to compare PRRT with cytotoxic chemotherapy (capecitabine and temozolomide) versus chemotherapy alone (NCT02358356) and a phase III randomized trial comparing PRRT with interferon (NCT01860742).

FUTURE DIRECTIONS

Considerable advances have been made in the treatment NETs over the last decade. SSAs have been applied primarily for the management of symptoms arising from various clinical syndromes in NETs, and various SSA formulations are now available that are long acting and provide sustained symptomatic benefit. Results from the PROMID and CLARINET studies have established the role of SSAs for controlling tumor growth in NETs. Prospective clinical trials are now underway to evaluate PRRT in SSTR-positive NETs.

REFERENCES

1. Lawrence B, Gustafsson BI, Chan A, et al. The epidemiology of gastroenteropancreatic neuroendocrine tumors. Endocrinol Metab Clin North Am 2011; 40(1):1–18, vii.

2. Yao JC, Hassan M, Phan A, et al. One hundred years after "carcinoid": epidemiology of and prognostic factors for neuroendocrine tumors in 35,825 cases in the United States. J Clin Oncol 2008;26(18):3063–72.
3. Garcia-Carbonero R, Capdevila J, Crespo-Herrero G, et al. Incidence, patterns of care and prognostic factors for outcome of gastroenteropancreatic neuroendocrine tumors (GEP-NETs): results from the National Cancer Registry of Spain (RGETNE). Ann Oncol 2010;21(9):1794–803.
4. Mocellin S, Nitti D. Gastrointestinal carcinoid: epidemiological and survival evidence from a large population-based study (n = 25 531). Ann Oncol 2013;24(12):3040–4.
5. Marx S, Spiegel AM, Skarulis MC, et al. Multiple endocrine neoplasia type 1: clinical and genetic topics. Ann Intern Med 1998;129(6):484–94.
6. Donis-Keller H, Dou S, Chi D, et al. Mutations in the RET proto-oncogene are associated with MEN 2A and FMTC. Hum Mol Genet 1993;2(7):851–6.
7. Rindi GAR, Bosman FT, Arnold R, et al. Nomenclature and classification of neuroendocrine neoplasms of the digestive system. WHO classification of tumours of the digestive system. 4th edition. Lyon: International Agency for Research on cancer (IARC); 2010. p. 13.
8. Kulke MH, Mayer RJ. Carcinoid tumors. N Engl J Med 1999;340(11):858–68.
9. Schnirer II, Yao JC, Ajani JA. Carcinoid–a comprehensive review. Acta Oncol 2003;42(7):672–92.
10. Oberg K, Knigge U, Kwekkeboom D, et al. Neuroendocrine gastro-enteropancreatic tumors: ESMO Clinical Practice Guidelines for diagnosis, treatment and follow-up. Ann Oncol 2012;23(Suppl 7):vii124–30.
11. Brazeau P, Vale W, Burgus R, et al. Hypothalamic polypeptide that inhibits the secretion of immunoreactive pituitary growth hormone. Science 1973;179(4068):77–9.
12. Lamberts SW, van der Lely AJ, de Herder WW, et al. Octreotide. N Engl J Med 1996;334(4):246–54.
13. Reichlin S. Secretion of somatostatin and its physiologic function. J Lab Clin Med 1987;109(3):320–6.
14. Nilsson O, Kolby L, Wangberg B, et al. Comparative studies on the expression of somatostatin receptor subtypes, outcome of octreotide scintigraphy and response to octreotide treatment in patients with carcinoid tumours. Br J Cancer 1998;77(4):632–7.
15. Modlin IM, Pavel M, Kidd M, et al. Review article: somatostatin analogues in the treatment of gastroenteropancreatic neuroendocrine (carcinoid) tumours. Aliment Pharmacol Ther 2010;31(2):169–88.
16. Theodoropoulou M, Stalla GK. Somatostatin receptors: from signaling to clinical practice. Front Neuroendocrinol 2013;34(3):228–52.
17. Reisine T, Bell GI. Molecular biology of somatostatin receptors. Endocr Rev 1995; 16(4):427–42.
18. Benuck M, Marks N. Differences in the degradation of hypothalamic releasing factors by rat and human serum. Life Sci 1976;19(8):1271–6.
19. Reichlin S. Somatostatin. N Engl J Med 1983;309(24):1495–501.
20. Larsson LI, Goltermann N, de Magistris L, et al. Somatostatin cell processes as pathways for paracrine secretion. Science 1979;205(4413):1393–5.
21. de Herder WW, Hofland LJ, van der Lely AJ, et al. Somatostatin receptors in gastroentero-pancreatic neuroendocrine tumours. Endocr Relat Cancer 2003; 10(4):451–8.
22. Fjallskog ML, Ludvigsen E, Stridsberg M, et al. Expression of somatostatin receptor subtypes 1 to 5 in tumor tissue and intratumoral vessels in malignant endocrine pancreatic tumors. Med Oncol 2003;20(1):59–67.

23. Thulin L, Samnegard H, Tyden G, et al. Efficacy of somatostatin in a patient with carcinoid syndrome. Lancet 1978;2(8079):43.
24. Guillemin R. Peptides in the brain: the new endocrinology of the neuron. Science 1978;202(4366):390–402.
25. Oberg K, Kvols L, Caplin M, et al. Consensus report on the use of somatostatin analogs for the management of neuroendocrine tumors of the gastroentero-pancreatic system. Ann Oncol 2004;15(6):966–73.
26. Kidd M, Drozdov I, Joseph R, et al. Differential cytotoxicity of novel somatostatin and dopamine chimeric compounds on bronchopulmonary and small intestinal neuroendocrine tumor cell lines. Cancer 2008;113(4):690–700.
27. Bruns C, Lewis I, Briner U, et al. SOM230: a novel somatostatin peptidomimetic with broad somatotropin release inhibiting factor (SRIF) receptor binding and a unique antisecretory profile. Eur J Endocrinol 2002;146(5):707–16.
28. Rubin J, Ajani J, Schirmer W, et al. Octreotide acetate long-acting formulation versus open-label subcutaneous octreotide acetate in malignant carcinoid syndrome. J Clin Oncol 1999;17(2):600–6.
29. Bajetta E, Procopio G, Catena L, et al. Lanreotide autogel every 6 weeks compared with Lanreotide microparticles every 3 weeks in patients with well differentiated neuroendocrine tumors: a Phase III Study. Cancer 2006;107(10):2474–81.
30. Ruszniewski P, Ish-Shalom S, Wymenga M, et al. Rapid and sustained relief from the symptoms of carcinoid syndrome: results from an open 6-month study of the 28-day prolonged-release formulation of lanreotide. Neuroendocrinology 2004; 80(4):244–51.
31. Khan MS, El-Khouly F, Davies P, et al. Long-term results of treatment of malignant carcinoid syndrome with prolonged release Lanreotide (Somatuline Autogel). Aliment Pharmacol Ther 2011;34(2):235–42.
32. O'Toole D, Ducreux M, Bommelaer G, et al. Treatment of carcinoid syndrome: a prospective crossover evaluation of lanreotide versus octreotide in terms of efficacy, patient acceptability, and tolerance. Cancer 2000;88(4):770–6.
33. Vinik A, Wolin E, Audry H, et al. ELECT: a phase 3 study of efficacy and safety of lanreotide autoge/depot (LAN) treatment for carcinoid syndrome in patient with neuroendocrine tumors (NETs). J Clin Oncol 2014;32(Suppl 3) [abstract: 268].
34. Hobday T, Rubin J, Holen K, et al. MC044h, a phase II trial of sorafenib in patients (pts) with metastatic neuroendocrine tumors (NET): a Phase II Consortium (P2C) study. ASCO Annual Meeting June 1–5, Chicago, Il, abstract # 4504, 2007.
35. Schmid HA, Schoeffter P. Functional activity of the multiligand analog SOM230 at human recombinant somatostatin receptor subtypes supports its usefulness in neuroendocrine tumors. Neuroendocrinology 2004;80(Suppl 1):47–50.
36. Wolin EM. A multicenter, randomized, blinded, phase III study of pasireotide LAR versus octreotide LAR in patients with metastatic neuroendocrine tumors (NET) with disease-related symptoms inadequately controlled by somatostatin analogs. J Clin Oncol 2013;31(Suppl) [abstract: 4031].
37. Boyd AE, DeFord LL, Mares JE, et al. Improving the success rate of gluteal intra-muscular injections. Pancreas 2013;42(5):878–82.
38. Strosberg JR, Benson AB, Huynh L, et al. Clinical benefits of above-standard dose of octreotide LAR in patients with neuroendocrine tumors for control of carcinoid syndrome symptoms: a multicenter retrospective chart review study. Oncologist 2014;19(9):930–6.
39. Shen C, Shih YC, Xu Y, et al. Octreotide long-acting repeatable use among elderly patients with carcinoid syndrome and survival outcomes: a population-based analysis. Cancer 2014;120(13):2039–49.

40. Schally AV. Oncological applications of somatostatin analogues. Cancer Res 1988;48(24 Pt 1):6977–85.
41. Susini C, Buscail L. Rationale for the use of somatostatin analogs as antitumor agents. Ann Oncol Dec 2006;17(12):1733–42.
42. Lawnicka H, Stepien H, Wyczolkowska J, et al. Effect of somatostatin and octreotide on proliferation and vascular endothelial growth factor secretion from murine endothelial cell line (HECa10) culture. Biochem Biophys Res Commun 2000; 268(2):567–71.
43. Rinke A, Muller HH, Schade-Brittinger C, et al. Placebo-controlled, double-blind, prospective, randomized study on the effect of octreotide LAR in the control of tumor growth in patients with metastatic neuroendocrine midgut tumors: a report from the PROMID Study Group. J Clin Oncol 2009;27(28):4656–63.
44. Caplin M, Ruszniewski P, Pavel M, et al. Progression-free survival (PFS) with lanreotide autogel/depot (LAN) in enteropancreatic NETs patients: the CLARINET extension study. J Clin Oncol 2014;32(Suppl 5s) [abstract: 4107].
45. Massimino K, Harrskog O, Pommier S, et al. Octreotide LAR and bolus octreotide are insufficient for preventing intraoperative complications in carcinoid patients. J Surg Oncol 2013;107(8):842–6.
46. Angeletti S, Corleto VD, Schillaci O, et al. Single dose of octreotide stabilize metastatic gastro-entero-pancreatic endocrine tumours. Ital J Gastroenterol Hepatol 1999;31(1):23–7.
47. Haug AR, Cindea-Drimus R, Auernhammer CJ, et al. The role of 68Ga-DOTATATE PET/CT in suspected neuroendocrine tumors. Journal of nuclear medicine : official publication. J Nucl Med 2012;53(11):1686–92.
48. Arnold R, Chen YJ, Costa F, et al. ENETS Consensus Guidelines for the Standards of Care in Neuroendocrine Tumors: follow-up and documentation. Neuroendocrinology 2009;90(2):227–33.
49. Heppeler A, Froidevaux S, Eberle AN, et al. Receptor targeting for tumor localisation and therapy with radiopeptides. Curr Med Chem 2000;7(9):971–94.
50. Waldherr C, Pless M, Maecke HR, et al. The clinical value of [90Y-DOTA]-D-Phe1-Tyr3-octreotide (90Y-DOTATOC) in the treatment of neuroendocrine tumours: a clinical phase II study. Ann Oncol 2001;12(7):941–5.
51. Waldherr C, Pless M, Maecke HR, et al. Tumor response and clinical benefit in neuroendocrine tumors after 7.4 GBq (90)Y-DOTATOC. Journal of nuclear medicine : official publication. J Nucl Med 2002;43(5):610–6.
52. Paganelli G, Bodei L, Handkiewicz Junak D, et al. 90Y-DOTA-D-Phe1-Try3-octreotide in therapy of neuroendocrine malignancies. Biopolymers 2002;66(6):393–8.
53. Bodei L, Cremonesi M, Zoboli S, et al. Receptor-mediated radionuclide therapy with 90Y-DOTATOC in association with amino acid infusion: a phase I study. Eur J Nucl Med Mol Imaging 2003;30(2):207–16.
54. Bushnell D, O'Dorisio T, Menda Y, et al. Evaluating the clinical effectiveness of 90Y-SMT 487 in patients with neuroendocrine tumors. Journal of nuclear medicine : official publication. J Nucl Med 2003;44(10):1556–60.
55. Kwekkeboom DJ, de Herder WW, Kam BL, et al. Treatment with the radiolabeled somatostatin analog [177 Lu-DOTA 0,Tyr3]octreotate: toxicity, efficacy, and survival. J Clin Oncol 2008;26(13):2124–30.
56. Wild D, Fani M, Fischer R, et al. Comparison of somatostatin receptor agonist and antagonist for peptide receptor radionuclide therapy: a pilot study. J Nucl Med 2014;55(8):1248–52.
57. Pavel ME, Hainsworth JD, Baudin E, et al. Everolimus plus octreotide long-acting repeatable for the treatment of advanced neuroendocrine tumours associated

with carcinoid syndrome (RADIANT-2): a randomised, placebo-controlled, phase 3 study. Lancet 2011;378(9808):2005–12.

58. Kulke M. A randomized open-label phase II study of everolimus alone or in combination with pasireotide LAR in advanced, progressive pancreatic neuroendocrine tumors: COOPERATE-2 Trial. Presented at 12th Annual ENETS Conference, March 11–13, Barcelona, Spain, 2015.

59. Yao J. SWOG S0518: phase III prospective randomized comparison of depot octreotide plus interferon alpha-2b versus depot octreotide plus bevacizumab (NSC #704865) in advanced, poor prognosis carcinoid patients (NCT00569127). J Clin Oncol 2015;33(Suppl) [abstract: 4004].

60. Kulke M. Randomized phase II study of everolimus (E) versus everolimus plus bevacizumab (E+B) in patients (Pts) with locally advanced or metastatic pancreatic neuroendocrine tumors (pNET), CALGB 80701 (Alliance). J Clin Oncol 2015; 33(Suppl) [abstract: 4005].

61. Hopfner M, Sutter AP, Gerst B, et al. A novel approach in the treatment of neuroendocrine gastrointestinal tumours. Targeting the epidermal growth factor receptor by gefitinib (ZD1839). Br J Cancer 2003;89(9):1766–75.

62. Eisenhauer EA, Therasse P, Bogaerts J, et al. New response evaluation criteria in solid tumours: revised RECIST guideline (version 1.1). Eur J Cancer 2009;45(2): 228–47.

63. Simon R. Optimal two-stage designs for phase II clinical trials. Control Clin Trials 1989;10(1):1–10.

64. Agus DB, Gordon MS, Taylor C, et al. Phase I clinical study of pertuzumab, a novel HER dimerization inhibitor, in patients with advanced cancer. J Clin Oncol 2005;23(11):2534–43.

65. Friess T, Scheuer W, Hasmann M. Combination treatment with erlotinib and pertuzumab against human tumor xenografts is superior to monotherapy. Clin Cancer Res 2005;11(14):5300–9.

Peptide Receptor Radionuclide Therapy in the Treatment of Neuroendocrine Tumors

Dik J. Kwekkeboom, MD, PhD*, Eric P. Krenning, MD, PhD

KEYWORDS

• Neuroendocrine tumor • Carcinoid • Radionuclide therapy • PRRT • Treatment

KEY POINTS

• Peptide receptor radionuclide therapy (PRRT) is a promising new treatment modality for inoperable or metastasized gastroenteropancreatic neuroendocrine tumors patients.
• Most studies report objective response rates in 15% to 35% of patients.
• Progression-free and overall survival compare favorably with that for somatostatin analogues, chemotherapy, or newer, "targeted" therapies.

INTRODUCTION

In patients with inoperable metastasized gastroenteropancreatic neuroendocrine tumors (GEPNETs), therapeutic options are limited. Treatment with somatostatin analogues decreases hormonal overproduction and can relieve symptoms in patients with GEPNETs.[1,2] Furthermore, more recent studies showed that treatment with somatostatin analogues prolongs progression-free survival (PFS) in patients with well-differentiated (grades 1 and 2) GEPNETs.[3,4]

The majority of GEPNETs express somatostatin receptors, mainly somatostatin receptor subtypes 2 and 5.[5] These can be visualized using radiolabeled somatostatin analogues. The first commercially available diagnostic somatostatin analogue was [^{111}Indium-DTPA^0]octreotide (Octreoscan; Mallinckrodt, St Louis, MO).[6] Nowadays, newer PET radiopharmaceuticals are available, such as [^{68}Ga-DOTA-Tyr^3]octreotide[7] and [^{68}Ga-DOTA-Tyr^3]octreotate.[8] A logical sequel to somatostatin receptor imaging for diagnostic purposes was to use the same receptor-binding concept for treatment (**Fig. 1**).

Disclosures: Both authors own shares in Advanced Accelerator Applications (AAA).
Department of Nuclear Medicine, Erasmus MC, University Medical Center, s-Gravendijkwal 230, Rotterdam 3015CE, The Netherlands
* Corresponding author.
E-mail address: d.j.kwekkeboom@erasmusmc.nl

Hematol Oncol Clin N Am 30 (2016) 179–191
http://dx.doi.org/10.1016/j.hoc.2015.09.009
0889-8588/16/$ – see front matter © 2016 Elsevier Inc. All rights reserved.

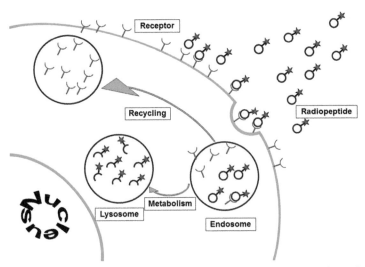

Fig. 1. Mechanism of action of peptide receptor radionuclide therapy. The radiolabeled somatostatin analogues are internalized, and the breakdown products of the radiolabeled peptides are stored in lysosomes, thus enabling a long irradiation of tumor cells.

PEPTIDE RECEPTOR RADIONUCLIDE THERAPY EFFICACY: OBJECTIVE RESPONSE AND SURVIVAL

Because at that time somatostatin analogues labeled with beta-emitting radionuclides were not available for clinical use, early studies in the 1990s used high activities of the Auger electron-emitting [^{111}In-DTPA^0]octreotide for peptide receptor radionuclide therapy (PRRT). These treatments often resulted in symptom relief in patients with metastasized GEPNETs, but objective tumor responses were rare (**Table 1**).[9,10]

The next generation of analogues used in PRRT consisted of a modified somatostatin analogue, [Tyr^3]octreotide, and a different chelator, DOTA instead of DTPA, which allows stable binding of the β-emitting radionuclide ^{90}yttrium (^{90}Y). Its maximal tissue penetration is 12 mm and its half-life is 2.7 days. [^{90}Y-DOTA^0,Tyr^3]octreotide (^{90}Y-DOTATOC) was used in several phase I and phase II PRRT trials in various countries (see **Table 1**).[11–18] The reported objective responses range from 4% to 33%. Differences in cycle doses and administered cumulative dose, as well as differences in patient characteristics (included tumor types, patient performance status) make it virtually impossible to compare these studies. Different studies report median PFS varying from 17 to 29 months, and median overall survival (OS) from 22 to 37 months (**Table 2**).[15–18] In a report on the treatment effects of ^{90}Y-DOTATOC in a large group of patients, the response to ^{90}Y-DOTATOC was associated with longer survival.[23]

^{177}Lutetium (^{177}Lu) is a medium energy β-emitter, with a maximal tissue penetration of 2 mm. ^{177}Lu also emits low-energy γ-rays, allowing scintigraphy after therapy (**Fig. 2**). The somatostatin analogue [DOTA^0,Tyr^3]octreotate differs from [DOTA^0,-Tyr^3]octreotide only in that the C-terminal threoninol is replaced with threonine, resulting in a higher affinity for the somatostatin receptor subtype 2 than octreotide.[24] The treatment effects of [^{177}Lu-DOTA^0,Tyr^3]octreotate (^{177}Lu-octreotate) therapy were described in a large group of GEPNET patients.[19] Complete remission (CR) was found in 5 (2%) patients, partial remission (PR) in 86 (28%), and minor response in 51 (16%; see **Table 2**). Prognostic factors for predicting tumor remission (CR, PR, or minor

Table 1
Tumor responses in patients with gastroenteropancreatic neuroendocrine tumors, treated with different radiolabeled somatostatin analogues

Center (Reference)	Ligand	Patient Number	Tumor Response					
			CR, n (%)	PR, n (%)	MR, n (%)	SD, n (%)	PD, n (%)	CR + PR (%)
Rotterdam (Valkema et al,[9] 2002)	[111In-DTPA0]octreotide	26	0	0	5 (19)	11 (42)	10 (38)	0
New Orleans (Anthony et al,[10] 2002)	[111In-DTPA0]octreotide	26	0	2 (8)	NA	21 (81)	3 (12)	8
Milan (Bodei et al,[11] 2003)	[90Y-DOTA0,Tyr3]octreotide	21	0	6 (29)	NA	11 (52)	4 (19)	29
Basel (Waldherr et al,[12,13] 2001/2002)	[90Y-DOTA0,Tyr3]octreotide	74	3 (4)	15 (20)	NA	48 (65)	8 (11)	24
Basel (Waldherr et al,[14] 2002)	[90Y-DOTA0,Tyr3]octreotide	33	2 (6)	9 (27)	NA	19 (57)	3 (9)	33
Multicenter (Valkema et al,[15] 2006)	[90Y-DOTA0,Tyr3]octreotide	58	0	5 (9)	7 (12)	33 (61)	10 (19)	9
Multicenter (Bushnell et al,[16] 2010)	[90Y-DOTA0,Tyr3]octreotide	90	0	4 (4)	NA	63 (70)	11 (12)	4
Copenhagen (Pfeifer et al,[17] 2011)	[90Y-DOTA0,Tyr3]octreotide	53	2 (4)	10 (19)	NA	34 (64)	7 (13)	23
Warsaw (Cwikla et al,[18] 2010)	[90Y-DOTA0,Tyr3]octreotate	58	0	13 (23)	NA	44 (73)	3 (5)	23
Rotterdam (Kwekkeboom et al,[19] 2008)	[177Lu-DOTA0,Tyr3]octreotate	310	5 (2)	86 (28)	51 (16)	107 (35)	61 (20)	29
Gothenburg (Sward et al,[20] 2010)	[177Lu-DOTA0,Tyr3]octreotate	26	0	6 (38)	NA	8 (50)	2 (13)	38
Lund (Garkavij et al,[21] 2010)	[177Lu-DOTA0,Tyr3]octreotate	12	0	2 (17)	3 (25)	5 (40)	2 (17)	17
Milan (Bodei et al,[22] 2011)	[177Lu-DOTA0,Tyr3]octreotate	42	1 (2)	12 (29)	9 (21)	11 (26)	9 (21)	31

Abbreviations: CR, complete remission; MR, minor response; PD, progressive disease; PR, partial response; SD, stable disease.
Data from Refs.[9–22]

Table 2
Survival data in patients with gastroenteropancreatic neuroendocrine tumors, treated with different radiolabeled somatostatin analogues

Center (Reference)	Ligand	Patient Number	PFS	OS
Multicenter (Valkema et al,[15] 2006)	[^{90}Y-DOTA^0,Tyr^3]octreotide	58	29	37
Multicenter (Bushnell et al,[16] 2010)	[^{90}Y-DOTA^0,Tyr^3]octreotide	90	16	27
Copenhagen (Pfeifer et al,[17] 2011)	[^{90}Y-DOTA^0,Tyr^3]octreotide	53	29	—
Warsaw (Cwikla et al,[18] 2010)	[^{90}Y-DOTA^0,Tyr^3]octreotate	58	17	22
Rotterdam (Kwekkeboom et al,[19] 2008)	[^{177}Lu-DOTA^0,Tyr^3]octreotate	310	33	46

Abbreviations: OS, overall survival; PFS, progression-free survival.
Data from Refs.[15–19]

response) as treatment outcome were high uptake on the Octreoscan, Karnofsky performance score of greater than 70, and low metastatic load to the liver. Median time to progression was 40 months from start of treatment. Progression of disease was more common in patients with extensive disease and in patients who were in a relatively poor general clinical condition (Karnofsky score of <70%, significant weight loss, presence of bone metastases). Several of these factors that had a significant impact on PFS were also found in another study.[22] Median OS was 46 months (see **Table 2**).

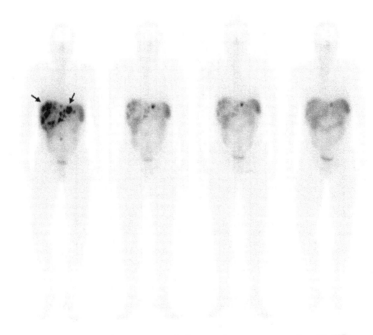

Fig. 2. Tumor responses can be monitored after each treatment cycle with ^{177}Lu-octreotate, using posttherapy scans. Scans made 1 day after each treatment cycle with ^{177}Lu-octreotate in a patient with metastatic carcinoid. The uptake in liver metastases (*arrows*) diminishes after each cycle, indicating a tumor response. (*Courtesy of* Erasmus Medical, Center Department of Nuclear Medicine, Rotterdam, The Netherlands.)

PEPTIDE RECEPTOR RADIONUCLIDE THERAPY: QUALITY OF LIFE

In a large group of (nearly 300) patients treated with PRRT and who had a long follow-up, it was shown that quality of life, but also symptomatology improved in 40% to 70% of cases, depending on the preexistence of a certain symptom (**Box 1**).[25] This is important because the months to years that are gained after PRRT can only be called promising if the time that is gained is free of serious side effects or symptomatology that affect quality of life. By contrast, it was shown that the years gained after PRRT had an improved quality of life, as judged by the patients themselves, using a validated questionnaire.[25]

PEPTIDE RECEPTOR RADIONUCLIDE THERAPY: ACUTE AND SUBACUTE SIDE EFFECTS

PRRT is generally well-tolerated. Acute side effects are usually mild and self-limiting. Nausea or, more rarely, vomiting is related to the concomitant administration of kidney-protective amino acids. Other, subacute side effects are related to the radio-peptide itself, such as bone marrow suppression, mild hair loss (observed with ^{177}Lu-octreotate), or, more rarely, an exacerbation of a clinical syndrome (**Box 2**). The most common subacute side effect of PRRT, occurring within 4 to 6 weeks after therapy is bone marrow suppression. Usually, the hematologic toxicity is mild and reversible. More serious, World Health Organization grade 3 or 4 toxicity may occur, but in less than 15% of patients.[11–13,15,17,22,23]

PEPTIDE RECEPTOR RADIONUCLIDE THERAPY: LONG-TERM SIDE EFFECTS

Long-term serious side effects of PRRT are renal failure or myelodysplastic syndrome (MDS)/leukemia. Proper kidney protection with the coinfusion of positively charged amino acids is mandatory in PRRT. With advances in expertise and knowledge about PRRT, cases of severe, end-stage renal damage are currently very rare. However, despite kidney protection, loss of kidney function can occur after PRRT, with a creatinine clearance loss of about 4% per year for ^{177}Lu-octreotate and 7% per year for ^{90}Y-DOTATOC.[26] Studies have demonstrated that a greater and more persistent decline in creatinine clearance is more frequent if risk factors for delayed renal toxicity are present, particularly long-standing and poorly controlled diabetes and hypertension.[27]

With adequate renal amino acid protection, grade 3 to 4 renal toxicity occurs in less than 3% of patients. One recent study, however, reports a grade 3 to 4 renal toxicity in 9% of their patients.[23] This relatively high incidence is probably related to the relatively high activities administered per cycle and to the fact that patients with preexisting

---

Box 1
Peptide receptor radionuclide therapy: quality of life

- [^{177}Lu-DOTA[0],Tyr[3]]octreotate: 265 Dutch patients; European Organization for Research and Treatment of Cancer Core Quality of Life-C30 Questionnaire:
  - Improved Global Health Score in 36% who scored suboptimal at baseline.
  - Improved symptomatology in 40% to 70% of patients who had certain symptoms.

Data from Khan S, Krenning EP, van Essen M, et al. Quality of life in 265 patients with gastroenteropancreatic or bronchial neuroendocrine tumors treated with [177Lu-DOTA0,Tyr3] octreotate. J Nucl Med 2011;52:1361–68.

<table>
<tr><td>

Box 2
Peptide receptor radionuclide therapy: acute and subacute side effects

- *Nausea* after 25% of administrations
- *Vomiting* after 10% of administrations
- *(Abdominal) pain* after 10% of administrations
- *Temporary hair loss* in 60% of patients after [^{177}Lu-DOTA^0,Tyr^3]octreotate
- *Grade 3/4 hematologic toxicity* in less than 15% of patients
- *Hormonal crises* in less than 1% of patients

</td></tr>
</table>

poor kidney function were not excluded from treatment. The possible lack of the use of amino acids in the first years of this study must also be taken into account.[28]

Serious side effects of PRRT on the bone marrow, such as MDS or leukemia, were reported by various groups. Many reports underestimate the occurrence of MDS because of the short follow-up of the patients and also the high loss to follow-up. In some cases, the causal relationship with PRRT may be questioned, because of previous treatments, such as chemotherapy with alkylating agents or radiotherapy. The frequency of MDS seems higher after ^{177}Lu-octreotate than after ^{90}Y-DOTATOC, but also in analyses with long patient follow-up it does not exceed 2% of patients (our unpublished results; **Box 3**).

PEPTIDE RECEPTOR RADIONUCLIDE THERAPY: VARIANTS

Over the past years, different approaches have been tried to improve PRRT.

Combination of Radionuclides

From experiments in rats, it became clear that ^{90}Y-labeled somatostatin analogues may be more effective for larger tumors, and ^{177}Lu-labeled somatostatin analogues may be more effective for smaller tumors, and that their combination may be the most effective.[29] Several retrospective, nonrandomized patient studies seem to indicate the same.[30–32] In a recent follow-up report on the efficacy of the combination of PRRT, Seregni and colleagues[33] reported an objective response rate in 43% of the cases, whereas in their initial report an objective response rate of 67% was reported.[31] This exemplifies the role of selection bias and the need for prospective, randomized

<table>
<tr><td>

Box 3
Peptide receptor radionuclide therapy: long-term serious adverse advents

- [^{90}Y-DOTA^0,Tyr^3]octreotide: Renal insufficiency in 1% to 4% of patients (3 studies); MDS in 2% of cases (1 study)
- [^{90}Y-DOTA^0,Tyr^3]octreotide: Renal insufficiency in 9% of patients in 1 study
  ○ Poor baseline kidney function not excluded
  ○ Not all had amino acid kidney protection
- [^{177}Lu-DOTA^0,Tyr^3]octreotate: Renal insufficiency in less than 1%; MDS in 1% (1 study)
- [^{177}Lu-DOTA^0,Tyr^3]octreotate: MDS in 2% (unpublished, long follow-up data Rotterdam)

Abbreviation: MDS, myelodysplastic syndrome.

</td></tr>
</table>

controlled studies to ultimately prove that PFS is better when using a combination of radionuclides.

Intraarterial Peptide Receptor Radionuclide Therapy

Several groups have investigated the feasibility of locoregional intraarterial, administration of radiolabeled somatostatin analogues for the treatment of livermetastases.[34–37] Intraarterial PRRT results in a greater uptake of radioactivity in liver metastases and tumor response rates seem higher than with intravenous administration. Long-term responses and toxicity data are not available yet. Randomised studies comparing intravenous to intraarterial PRRT are lacking.

Radiosensitizing Drugs and Peptide Receptor Radionuclide Therapy

The application of radiosensitizing chemotherapeutical agents in combination with external beam radiotherapy may lead to increased antitumoral effects. It could therefore be of interest also with PRRT. After proving the safety of the combined therapy, a randomized trial was started comparing treatment with ^{177}Lu-octreotate with and without capecitabine (the oral prodrug of 5-fluoracil; Xeloda; Roche, Basel, Switzerland) in patients with GEPNETs.[38] Results of another nonrandomized phase II study treating patients with a combination of capecitabine and ^{177}Lu-octreotate demonstrated tumor control and stabilization in 94% of the 33 included patients. However, owing to grade 3 capecitabine-induced angina 3 patients discontinued the drug, but were able to complete the intended 4 cycles of PRRT.[39]

Claringbold and colleagues[40] treated GEPNET patients with a combination of ^{177}Lu-octreotate and capecitabine and temozolomide. Thirty-four patients were evaluable for tumor response. Overall, CR was found in 15%, PR in 38%, stable disease (SD) in 38%, and progressive disease (PD) in 9%. Median PFS was 31 months. The study had no control group.

Neoadjuvant Peptide Receptor Radionuclide Therapy

The use of PRRT in patients with inoperable pancreatic NETs who, after tumor shrinkage, may become candidates for surgery is very promising. There are some case reports describing the neoadjuvant use of PRRT in patients with pancreatic NETs who could be operated on successfully after PRRT.[41,42] Van Vliet and colleagues[43] studied 29 patients with a pathology-proven nonfunctioning pancreatic NET treated with ^{177}Lu-octreotate. All patients had a borderline or unresectable pancreatic tumor or oligometastatic disease (defined as ≤3 liver metastases). After the treatment with ^{177}Lu-octreotate, successful surgery was performed in 9 of the 29 patients (31%). The median PFS was 69 months for patients with successful surgery and 49 months for the other patients. The authors conclude that neoadjuvant treatment with ^{177}Lu-octreotate is a valuable option for patients with initially unresectable pancreatic NETs.

Adjuvant Peptide Receptor Radionuclide Therapy

PRRT may also be used in an adjuvant setting after surgery of GEPNETs, preventing tumor growth after spread owing to manipulation of the tumor during surgery or preventing further growth of already present micrometastases. In an animal study, therapy with ^{177}Lu-octreotate prevented or significantly reduced the growth of tumor deposits in the liver after injection of tumor cells via the portal vein mimicking perioperative tumor spill.[44] No data on adjuvant PRRT in man have been published. To detect a difference in survival and/or tumor recurrence rate in patients treated with and without adjuvant PRRT, a large, multicenter trial with years of follow-up would be needed.

Peptide Receptor Radionuclide Therapy As Salvage Therapy

Although tumor response rates after initial treatment with PRRT are encouraging, CR is rare and eventually tumor progression occurs in the majority of patients. Retreatment with extra cycles of PRRT as salvage therapy may then be considered when better alternatives are not available. We reported that "salvage" therapy with 2 additional cycles of ^{177}Lu-octreotate does not lead to serious hematologic or nephrotoxic side effects. However, the tumor response rate was less compared with initial treatment.[45] Also, another report states that long PFS after the initial treatment with PRRT predicts a prolonged PFS after salvage therapy.[46] For that reason, retreatment seems a welcome option for patients who responded well after the initial cycles of PRRT.

Peptide Receptor Radionuclide Therapy with Alpha-Emitters

Several oncologic studies with alpha-particle–emitting radionuclides have been reported, including the treatment of myeloid leukemia with an anti-CD33 monoclonal antibody labeled with [213]bismuth ([213]Bi),[47] the therapy of patients with bone metastases from hormone-refractory prostate cancer with [223]radium,[48] and the locoregional targeted radiotherapy with [211]astatine-labeled antitenascin monoclonal antibody in patients with recurrent malignant brain tumors.[49] Only limited research has been performed on somatostatin analogues labeled with alpha-emitters. Nayak and colleagues[50,51] demonstrated in 2 preclinical studies the advantages of [213]Bi-octreotate over ^{177}Lu-octreotate in a somatostatin receptor-positive cell line. Kratochwil and colleagues[34] reported preliminary data on the therapeutic application of the intraarterial administration of [213]Bi-octreotate. In a dose-escalation study, 10 patients with liver metastases from NET were injected intraarterially with [213]Bi-octreotate. No acute kidney, endocrine or hematologic toxicity was observed during the first escalation steps. Alpha particles have a short path length and are potentially ideal to treat small tumor volumes effectively. Despite the conceptual appeal and the theoretic advantages, the translation of targeted alpha particle therapy into the clinical domain has been slow, on the one hand because of limited radionuclide availability and on the other hand because of the lack of alpha-emitters with physical half-lives practicable in clinical use.

PEPTIDE RECEPTOR RADIONUCLIDE THERAPY: RANDOMISED TRIALS

There is a need for randomised controlled trials comparing PRRT with "standard" treatment, that is, treatment with agents that have proven benefit when tested in randomised trials. A randomised study (NETTER-1 [A Study Comparing Treatment With 177Lu-DOTA0-Tyr3-Octreotate to Octreotide LAR in Patients With Inoperable, Progressive, Somatostatin Receptor Positive Midgut Carcinoid Tumours]) comparing PRRT with ^{177}Lu-octreotate with high-dose sandostatin long-acting release treatment in patients with progressive metastatic midgut carcinoids stopped patient enrollment according to plan in Europe and the United States in early 2015. A study comparing PRRT with sunitinib or everolimus in patients with pancreatic NETs may be expected to follow soon.

COMBINING PEPTIDE RECEPTOR RADIONUCLIDE THERAPY WITH OTHER TREATMENTS

In the past years, new targeted therapies for the treatment of GEPNETs became available. Treatment with sunitinib (Sutent; Pfizer Inc, New York, NY), a tyrosine kinase inhibitor, resulted in a longer median PFS than placebo (11 vs 5 months) in patients with pancreatic NETs.[52] Also, treatment with everolimus (Afinitor; Novartis Pharmaceuticals, Basel, Switzerland), an inhibitor of the mammalian target of rapamycin,

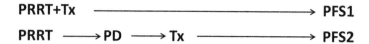

Fig. 3. Scheme for comparing a combination of therapies to their sequential use. PFS, progression-free survival; PRRT, peptide receptor radionuclide therapy; Tx, treatment.

resulted in a longer median PFS than placebo (11 vs 5 months) in patients with pancreatic NETs.[53] The combination of PRRT with sunitinib or everolimus, or the sequential use of PRRT with one of these drugs may therefore be of interest in the treatment of patients with pancreatic NETs.

The next question to be addressed, then, is whether combining PRRT with targeted therapies, such as treatment with everolimus or sunitinib, could improve treatment results in terms of percentage objective responses, or, preferentially, PFS and OS. The question to be answered, however, is whether a combination of PRRT and other therapies performed within a limited time span from one another (for instance, 3–4 months), results in a better PFS than a strategy in which the other therapy is reserved until after (renewed) tumor progression. This may hold true for the combination of PRRT with chemotherapy with, for instance, temozolomide and capecitabine or with everolimus or sunitinib. Such combinations, in our view, are promising only of they result in a longer PFS than when using a sequential approach, in which the second treatment is only started if the disease progresses after the first (**Fig. 3**). A higher percentage of objective responses with a combinatorial approach should not be mistaken for a better treatment outcome, because with any of the 2 single treatments a certain percentage of patients can be expected to have an objective response anyhow, and the added responses will always exceed the response of any single treatment (**Fig. 4**). Also, it was shown in a large multivariate analysis that tumor response other than PD did not result in significant differences in PFS or OS (ie, patients with PR had no longer PFS than those with SD).[19] It should also be kept in mind that in the vast majority of patients the goal of treatment is not cure, but prevention of disease progression. With a limited number of treatment options, combining treatment modalities at the beginning may leave the attending physician empty handed later on.

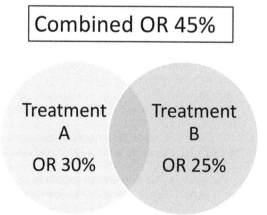

Fig. 4. Venn diagram illustrating that combining treatments will always result in improved response rates. OR, objective response.

SUMMARY

PRRT is a new and valuable treatment for patients with inoperable or metastasized GEPNETs. In general, PRRT is well-tolerated and acute side effects are usually mild and self-limiting. Reported objective response rates range from 15% to 35%, and in terms of PFS and OS PRRT compares favorably with accepted therapies.

Attempts to improve the antitumoral efficacy of PRRT include combining PRRT with radiosensitizing chemotherapeutic agents or combining Y90 and 177Lu as tandem treatment. Another way to improve the uptake of the radiopharmaceutical is by intra-arterial administration of PRRT and is especially suitable in case of high tumor load in the liver. Additional cycles of PRRT as "salvage" therapy may be considered in case of renewed disease progression after PRRT in selected patients. Although PRRT is seldom given with curative intent, neoadjuvant treatment can be of value in patients with initially inoperable pancreatic NETs and PRRT may make these patients candidates for surgery.

Data from randomised controlled trials for PRRT are lacking at the time that this review was written (July 2015). The NETTER-1 study on PRRT with ^{177}Lu-octreotate is the first multicenter, randomized controlled phase III trial that stopped patient enrollment early 2015, and will provide further insights in the safety and efficacy of PRRT by comparing treatment with 177-Lu-octreotate to treatment with high dose somatostatin analogues.

REFERENCES

1. Janson ET, Oberg K. Long-term management of the carcinoid syndrome. Treatment with octreotide alone and in combination with alpha-interferon. Acta Oncol 1993;32:225–9.
2. Ruszniewski P, Ducreux M, Chayvialle JA, et al. Treatment of the carcinoid syndrome with the longacting somatostatin analogue lanreotide: a prospective study in 39 patients. Gut 1996;39:279–83.
3. Rinke A, Müller HH, Schade-Brittinger C, et al. Placebo-controlled, double-blind, prospective, randomized study on the effect of octreotide LAR in the control of tumor growth in patients with metastatic neuroendocrine midgut tumors: a report from the PROMID Study Group. J Clin Oncol 2009;27:4656–63.
4. Caplin ME, Pavel M, Ćwikła JB, et al. Lanreotide in metastatic enteropancreatic neuroendocrine tumors. N Engl J Med 2014;371:224–33.
5. Reubi JC, Waser B, Schaer JC, et al. Somatostatin receptor sst1-sst5 expression in normal and neoplastic human tissues using receptor autoradiography with subtype-selective ligands. Eur J Nucl Med 2001;28:836–46.
6. Balon HR, Goldsmith SJ, Siegel BA, et al. Procedure guideline for somatostatin receptor scintigraphy with (111)In-pentetreotide. J Nucl Med 2001;42:1134–8.
7. Gabriel M, Decristoforo C, Kendler D, et al. 68Ga-DOTA-Tyr3-octreotide PET in neuroendocrine tumors: comparison with somatostatin receptor scintigraphy and CT. J Nucl Med 2007;48:508–18.
8. Kayani I, Bomanji JB, Groves A, et al. Functional imaging of neuroendocrine tumors with combined PET/CT using 68Ga-DOTATATE (DOTA-DPhe1,Tyr3-octreotate) and 18F-FDG. Cancer 2008;112:2447–55.
9. Valkema R, De Jong M, Bakker WH, et al. Phase I study of peptide receptor radionuclide therapy with [In-DTPA]octreotide: the Rotterdam experience. Semin Nucl Med 2002;32:110–22.
10. Anthony LB, Woltering EA, Espenan GD, et al. Indium-111-pentetreotide prolongs survival in gastroenteropancreatic malignancies. Semin Nucl Med 2002;32:123–32.

11. Bodei L, Cremonesi M, Zoboli S, et al. Receptor-mediated radionuclide therapy with 90Y-DOTATOC in association with amino acid infusion: a phase I study. Eur J Nucl Med Mol Imaging 2003;30:207–16.

12. Waldherr C, Pless M, Maecke HR, et al. The clinical value of [90Y-DOTA]-D-Phe1-Tyr3-octreotide (90Y-DOTATOC) in the treatment of neuroendocrine tumours: a clinical phase II study. Ann Oncol 2001;12:941–5.

13. Waldherr C, Pless M, Maecke HR, et al. Tumor response and clinical benefit in neuroendocrine tumors after 7.4 GBq (90)Y-DOTATOC. J Nucl Med 2002;43: 610–6.

14. Waldherr C, Schumacher T, Maecke H, et al. Does tumor response depend on the number of treatment sessions at constant injected dose using 90Yttrium-DOTATOC in neuroendocrine tumors? [abstract]. Eur J Nucl Med Mol Imaging 2002;29(Suppl 1):S100.

15. Valkema R, Pauwels S, Kvols LK, et al. Survival and response after peptide receptor radionuclide therapy with [90Y-DOTA0,Tyr3]octreotide in patients with advanced gastroenteropancreatic neuroendocrine tumors. Semin Nucl Med 2006;36:147–56.

16. Bushnell DL Jr, O'Dorisio TM, O'Dorisio MS, et al. 90Y-edotreotide for metastatic carcinoid refractory to octreotide. J Clin Oncol 2010;28:1652–9.

17. Pfeifer AK, Gregersen T, Gronbaek H, et al. Peptide receptor radionuclide therapy with Y-DOTATOC and (177)Lu-DOTATOC in advanced neuroendocrine tumors: results from a Danish cohort treated in Switzerland. Neuroendocrinology 2011;93:189–96.

18. Cwikla JB, Sankowski A, Seklecka N, et al. Efficacy of radionuclide treatment DOTATATE Y-90 in patients with progressive metastatic gastroenteropancreatic neuroendocrine carcinomas (GEP-NETs): a phase II study. Ann Oncol 2010;21: 787–94.

19. Kwekkeboom DJ, de Herder WW, Kam BL, et al. Treatment with the radiolabeled somatostatin analog [177 Lu-DOTA 0,Tyr3]octreotate: toxicity, efficacy, and survival. J Clin Oncol 2008;26:2124–30.

20. Sward C, Bernhardt P, Ahlman H, et al. [177Lu-DOTA 0-Tyr 3]-octreotate treatment in patients with disseminated gastroenteropancreatic neuroendocrine tumors: the value of measuring absorbed dose to the kidney. World J Surg 2010;34:1368–72.

21. Garkavij M, Nickel M, Sjogreen-Gleisner K, et al. 177Lu-[DOTA0,Tyr3] octreotate therapy in patients with disseminated neuroendocrine tumors: analysis of dosimetry with impact on future therapeutic strategy. Cancer 2010;116:1084–92.

22. Bodei L, Cremonesi M, Grana CM, et al. Peptide receptor radionuclide therapy with (1)(7)(7)Lu-DOTATATE: the IEO phase I-II study. Eur J Nucl Med Mol Imaging 2011;38:2125–35.

23. Imhof A, Brunner P, Marincek N, et al. Response, survival, and long-term toxicity after therapy with the radiolabeled somatostatin analogue [90Y-DOTA]-TOC in metastasized neuroendocrine cancers. J Clin Oncol 2011;29:2416–23.

24. Reubi JC, Schar JC, Waser B, et al. Affinity profiles for human somatostatin receptor subtypes SST1-SST5 of somatostatin radiotracers selected for scintigraphic and radiotherapeutic use. Eur J Nucl Med 2000;27:273–82.

25. Khan S, Krenning EP, van Essen M, et al. Quality of life in 265 patients with gastroenteropancreatic or bronchial neuroendocrine tumors treated with [177Lu-DOTA0,Tyr3]octreotate. J Nucl Med 2011;52:1361–8.

26. Valkema R, Pauwels SA, Kvols LK, et al. Long-term follow-up of renal function after peptide receptor radiation therapy with (90)Y-DOTA(0),Tyr(3)-octreotide and (177)Lu-DOTA(0), Tyr(3)-octreotate. J Nucl Med 2005;46(Suppl 1):83S–91S.

27. Bodei L, Cremonesi M, Ferrari M, et al. Long-term evaluation of renal toxicity after peptide receptor radionuclide therapy with 90Y-DOTATOC and 177Lu-DOTATATE: the role of associated risk factors. Eur J Nucl Med Mol Imaging 2008;35:1847–56.

28. Otte A, Herrmann R, Heppeler A, et al. Yttrium-90 DOTATOC: first clinical results. Eur J Nucl Med 1999;26:1439–47.

29. de Jong M, Breeman WA, Valkema R, et al. Combination radionuclide therapy using 177Lu- and 90Y-labeled somatostatin analogs. J Nucl Med 2005;46(Suppl 1): 13S–7S.

30. Kunikowska J, Królicki L, Hubalewska-Dydejczyk A, et al. Clinical results of radionuclide therapy of neuroendocrine tumours with 90Y-DOTATATE and tandem 90Y/177Lu-DOTATATE: which is a better therapy option? Eur J Nucl Med Mol Imaging 2011;38:1788–97.

31. Seregni E, Maccauro M, Coliva A, et al. Treatment with tandem [(90)Y]DOTA-TATE and [(177)Lu] DOTA-TATE of neuroendocrine tumors refractory to conventional therapy: preliminary results. Q J Nucl Med Mol Imaging 2010;54:84–91.

32. Villard L, Romer A, Marincek N, et al. Cohort study of somatostatin-based radiopeptide therapy with [(90)Y-DOTA]-TOC versus [(90)Y-DOTA]-TOC plus [(177)Lu-DOTA]-TOC in neuroendocrine cancers. J Clin Oncol 2012;30:1100–6.

33. Seregni E, Maccauro M, Chiesa C, et al. Treatment with tandem [90Y]DOTA-TATE and [177Lu]DOTA-TATE of neuroendocrine tumours refractory to conventional therapy. Eur J Nucl Med Mol Imaging 2014;41:223–30.

34. Kratochwil C, Giesel FL, Lopez-Benitez R, et al. Intraindividual comparison of selective arterial versus venous 68Ga-DOTATOC PET/CT in patients with gastroenteropancreatic neuroendocrine tumors. Clin Cancer Res 2010;16:2899–905.

35. Pool SE, Kam BL, Koning GA, et al. [(111)In-DTPA]octreotide tumor uptake in GEPNET liver metastases after intra-arterial administration: an overview of preclinical and clinical observations and implications for tumor radiation dose after peptide radionuclide therapy. Cancer Biother Radiopharm 2014;29:179–87.

36. Limouris GS, Chatziioannou A, Kontogeorgakos D, et al. Selective hepatic arterial infusion of In-111-DTPA-Phe1-octreotide in neuroendocrine liver metastases. Eur J Nucl Med Mol Imaging 2008;35:1827–37.

37. Kratochwil C, Giesel FL, Bruchertseifer F. 213Bi-DOTATOC receptor-targeted alpha-radionuclide therapy induces remission in neuroendocrine tumours refractory to beta radiation: a first-in-human experience. Eur J Nucl Med Mol Imaging 2014;41:2106–19.

38. van Essen M, Krenning EP, Kam BL, et al. Report on short-term side effects of treatments with 177Lu-octreotate in combination with capecitabine in seven patients with gastroenteropancreatic neuroendocrine tumours. Eur J Nucl Med Mol Imaging 2008;35:743–8.

39. Claringbold PG, Brayshaw PA, Price RA, et al. Phase II study of radiopeptide 177Lu-octreotate and capecitabine therapy of progressive disseminated neuroendocrine tumours. Eur J Nucl Med Mol Imaging 2011;38:302–11.

40. Claringbold PG, Price RA, Turner JH. Phase I-II study of radiopeptide 177Lu-octreotate in combination with capecitabine and temozolomide in advanced low-grade neuroendocrine tumors. Cancer Biother Radiopharm 2012;27:561–9.

41. Kaemmerer D, Prasad V, Daffner W, et al. Neoadjuvant peptide receptor radionuclide therapy for an inoperable neuroendocrine pancreatic tumor. World J Gastroenterol 2009;15:5867–70.

42. Stoeltzing O, Loss M, Huber E, et al. Staged surgery with neoadjuvant 90Y-DOTATOC therapy for down-sizing synchronous bilobular hepatic metastases from a neuroendocrine pancreatic tumor. Langenbecks Arch Surg 2010;395:185–92.

43. Van Vliet EI, Van Eijck CH, De Krijger RR, et al. Neoadjuvant treatment of nonfunctioning pancreatic neuroendocrine tumors with [^{177}Lu-DOTA^0,Tyr^3]octreotate. J Nucl Med 2015. [Epub ahead of print].

44. Breeman WA, Mearadji A, Capello A, et al. Anti-tumor effect and increased survival after treatment with [177Lu-DOTA0,Tyr3]octreotate in a rat liver micrometastases model. Int J Cancer 2003;104:376–9.

45. van Essen M, Krenning EP, Kam BL, et al. Salvage therapy with (177)Lu-octreotate in patients with bronchial and gastroenteropancreatic neuroendocrine tumors. J Nucl Med 2010;51:383–90.

46. Sabet A, Haslerud T, Pape UF, et al. Outcome and toxicity of salvage therapy with 177Lu-octreotate in patients with metastatic gastroenteropancreatic neuroendocrine tumours. Eur J Nucl Med Mol Imaging 2014;41:205–10.

47. Jurcic JG, Larson SM, Sgouros G, et al. Targeted alpha particle immunotherapy for myeloid leukemia. Blood 2002;100:1233–9.

48. Nilsson S, Franzén L, Parker C, et al. Bone-targeted radium-223 in symptomatic, hormone-refractory prostate cancer: a randomised, multicentre, placebo-controlled phase II study. Lancet Oncol 2007;8:587–94.

49. Zalutsky MR, Reardon DA, Akabani G, et al. Clinical experience with alpha-particle emitting 211At: treatment of recurrent brain tumor patients with 211At-labeled chimeric antitenascin monoclonal antibody 81C6. J Nucl Med 2008;49:30–8.

50. Nayak T, Norenberg J, Anderson T, et al. A comparison of high- versus low-linear energy transfer somatostatin receptor targeted radionuclide therapy in vitro. Cancer Biother Radiopharm 2005;20:52–7.

51. Nayak TK, Norenberg JP, Anderson TL, et al. Somatostatin-receptor-targeted alpha-emitting 213Bi is therapeutically more effective than beta(-)-emitting 177Lu in human pancreatic adenocarcinoma cells. Nucl Med Biol 2007;34:185–93.

52. Raymond E, Dahan L, Raoul JL, et al. Sunitinib malate for the treatment of pancreatic neuroendocrine tumors. N Engl J Med 2011;364:501–13.

53. Yao JC, Shah MH, Ito T, et al. Everolimus for advanced pancreatic neuroendocrine tumors. N Engl J Med 2011;364:514–23.

Hepatic-directed Therapies in Patients with Neuroendocrine Tumors

Andrew S. Kennedy, MD[a,b]

KEYWORDS

- Hepatic-directed therapies • Neuroendocrine tumors
- Therapy response and survival • Metastases • Intra-arterial

KEY POINTS

- Intra-arterial therapies for unresectable liver metastases from neuroendocrine primary tumors are supported by level 2a medical evidence (National Cancer Institute) regarding symptom control and imaging response.
- There is insufficient medical evidence showing which intra-arterial therapy (transarterial embolization [TAE], transarterial chemoembolization [TACE], transarterial radioembolization [TARE]) provides the highest response rate, progression-free survival, or overall survival.
- TARE produces less toxicity and has similar efficacy to TAE and TACE.
- Intra-arterial therapies are an important aspect of managing metastases from neuroendocrine tumor liver disease in all stages of disease, including asymptomatic, first-line, salvage, and palliation scenarios.

INTRODUCTION

Neuroendocrine tumors (NETs) of the gastrointestinal (GI) tract have a propensity for producing hepatic metastases. The liver is the most common site of metastatic dissemination from NETs and this occurs in from 10% to 65% of cases.[1,2] Most GI NETs arise from the foregut or midgut, are malignant, and can cause severe debilitating symptoms adversely affecting quality of life.[3–5] Aggressive treatments to reduce symptoms have an important role in therapy.

Patients with GI NETs usually present with inoperable metastatic disease and severe symptoms from a variety of hormones and biogenic amines. Less than 10% of patients with small bowel and colon NETs experience what is referred to as carcinoid syndrome,[5] the symptoms of which are episodic flushing, bronchoconstriction

[a] Radiation Oncology Research, Sarah Cannon Research Institute, Nashville, TN, USA;
[b] Department of Biomedical Engineering, Department of Mechanical and Aerospace Engineering, North Carolina State University, Raleigh, NC, USA
E-mail address: Andrew.Kennedy@sarahcannon.com

Hematol Oncol Clin N Am 30 (2016) 193–207
http://dx.doi.org/10.1016/j.hoc.2015.09.010
0889-8588/16/$ – see front matter © 2016 Elsevier Inc. All rights reserved.

(wheezing), diarrhea, and eventually heart valve dysfunction. Disease progression differs widely[4] but the overall median survival is 75 months.[6] With metastatic disease, 5-year survival rates are less than 20%.[7,8] In patients with advanced, unresectable liver metastases the treatment challenge is directed toward palliating symptoms and slowing down or stabilizing tumor growth.

Metastases from NETs (mNETs) to the liver represent a significant clinical entity, and multiple treatment modalities have been used, engaging multidisciplinary teams of gastroenterologists, diagnostic radiologists, oncologists, surgeons, and interventional radiologists. Management modalities used in patients with unresectable metastatic disease, described in other articles of this issue, include systemic chemotherapy, somatostatin analogues, cryotherapy, radiofrequency ablation, peptide receptor radiation therapy, percutaneous alcohol injection, and hepatic transplantation.[3,9–19]

This article describes intra-arterial hepatic-directed therapies for mNETs, a group of treatments in which the therapeutic and/or embolic agents are released intra-arterially in specific hepatic vessels to target tumors.

HEPATIC ANATOMY AND RATIONALE FOR INTRA-ARTERIAL THERAPIES

The unique double vascular supply of the liver, through the portal vein and the hepatic artery, and the predominantly arterial irrigation of liver tumors are the basis for intra-arterial therapies.[20] Three types of hepatic arterial embolization techniques are currently in use: transarterial embolization (TAE); transarterial chemoembolization (TACE), which includes using drug-eluting beads (DEBs); and radioactive microsphere release into arteries. Radioactive microsphere release is also known as radioembolization, transarterial radioembolization (TARE), and selective internal radiation therapy (SIRT).[8,21–23] TARE is a form of brachytherapy in which intra-arterially injected microspheres loaded with yttrium 90 (^{90}Y) serve as sealed sources for internal radiation via a near-pure beta-decay isotope with limited tissue penetrance in the range of 2 to 3 mm.[21,22]

A well-established body of literature has described the process of tumoral angiogenesis occurring exclusively from the hepatic arterial supply.[20,24,25] Circulation from the portal vein does not provide a significant contribution to tumor perfusion. Catheter-based hepatic arterial administration of therapy therefore results in a preferential deposition of a drug/particle into the tumor vasculature, which minimizes liver parenchymal exposure. Carrier-based delivery of chemotherapeutics is achieved via either the infusion of a lipiodol/water-based emulsion or via statically charged DEBs.

INTRA-ARTERIAL THERAPIES REVIEW

The various facets of intra-arterial therapies are discussed here, including their mechanisms of action, patient eligibility factors, and common toxicities arising from liver treatment, as well as therapy response evaluations and retreatment factors.

Mechanisms of Action

Arterial embolization, or TAE, is the general term for the procedure by which a catheter is inserted into an artery percutaneously, eventually directly accessing the hepatic artery. Contrast is subsequently injected via the catheter to verify its position relative to the vascular distribution of the target tumor. Contrast is frequently used during and after delivery of the therapeutic agent to monitor progress of treatment and verify completion of intended effect (ie, stasis or pruning of tumor arteries).

Transarterial embolization

In hepatic transarterial (bland) embolization, catheterization is typically followed by the injection of 50 μm of polyvinyl alcohol (PVA) particles, with or without ethiodized oil. No chemotherapeutic agents are used. The PVA particles physically occlude blood flow through the selected hepatic artery, thereby inducing ischemic injury; if stasis remains unachieved, then larger PVA particles of 200 to 500 μm can be used.[15,26,27] Hypoxia is the goal of TAE with subsequent ischemic tumor cell death.

Transarterial chemoembolization

TACE follows the same principles as TAE, but an intra-arterial chemotherapeutic agent is added at the time of embolization. TACE has the potential to result in intratumoral drug concentrations more than 20 times greater than those afforded by the systemic administration of the same drug.[28] In addition, TACE affords the potential clinical benefit of tumor ischemia following embolization. Drugs that are commonly used for this purpose include doxorubicin, irinotecan, mitomycin C, and streptozocin.

Overall, TACE embraces different procedures that share 2 different aims: (1) to increase the exposure of tumor cells to cytotoxic agents, and (2) to induce ischemic necrosis. This aim is usually accomplished by the sequential intra-arterial injection of chemotherapeutic agents and embolizing particles. The wide variety of drug vehicles, cytotoxic agents, and embolizing particles has introduced numerous variations worldwide and no standard protocol has been uniformly adopted. Centers have different choices regarding type and/or dose of the anticancer agents used, use of lipiodol as a vehicle, embolizing material, selectivity of catheter positioning, embolization end points, and schedule and/or interval of retreatment.

Although the most popular technique used in conventional TACE has been the administration of an anticancer-in-lipiodol emulsion followed by embolic agents, bland embolization is still preferred in some centers, and TACE with drug-eluting particles (DEB-TACE) has replaced conventional regimens in others.[19,23,25,29,30]

Transarterial chemoembolization using drug-eluting beads

The concept of DEB-TACE is to intra-arterially inject embolizing particles that have been loaded in vitro with cytotoxic agents and slowly release them into the tumor environment. These beads are composed of either a sulfonate-modified PVA hydrogel (DC-Beads, Biocompatibles, Surrey, United Kingdom) or a sodium acrylate and vinyl alcohol copolymer (HepaSphere, BioSphere Medical, Inc, Rockland, MA). DEB-TACE provides a way of performing TACE in a more standardized way and has shown that when the optimal patients are selected, the beneficial effect of TACE can challenge that of percutaneous ablation.[10,23]

The 2 most common DEB platforms are based on PVA (DC/LC Bead, BTG, UK Ltd) and acryl-amine polymer (AAP; Quadrasphere, Merit Medical, South Jordan, UT) substrates that possess static charge. This charge allows oppositely charged molecules to bind and release via ion exchange.[25,31,32] For PVA, the ionic interaction occurs between the positively charged chemotherapy, typically doxorubicin or an irinotecan (IRI) salt, and the negatively charged sulfonic acid group. In AAP, the drug binds to carboxylate groups.[33,34] When DEBs are loaded with IRI, the procedure, platform, and technique are collectively termed DEBIRI. Dose intensity of IRI varies widely in the literature, with a reported dose range of 50 to 200 mg of IRI loaded onto 2 to 4 mL of DEBs.

DEBs possess a pharmacologic advantage by offering simultaneous embolization and sustained release of the drug to the tumor.[10] Some studies have shown that the pharmacokinetics of chemotherapy delivery trend toward controlled release in some configurations of DEB.[10,31,34] However, DEBs have a significant cost compared with non–DEB-TACE.[35] More importantly, the drugs currently used in DEBs have not been specifically proved to be active against mNETs.

Radioembolization (transarterial radioembolization)

TARE comprises those procedures in which intra-arterially injected radioactive microspheres are used for internal radiation treatment.[8,22,23,25,36] There are 2 types of commercially available radioactive microspheres: a ceramic/glass composition (TheraSphere, BTG International Ltd, London, United Kingdom) and resin polymer microsphere (SIR-Spheres; Sirtex Medical Limited, Sydney, Australia). Both use ^{90}Y as the radiation-emitting isotope. ^{90}Y is a pure beta emitter with half-life of 64.2 hours (94% of the energy is emitted in the first 11 days) and average tissue penetration of 2.5 mm (isolation for radiation protection is not needed after implantation). Because of their small size (25–45 μm), they produce no significant ischemic effect, as opposed to the greater than 100-μm particles used in TACE. To avoid misplacement of particles in extrahepatic territories, a thorough angiographic evaluation is performed 1 to 2 weeks before treatment to detect and eventually occlude aberrant vessels arising from hepatic arteries that may feed the gastrointestinal tract, and to measure the hepatopulmonary shunting using technetium-99m–labeled macroaggregated albumin.

TACE and TARE should not be considered competing therapies, but complementary tools. For many patients, their individual tumor and normal liver characteristics are such that they are candidates for either TACE/TAE or TARE. There are potential advantages and disadvantages with each approach.[21] Overall, TARE does not have the two main contraindications for use that limit use of TACE, mainly limited use in bulky disease and portal vein thrombosis, but still have a good liver function.

Fundamentally, embolic therapy is designed to exploit and preferentially deposit therapeutic particles into the blood vessels feeding the tumor. In the setting of TARE, this technique is justified because the preferential deposition of radiation into the tumor vascular bed results in targeted delivery of therapy and cell killing by radiation not ischemia.[37] In contrast, given the mechanism of action and metabolism associated with DEBIRI, trials indicate that the metabolism or conversion into its active metabolite occurs within the normal hepatic parenchyma, not the tumor.[25] Therefore embolic effects may predominate in TACE/DEB-TACE approaches, whereas ischemia is not a factor in radiation-mediated TARE tumor cell kill. Hypoxia is a critically important inhibitor of radiation effectiveness and thus is actively avoided.

Patient Selection Factors: Eligibility

Indications for eligibility include nonoperative candidates with symptomatic or asymptomatic tumors, with dominant metastatic burden in the liver. Contraindications include main portal vein thrombosis (TAE/TACE), bilirubin level greater than 2 mg/dL, inability to adequately prevent significant extrahepatic deposition of therapeutic agents, and contraindications to angiography.

Transarterial embolization/transarterial chemoembolization: classic and drug-eluting beads

To be selected for TAE or TACE, patients generally must meet the criteria discussed earlier with additional contraindications to treatment that include pregnancy, myelosuppression, and renal failure.[19]

Radioembolization (transarterial radioembolization)

Patients can only be considered for TARE if they have sufficiently compensated liver function with main factors of normal or near-normal serum total bilirubin level

(<2 mg/dL), no coagulopathy, and if they have minimal ascites and no hepatic enceph-alopathy.[8] Patients are included or excluded by well-established and accepted pa-rameters regarding liver reserve and vascular access. Vascular issues of import include the ability to isolate the liver arterial tree from gastric and small bowel branches. Also excluded for safety reasons are patients with arteriovenous fistulas in tumors that allow a high percentage of microspheres to pass through the liver capil-lary bed to the lung vascular bed. Controversy exists as to what percentage of shunt-ing excludes patients from TARE, which is based on a few case reports involving hepatocellular carcinoma tumors. A guideline from both manufacturers of TARE mi-crospheres has limited the total lung absorbed dose of radiation to 30 Gy (instruction documents, SirSphere and TheraSphere).[22] Subsequent reports have called this dose level in lungs into question.[38] No patient with mNET has been reported to have expe-rienced pneumonitis or severe pulmonary side effects. Absolute contraindications have been: pregnant women, heavily previously irradiated liver volumes, and predicted normal liver volume remaining after TARE to be less than 700 cm^3.

Common Toxicities of Liver Treatment by Intra-arterial Therapy

Toxicities resulting most often from the use of TAE, TACE, and TARE are similar but have some significant and important different entities based on the mechanisms of action.

Transarterial embolization/classic transarterial chemoembolization and drug-eluting beads transarterial chemoembolization

Posttreatment side effects reported from TAE, TACE, or both may include nausea, vomiting, abdominal pain, diarrhea, weight loss, fever, hepatorenal syndrome, sepsis, transient myelosuppression, as well as the more rare complications of anasarca, cortical blindness, necrotizing cholecystitis, pancreatitis, and hepatic abscess (**Table 1**).[21,35,39–41] Commonly referred to as postembolization syndrome after TAE/TACE, up to 40% of patients remain as inpatients on the day of treatment, for an average of 3 days to receive intravenous medications for pain, nausea, and dehydra-tion. Once it resolves, it does not recur and has been described as an ischemic phenomenon.

Doxorubicin has shown a narrow window of activity with significant toxicities, including liver failure, in its use with colorectal metastases in animal models.[42] In colo-rectal metastases, when this toxicity profile is considered with the well-documented resistance of colorectal metastases to doxorubicin,[43,44] its application in intra-arterial and liver-directed therapies of NETs is unsubstantiated and may potentially be harm-ful.[25] Guiu and colleagues[45] reported on consecutive patients treated with DEBs (irinotecan) and evaluated each for liver or biliary injuries as seen on MRI or computed tomography (CT) scans. A total of 120 patients with mNETs and 88 patients with he-patocellular carcinoma were studied. Liver/biliary injury followed 17.2% (82 of 476) of sessions in 30.8% (64 of 208) of patients. The occurrence of liver/biliary injury was associated with DEBs (odds ratio [OR], 6.63; P<.001) not dependent on the tumor type. Biloma/parenchymal infarct was strongly associated with both DEBs (OR, 9.78; P = .002) and mNET histology (OR, 8.13; P = .04). Biloma/liver infarcts were managed conservatively but were associated with an increase in serum levels of aspartate aminotransferase, alanine aminotransferase, alkaline phosphatases, and gamma glutamyl transpeptidase (P = .005, P = .005, P = .012, and P = .006, respectively).[45]

Fiore and colleagues[46] retrospectively investigated 30 patients with gastroentero-pancreatic NETs with liver metastases. Seventeen patients underwent TAE and

Table 1
Toxicities after TAE or TACE (classic and DEBs)

Study	N	Device Used	Toxicity
Dong	123	TACE	Abdominal pain (44%), diarrhea (30%), weight loss (22%)
de Baere	20	TACE with doxorubicin-eluting beads	Nausea (61%), fever (36%)
Vogl	48	TACE with mitomycin C / TACE with mitomycin C + gemcitabine	Nausea and vomiting (27.8%), abdominal pain (11.1%) / Nausea and vomiting (16.7%), abdominal pain (10%)
Loewe	23	Bland embolization	Not reported
Eriksson	41	Bland embolization	Postembolization syndrome (all), nausea (33%), fever (7 patients), median hospitalization: 12 d
Pitt	100	Bland[51] vs TACE[49]	Bland: 7 of 51, (3 liver abscesses, 1 groin hematoma, 2 ileus, 1 hypotension) TACE: none
Ruutiainen	67	Bland[23] vs TACE[44]	Grade 3 or worse toxicity in 25% of TACE and 22% of bland TACE ($\geq$grade 3): pain (3), nausea (1), GGT/ALP (4), AST (1), infection (1) Bland ($\geq$grade 3): GGT/ALP (3), AST (1), cardiac (1)
Gupta	49	TACE[27] vs bland[42]	Serious adverse events in 19 patients (8.5%), hepatorenal syndrome (7), sepsis (6), transient myelosuppression (1), anasarca (1), cortical blindness (1), necrotizing cholecystitis (1), hepatic abscess (2), overall complications in TACE, 20%; bland, 12%
Maire	26	TACE[12] vs bland[14]	TACE: postembolization syndrome (10), carcinoid crisis (2), acute liver failure (1), neutropenia (2) Bland: postembolization syndrome (10), carcinoid crisis (0), acute liver failure (2), neutropenia (0)
Guiu	120 NET 88 HCC	DEB-TACE in HCC (cirrhotic) and NETs (noncirrhotic)	Liver biliary injury occurred in 64 of 208 patients. Occurrence associated with DEB-TACE $P<.001$ irrespective of tumor type
Ruszniewski	23	TACE	Bleeding peptic ulcer (1), oligoanuric renal failure (1), abdominal pain (50%), fever (6 patients), nausea and vomiting (5)

Abbreviations: AST, aspartate transaminase; ALP, alkaline phosphatase; GGT, gamma-glutamyl transferase; HCC, hepatocellular carcinoma.
Data from Refs.[26,30,39,45,53–55,59–62]

13 patients underwent TACE. These investigators concluded that although TAE and TACE are both effective in patients with mNETs, TAE is preferred to TACE in light of its similar antitumor effects and slightly better toxicity profile.[46] The choice of TAE versus TACE continues to be controversial without definitive medical evidence and is therefore driven by institutional experience and preference.

Radioembolization (transarterial radioembolization)

Patients are evaluated at least during the 6th and 12th weeks after TARE treatment, with some patients needing more frequent evaluations (**Table 2**). During follow-up visits, laboratory data are obtained, including liver function tests; tumor markers if levels are increased before treatment; abdominal imaging with CT, MRI, or PET/OctreoScan; and a physical examination with recent history taken for side effects. After 12 weeks, patients resume a routine schedule of laboratory tests and imaging at 3-month intervals. Acute toxicities are most often mild abdominal pain lasting from day 1 to day 3, and rarely needing narcotics to control discomfort. Nausea and emesis are typically mild and controlled with antiemetics. Fatigue can last up to 14 days after treatment. Serious injuries are rare, with gastric or duodenal ulcer formation in 2% to 5% and radioembolization-induced liver disease occurring in less than 1% of all patients.

Kalinowski and colleagues[47] completed the only quality-of-life study in liver embolotherapy on NETs, but that study investigated only resin TARE treatments and included a sample of just 9 patients. However, coupled with other prospective and retrospective studies,[8,36,48–52] the report suggests that the acute toxicity profile of TARE is lower than those of TAE or TACE.

Therapy Response and Survival

Patients with extensive liver tumor burden experience poorer imaging response to embolization, as well as a greater rate of major complications. For patients who are not candidates for surgery, selective TAE, TACE, or TARE can produce objective responses, decreased levels of tumor markers, and control of symptoms. However, none of these techniques has been shown to be clearly superiority to the others in a

Table 2			
Toxicities after radioembolization (TARE)			
Study	**N**	**Device Used**	**Toxicity**
Rhee[51]	42	Yttrium 90 (glass) Yttrium 90 (resin)	Grade III/IV (14%)
Kennedy[8]	148	Yttrium 90 (resin)	33% (grade III), fatigue (6.5%)
King[36]	58	Yttrium 90 (resin) plus 5-FU	Radiation gastritis (2 patients), duodenal ulcer (1 patient),
Saxena[52]	48	Yttrium 90 (resin)	0.5% (grade III) 1 patient (biliary obstruction)
Cao[48]	58	Yttrium 90 (resin) plus 5-FU	Not reported
Paprottka[50]	42	Yttrium 90 (resin)	0% grade III
Memon[49]	40	Yttrium 90 (glass)	Fatigue (63%, all grades); nausea/vomiting (40%, all grades); grade III, IV (bilirubin, 8%; albumin, 2%; lymphocyte, 38%)

Abbreviations: 5-FU, 5-fluorouracil; HCC, hepatocellular carcinoma.
  Data from Refs.[8,36,48–52]

randomized controlled trial. Therefore, no statement on which intra-arterial therapy offers the best progression-free survival (PFS) and overall survival (OS) can be made. Bearing in mind the heterogeneity of metastases from NETs and the difficulty of defining cohorts of patients with the same pathologic classification of disease, rates of symptomatic response to TAE, TACE, and TARE in most studies seem to be 39% to 95% within a time period of 1 to 18 months from treatment.[21] Most patients therefore experience improvements in hormonal syndromes and the symptoms caused by the disease burden.

Transarterial embolization/transarterial chemoembolization: classic and drug-eluting beads

Hepatic arterial therapy in the management of mNETs has shown a response rate as high as 70% to 90% in retrospective, uncontrolled case study reports (**Table 3**).[35] TACE produces symptomatic responses in 53% to 100% of patients (10–55 months) and morphologic responses in 35% to 74% (6–63 months), with PFS of about 18 months and 5-year survival of 40% to 83%. Mortality varies from 0% to 5% and morbidity (ie, postembolization syndrome) varies from 28% to 90%.[40]

Dong and Carr[53] reported their experience of TACE in 123 patients with mNET; a 62% radiologic response was recorded with a mean survival of 3.3 years, and 3-year, 5-year, and 10-year survivals reported as 59%, 36%, and 20%, respectively. Few reports have such detailed long-term data on survival.

Because embolization stimulates release of vascular endothelial growth factor (VEGF) into the circulation, Strosberg and colleagues[27] investigated the use of sunitinib, an oral VEGF receptor inhibitor, in hepatic TAE for mNETs. They hypothesized that sunitinib could be safely administered after embolization. In their phase II clinical trial (n = 39), they concluded that the observed median PFS of 15.2 months and 59% 4-year OS (95% confidence interval, 0.38–0.80) associated with this sequence were encouraging.[27]

Pitt and colleagues[26] evaluated 100 patients using conventional TACE, and showed acceptable morbidity and mortality and an 88% improvement in symptoms, with a reasonable and well-established median OS. Median from diagnosis: TACE (n = 49), 50.1 months; bland, 39.1 months. One-year, 2-year, and 5-year survival: TACE, 69%, 52%, 19%, respectively; TAE (n = 51), 19%, 70%, 13%, respectively.

Ruutiainen and colleagues[54] investigated 219 embolization procedures in 67 patients: 23 patients received primarily bland embolization with PVA with or without iodized oil and 44 primarily received chemoembolization with cisplatin, doxorubicin, mitomycin C, iodized oil, and PVA. Radiologic response in TACE was 22% and in TAE was 38%. TACE was not associated with a higher degree of toxicity than TAE. TACE trended toward improvement in time to progression, symptom control, and survival. Survival for 1-year, 3-year, and 5-year survival for TACE was 86%, 67%, and 50%, respectively; for TAE it was 68%, 46%, and 33%, respectively.

Ruszniewski and colleagues[55] conducted one of the few prospective studies of intra-arterial therapies in the literature, randomizing and comparing TAE and TACE. The partial response (PR), stable disease (SD), progressive disease (PD), and time to progression (TTP) were 61, 22, 17, and 14 months, respectively. Eight of the 23 patients died at a median of 12.5 months after receiving their final TACE procedure.

Vogl and colleagues[39] studied TACE alone with either mitomycin C (group 1) or mitomycin C plus gemcitabine (group 2). Group 1 had a radiologic response of 11.1% (RECIST 1.0 [response evaluation criteria in solid tumors]) and a median survival of 38.7 months; 11.11% survived 5 years. Group 2 response was 23.3%, with a median survival of 57.1 months; 5-year survival was 46.67%.

Table 3
Response and survival after TAE or TACE (classic and DEB)

Study	N	Device Used	Radiologic Response; RECIST 1.0 (%)	Survival Times and Rates
Dong & Carr[53]	123	TACE	62	Mean: 3.3 y 3-y, 5-y, and 10-y survival: 59%, 36%, and 20%
de Baere[59]	20	TACE with doxorubicin-eluting beads	80	Not reported
Vogl[39]	48	TACE with mitomycin C	11.1	Median: 38.6 7 mo 5 y: 11.11%
		TACE with mitomycin C + gemcitabine	23.33	Median: 57.1 5 y: 46.67%
Loewe[30]	23	Bland embolization	73	Median: 69 mo 1-y and 5-y survival: 95.7% and 65.4%
Eriksson[60]	41	Bland embolization	50	Median: 80 mo 5 y: 60%
Pitt[26]	100	Bland[51] vs TACE[49]	NA	Median from dx: TACE, 50.1 mo; bland, 39.1 TACE 1-y, 2-y, 5-y survival: 69%, 52%, 19%. Bland: 19%, 70%, 13%
Ruutiainen[54]	67	Bland[23] vs TACE[44]	TACE: 22 Bland: 38	Survival of 1, 3, and 5 y TACE: 86%, 67%, 50% Bland: 68%, 46%, 33%
Gupta[61]	49	TACE[27] vs bland[42]	TACE: 50 Bland: 25	Median survival for carcinoid tumors: TACE 33.8 vs bland 33.2. Islet TACE 31.5 vs bland 18.2
Maire[62]	26	TACE[12] vs bland[14]	TACE: 100 Bland: 92	2-y survival: TACE, 80%; bland, 100%. Median PFS: TACE, 19.2 mo; bland, 23.6 mo
Guiu[45]	120 NET 88 HCC	DEB-TACE in HCC (cirrhotic) and NETs (noncirrhotic)	NA	NA
Ruszniewski[55]	23	TACE	PR, SD, PD, TTP HACE: 61, 22, 17,14 HAE: 20, 40, 40,12	8 of 23 died median of 12.5 mo after final TACE

Abbreviations: dx, diagnosis; NA, not available; PD, progressive disease; PR, partial response; RECIST, response evaluation criteria in solid tumors; SD, stable disease; TTP, time to progression.
Data from Refs.[26,30,39,45,53–55,59–62]

Radioembolization (transarterial radioembolization)

Tumor marker changes are known to fluctuate for a variety of non–cancer-related and non–treatment-related factors (**Table 4**). When levels are increased before TARE, most patients are noted to have a reduction in serum and urinary tumor markers. Chromogranin A and serotonin were most commonly reviewed; however, 24-hour 5-hydroxyindoleacetic acid (5-HIAA) is frequently used.[8] Imaging response is often reported post-TARE using RECIST via CT or MRI, with correlation in most cases of decline in levels of tumor markers and decreased tumor diameters, which may or may not meet the criteria of PR.

In a multicenter retrospective study, Kennedy and colleagues[8] reported that SD revealed by imaging was reported in 22.7% of patients, PR in 60.5%, and complete response in 27%. A 70-month median survival was recorded.[8] Memon and colleagues[49] carefully recorded long-term outcomes after TARE, which indicated treatment response in 62.7%; disease stabilization in 32.5%; and survival of 72.5% at 1 year, 62.5% at 2 years, and 45.0% at 3 years.

Studies of TARE using [90]Y (both glass and resin microspheres) in patients with mNETs have been performed at several centers.[8,36,48–52] Sample numbers ranged from 40 to 148.

Memon and colleagues,[49] with 40 patients, using glass spheres, showed a radiologic response (World Health Organization criteria) of 64% and 71.4% (European Association for the Study of the Liver [EASL] criteria); median survival was 34.4 months; and 1-year, 2-year, and 3-year survival we evaluated at 72.5%, 62.5%, 45.0%, respectively.[49]

King and colleagues[36] studied 58 patients using ^{90}Y resin microspheres and concurrent 5-fluorouracil (5-FU). Radiologic response was reported at 39%; median survival was 36 months; with 1-year, 2-year, and 3-year survival reported at 86%, 58%, and 47%, respectively.

Additional response and survival times are summarized elsewhere.[21]

Table 4
Response and survival after radioembolization (TARE)

Study	N	Device Used	Radiologic Response; RECIST 1.0 (%)	Survival
Rhee[51]	42	Yttrium 90 (glass)	54	Median: 22 mo
		Yttrium 90 (resin)	50	Median: 28 mo
Kennedy[8]	148	Yttrium 90 (resin)	63	Median: 70 mo
King[36]	58	Yttrium 90 (resin) plus 5-FU	39	Median: 36 mo; 1-y, 2-y, 3-y survival: 86%, 58%, and 47%
Saxena[52]	48	Yttrium 90 (resin)	54	Median: 35 mo; 1-y, 2-y, 3-y survival: 87%, 62%, and 42%
Cao[48]	58	Yttrium 90 (resin) plus 5-FU	39.2	Median: 36 mo
Paprottka[50]	42	Yttrium 90 (resin)	22.5	Median: 95% at 16.2 mo
Memon[49]	40	Yttrium 90 (glass)	WHO, 64; EASL, 71.4	Median: 34.4 mo; 1-y, 2-y, 3-y survival: 72.5%, 62.5%, 45%

Abbreviations: EASL, European Association for the Study of the Liver; WHO, World Health Organization.
Data from Refs.[8,36,48–52]

CONSENSUS GUIDELINES

Guidelines for use of TAE, TACE, and radioembolization for metastatic NETs have been produced by major multinational societies dedicated to NETs in the last 5 years. Brief summaries of their evaluations are described here.

European Neuroendocrine Tumor Society Consensus Guidelines (2012)

The European Neuroendocrine Tumor Society (ENETS) Consensus Guidelines determined that TAE or TACE should be used in patients with either liver-only disease or those with limited extrahepatic metastases.[21,56] The guidelines state that TAE and TACE are effective in symptom control and tumor growth and result in a significant decrease in levels of biochemical markers with objective tumor responses in about half of the patients.[56] ENETS guidelines report that no current evidence finds TACE superior to TAE and advocate that the cytotoxics used should include either doxorubicin or streptozotocin in mixtures with lipiodol. Because a common side effect is postembolization syndrome, TAE or TACE should be performed in experienced centers. Major side effects are rare and the procedure is contraindicated in cases of complete portal vein thrombosis, hepatic insufficiency, and Whipple procedure. TARE is listed as an investigational method in treating mNETs.[56]

The North American Neuroendocrine Tumor Society Guidelines (2010)

The 2010 North American Neuroendocrine Tumor Society guidelines represent the views from an international conference, for which 15 expert working groups prepared evidence-based assessments addressing specific questions, and from which an independent jury derived final recommendations.[57] In the area of imaging and liver-directed therapies, a paucity of biological, molecular, and genomic information is noted; and an absence of data from rigorous trials limits the validity of many publications detailing management. Recommendations for the use of TAE, TACE, and SIRT state that they should be used as part of a treatment panel. A weaker recommendation calls for their use within a clinical study protocol, with the aim of achieving a higher level of evidence regarding patient selection and treatment efficacy. These guidelines evaluate the benefit and harm as roughly equal and the cost as high.[57]

Neuroendocrine Tumor: Liver Metastases Consensus Conference (2012)

In 2012 an international conference endorsed and represented by 8 NET-related societies convened 15 expert working groups that prepared evidence-based assessments addressing specific questions in the management of liver metastases from NETs. An independent jury derived final recommendations. Regarding the specific workgroup of intra-arterial therapy, a multidisciplinary panel of experts selected the most appropriate reports in the literature and found 115 articles using intra-arterial therapy for mNET liver disease. Of those, they chose to base their report on 18 peer-reviewed published reports that met predefined measures in mNET liver therapy via TAE, TACE, and TARE. Eleven articles (see **Tables 1** and **3**) detailed TAE/TACE therapy and there were 7 for TARE (see **Tables 2** and **4**). The full conference report by Frilling and colleagues[57] and a separate detailed section report by Kennedy and colleagues[21] used both the US National Cancer Institute system of medical evidence and the GRADE (grading of recommendations assessment, development, and evaluation) by Guyatt and colleagues.[58]

Studies of moderate quality support the use of TAE, TACE, and TARE for mNETs.[8,36,48–52] The quality and strength of the reports available do not allow any modality to be determined as superior in terms of imaging response, symptomatic response, or impact on survival. The use of TARE may be advantageous compared with TAE and TACE because it causes fewer side effects and requires fewer treatments. The use of TARE with ^{90}Y is now accepted and endorsed by all the societies as a suitable replacement for TAE/TACE in liver mNETs.[21,57]

REFERENCES

1. Bax ND, Woods HF, Batchelor A, et al. Clinical manifestations of carcinoid disease. World J Surg 1996;20(2):142–6.
2. Proye C. Natural history of liver metastasis of gastroenteropancreatic neuroendocrine tumors: place for chemoembolization. World J Surg 2001;25(6): 685–8.
3. van der Lely AJ, de Herder WW. Carcinoid syndrome: diagnosis and medical management. Arq Bras Endocrinol Metabol 2005;49(5):850–60.
4. Kulke M. Advances in the treatment of neuroendocrine tumors. Curr Treat Options Oncol 2005;6(5):397–409.
5. Kulke MH, Mayer RJ. Carcinoid tumors. N Engl J Med 1999;340(11):858–68.
6. Yao JC, Hassan M, Phan A, et al. One hundred years after "carcinoid": epidemiology of and prognostic factors for neuroendocrine tumors in 35,825 cases in the United States. J Clin Oncol 2008;26(18):3063–72.
7. Oberg K. Neuroendocrine gastrointestinal tumors–a condensed overview of diagnosis and treatment. Ann Oncol 1999;10(Suppl 2):S3–8.
8. Kennedy AS, Dezarn WA, McNeillie P, et al. Radioembolization for unresectable neuroendocrine hepatic metastases using resin 90Y-microspheres: early results in 148 patients. Am J Clin Oncol 2008;31(3):271–9.
9. Florman S, Toure B, Kim L, et al. Liver transplantation for neuroendocrine tumors. J Gastrointest Surg 2004;8(2):208–12.
10. Gaur SK, Friese JL, Sadow CA, et al. Hepatic arterial chemoembolization using drug-eluting beads in gastrointestinal neuroendocrine tumor metastatic to the liver. Cardiovasc Intervent Radiol 2011;34(3):566–72.
11. Siperstein AE, Berber E. Cryoablation, percutaneous alcohol injection, and radiofrequency ablation for treatment of neuroendocrine liver metastases. World J Surg 2001;25(6):693–6.
12. Woodside KJ, Townsend CM Jr, Mark Evers B. Current management of gastrointestinal carcinoid tumors. J Gastrointest Surg 2004;8(6):742–56.
13. Yao KA, Talamonti MS, Nemcek A, et al. Indications and results of liver resection and hepatic chemoembolization for metastatic gastrointestinal neuroendocrine tumors. Surgery 2001;130(4):677–82 [discussion: 82–5].
14. Sutcliffe R, Maguire D, Ramage J, et al. Management of neuroendocrine liver metastases. Am J Surg 2004;187(1):39–46.
15. Chamberlain RS, Canes D, Brown KT, et al. Hepatic neuroendocrine metastases: does intervention alter outcomes? J Am Coll Surg 2000;190(4):432–45.
16. Berber E, Flesher N, Siperstein AE. Laparoscopic radiofrequency ablation of neuroendocrine liver metastases. World J Surg 2002;26(8):985–90.
17. Eriksson J, Stalberg P, Nilsson A, et al. Surgery and radiofrequency ablation for treatment of liver metastases from midgut and foregut carcinoids and endocrine pancreatic tumors. World J Surg 2008;32(5):930–8.
18. Kim YH, Ajani JA, Carrasco CH, et al. Selective hepatic arterial chemoembolization for liver metastases in patients with carcinoid tumor or islet cell carcinoma. Cancer Invest 1999;17(7):474–8.

19. McStay MK, Maudgil D, Williams M, et al. Large-volume liver metastases from neuroendocrine tumors: hepatic intraarterial 90Y-DOTA-lanreotide as effective palliative therapy. Radiology 2005;237(2):718–26.

20. Breedis C, Young G. The blood supply of neoplasms in the liver. Am J Pathol 1954;30:969–84.

21. Kennedy A, Bester L, Salem R, et al. Role of hepatic intra-arterial therapies in metastatic neuroendocrine tumours (NET): guidelines from the NET-Liver-Metastases Consensus Conference. HPB (Oxford) 2015;17(1):29–37.

22. Kennedy A, Nag S, Salem R, et al. Recommendations for radioembolization of hepatic malignancies using yttrium-90 microsphere brachytherapy: a consensus panel report from the radioembolization brachytherapy oncology consortium. Int J Radiat Oncol Biol Phys 2007;68(1):13–23.

23. Kennedy AS, Sangro B. Nonsurgical treatment for localized hepatocellular carcinoma. Curr Oncol Rep 2014;16:373–81.

24. Lien WM, Ackerman NB. The blood supply of experimental liver metastases II: a microcirculatory study of the normal and tumor vessels of the liver with the use of perfused silicone rubber. Surgery 1970;68(2):334–40.

25. Liu DM, Thakor AS, Baerlocher M, et al. A review of conventional and drug-eluting chemoembolization in the treatment of colorectal liver metastases: principles and proof. Future Oncol 2015;11(9):1421–8.

26. Pitt SC, Knuth J, Keily JM, et al. Hepatic neuroendocrine metastases: chemo- or bland embolization? J Gastrointest Surg 2008;12(11):1951–60.

27. Strosberg JR, Weber JM, Choi J, et al. A phase II clinical trial of sunitinib following hepatic transarterial embolization for metastatic neuroendocrine tumors. Ann Oncol 2012;23(9):2335–41.

28. Roche A, Girish BV, de Baere T, et al. Trans-catheter arterial chemoembolization as first-line treatment for hepatic metastases from endocrine tumors. Eur Radiol 2003;13(1):136–40.

29. Bloomston M, Al-Saif O, Klemanski D, et al. Hepatic artery chemoembolization in 122 patients with metastatic carcinoid tumor: lessons learned. J Gastrointest Surg 2007;11(3):264–71.

30. Loewe C, Schindl M, Cejna M, et al. Permanent transarterial embolization of neuroendocrine metastases of the liver using cyanoacrylate and lipiodol: assessment of mid- and long-term results. AJR Am J Roentgenol 2003;180(5):1379–84.

31. Lewis AL, Gonzalez MV, Leppard SW, et al. Doxorubicin eluting beads - 1: effects of drug loading on bead characteristics and drug distribution. J Mater Sci Mater Med 2007;18(9):1691–9.

32. Liu DM, Kos S, Buczkowski A, et al. Optimization of doxorubicin loading for superabsorbent polymer microspheres: in vitro analysis. Cardiovasc Intervent Radiol 2012;35(2):391–8.

33. Jones RP, Sutton P, Greensmith RM, et al. Hepatic activation of irinotecan predicts tumour response in patients with colorectal liver metastases treated with DEBIRI: exploratory findings from a phase II study. Cancer Chemother Pharmacol 2013;72(2):359–68.

34. Lewis AL, Holden RR, Chung ST, et al. Feasibility, safety and pharmacokinetic study of hepatic administration of drug-eluting beads loaded with irinotecan (DEBIRI) followed by intravenous administration of irinotecan in a porcine model. J Mater Sci Mater Med 2013;24(1):115–27.

35. Whitney R, Valek V, Fages JF, et al. Transarterial chemoembolization and selective internal radiation for the treatment of patients with metastatic neuroendocrine tumors: a comparison of efficacy and cost. Oncologist 2011;16(5):594–601.

36. King J, Quinn R, Glenn DM, et al. Radioembolization with selective internal radiation microspheres for neuroendocrine liver metastases. Cancer 2008;113(5):921–9.
37. Wang LM, Jani AR, Hill EJ, et al. Anatomical basis and histopathological changes resulting from selective internal radiotherapy for liver metastases. J Clin Pathol 2013;66(3):205–11.
38. Salem R, Parikh P, Atassi B, et al. Incidence of radiation pneumonitis after hepatic intra-arterial radiotherapy with yttrium-90 microspheres assuming uniform lung distribution. Am J Clin Oncol 2008;31(5):431–8.
39. Vogl TJ, Gruber T, Naguib NN, et al. Liver metastases of neuroendocrine tumors: treatment with hepatic transarterial chemotherapy using two therapeutic protocols. AJR Am J Roentgenol 2009;193(4):941–7.
40. Vogl TJ, Naguib NN, Zangos S, et al. Liver metastases of neuroendocrine carcinomas: interventional treatment via transarterial embolization, chemoembolization and thermal ablation. Eur J Radiol 2009;72(3):517–28.
41. Lee E, Leon Pachter H, Sarpel U. Hepatic arterial embolization for the treatment of metastatic neuroendocrine tumors. Int J Hepatol 2012;2012:471203.
42. Eyol E, Boleij A, Taylor RR, et al. Chemoembolisation of rat colorectal liver metastases with drug eluting beads loaded with irinotecan or doxorubicin. Clin Exp Metastasis 2008;25(3):273–82.
43. McCubrey JA, Steelman LS, Chappell WH, et al. Roles of the Raf/MEK/ERK pathway in cell growth, malignant transformation and drug resistance. Biochim Biophys Acta 2007;1773(8):1263–84.
44. Zheng Y, Zhou J, Tong Y. Gene signatures of drug resistance predict patient survival in colorectal cancer. Pharmacogenomics J 2015;15(2):135–43.
45. Guiu B, Deschamps F, Aho S, et al. Liver/biliary injuries following chemoembolisation of endocrine tumours and hepatocellular carcinoma: lipiodol vs. drug-eluting beads. J Hepatol 2012;56(3):609–17.
46. Fiore F, Del Prete M, Franco R, et al. Transarterial embolization (TAE) is equally effective and slightly safer than transarterial chemoembolization (TACE) to manage liver metastases in neuroendocrine tumors. Endocrine 2014;47(1):177–82.
47. Kalinowski M, Dressler M, Konig A, et al. Selective internal radiotherapy with yttrium-90 microspheres for hepatic metastatic neuroendocrine tumors: a prospective single center study. Digestion 2009;79(3):137–42.
48. Cao CQ, Yan TD, Bester L, et al. Radioembolization with yttrium microspheres for neuroendocrine tumour liver metastases. Br J Surg 2010;97(4):537–43.
49. Memon K, Lewandowski RJ, Mulcahy MF, et al. Radioembolization for neuroendocrine liver metastases: safety, imaging, and long-term outcomes. Int J Radiat Oncol Biol Phys 2012;83(3):887–94.
50. Paprottka PM, Hoffmann RT, Haug A, et al. Radioembolization of symptomatic, unresectable neuroendocrine hepatic metastases using yttrium-90 microspheres. Cardiovasc Intervent Radiol 2012;35(2):334–42.
51. Rhee TK, Lewandowski RJ, Liu DM, et al. 90Y Radioembolization for metastatic neuroendocrine liver tumors: preliminary results from a multi-institutional experience. Ann Surg 2008;247(6):1029–35.
52. Saxena A, Chua TC, Bester L, et al. Factors predicting response and survival after yttrium-90 radioembolization of unresectable neuroendocrine tumor liver metastases: a critical appraisal of 48 cases. Ann Surg 2010;251(5):910–6.
53. Dong XD, Carr BI. Hepatic artery chemoembolization for the treatment of liver metastases from neuroendocrine tumors: a long-term follow-up in 123 patients. Med Oncol 2011;28(Suppl 1):S286–90.

54. Ruutiainen AT, Soulen MC, Tuite CM, et al. Chemoembolization and bland embolization of neuroendocrine tumor metastases to the liver. J Vasc Interv Radiol 2007;18(7):847–55.
55. Ruszniewski P, Rougier P, Roche A, et al. Hepatic arterial chemoembolization in patients with liver metastases of endocrine tumors. A prospective phase II study in 24 patients. Cancer 1993;71(8):2624–30.
56. Pavel M, Baudin E, Couvelard A, et al. ENETS consensus guidelines for the management of patients with liver and other distant metastases from neuroendocrine neoplasms of foregut, midgut, hindgut, and unknown primary. Neuroendocrinology 2012;95(2):157–76.
57. Frilling A, Modlin IM, Kidd M, et al. Recommendations for management of patients with neuroendocrine liver metastases. Lancet Oncol 2014;15(1):e8–21.
58. Guyatt GH, Oxman AD, Kunz R, et al. Going from evidence to recommendations. BMJ 2008;336(7652):1049–51.
59. de Baere T, Deschamps F, Teriitheau C, et al. Transarterial chemoembolization of liver metastases from well differentiated gastroenteropancreatic endocrine tumors with doxorubicin-eluting beads: preliminary results. J Vasc Interv Radiol 2008;19(6):855–61.
60. Eriksson BK, Larsson EG, Skogseid BM, et al. Liver embolizations of patients with malignant neuroendocrine gastrointestinal tumors. Cancer 1998;83(11):2293–301.
61. Gupta S, Johnson MM, Murthy R, et al. Hepatic arterial embolization and chemoembolization for the treatment of patients with metastatic neuroendocrine tumors: variables affecting response rates and survival. Cancer 2005;104(8):1590–602.
62. Maire F, Lombard-Bohas C, O'Toole D, et al. Hepatic arterial embolization versus chemoembolization in the treatment of liver metastases from well-differentiated midgut endocrine tumors: a prospective randomized study. Neuroendocrinology 2012;96(4):294–300.

Clinical Trial Design in Neuroendocrine Tumors

Daniel M. Halperin, MD, James C. Yao, MD*

KEYWORDS

- Neuroendocrine tumors • Clinical trials • Patient homogeneity
- Standardized response assessment • Study design and interpretation

KEY POINTS

- Neuroendocrine tumors (NETs) present tremendous opportunities for productive clinical investigation, but substantial challenges as well.
- NETs are relatively rare, heterogeneous, and typically indolent tumors that are imperfectly visualized by most common imaging techniques, and have historically had minimal standardization of care.
- Investigators must be aware of common pitfalls in study design, informed by an understanding of the history of trials in the field, to make the best use of available data and our patient volunteers.
- When previous studies are considered as instructive not only about disease biology and management, but also about study design and interpretation, investigators are poised to continue iteratively refining our methods for the benefit of our patients with these diseases.
- We believe the salient issues in clinical trial design and interpretation in the NET field are patient homogeneity, standardized response assessment, and rigorous design and execution. Whether designing or interpreting a study in patients with NET, these principles should drive assessment.

INTRODUCTION

The field of neuroendocrine oncology has grown significantly over the past decade. Over that time, substantial collaborative efforts have allowed the successful conduct of multiple randomized controlled trials that have changed both the clinical practice of oncology and the scientific practice of conducting future studies. These studies provide ample opportunity for learning in study design and execution, and our intent in this article is to consolidate the lessons learned and offer direction as the field continues to advance.

Disclosure: The authors have nothing to disclose.
Department of Gastrointestinal Medical Oncology, The University of Texas MD Anderson Cancer Center, Unit 426, 1515 Holcombe Boulevard, Houston, TX 77030, USA
* Corresponding author.
E-mail address: jyao@mdanderson.org

Hematol Oncol Clin N Am 30 (2016) 209–217
http://dx.doi.org/10.1016/j.hoc.2015.09.011
0889-8588/16/$ – see front matter © 2016 Elsevier Inc. All rights reserved.

We would submit that the key principles for neuroendocrine tumor (NET) clinical trials moving forward are the selection of homogeneous patient populations, assessment of standardized criteria for progression and response by real-time centralized review, and rigorous study design. These principles arise from a history of rigorous clinical investigation that has evolved together with improvements in technology that enable us to conduct ever more sophisticated investigations. Similarly, we believe that these issues are central to interpretation of any given study, and should be reviewed when considering the results of any clinical trial.

HISTORICAL OVERVIEW

The earliest clinical trials for patients with NET evaluated conventional chemotherapy, and highlight many of the salient issues of clinical trial design in this patient population. These issues include grouping tumors by primary site and clinical aggressiveness, selection of response criteria, and assessment of those criteria.

One of the first studies tested streptozocin in 52 patients with metastatic pancreatic NETs (pNETs) in the 1970s.[1] This relatively large study for the era was conducted after an initial evaluation of the drug in 4 patients with pNET and 4 patients with extrapancreatic NET (carcinoid) revealed 1 response in a patient with pNET and no responses in the carcinoid patients.[2] This later study required the collaboration of 50 investigators to accrue 52 patients, and is notable for its inclusion of exclusively patients with pNET. Following their accrual, patients received standardized doses of the therapy and were followed for response. Response criteria were strictly defined to incorporate both improvements in hormone secretion and tumor volume assessed by physical examination of the assessing investigator. By its nature, this study was uncontrolled, but given the lack of alternative therapies, evidence of relevant activity established streptozocin as the standard therapy for advanced pNET.

Subsequently, 2 randomized studies of approximately 100 patients each were conducted by the Eastern Cooperative Oncology Group (ECOG) to develop streptozocin-based chemotherapy further.[3,4] The first demonstrated superiority of 5-fluorouracil combined with streptozocin over streptozocin alone[3] in a population of patients with pNET, although it continued to use a composite endpoint of biochemical and measureable response, with approximately one-third of patients eligible for classification of response based on biochemical parameters, and an unknown proportion eligible based on physical examination. Secondary endpoints of progression-free survival (PFS) and overall survival were not statistically different between the 2 arms. The second study evaluated 3 regimens: streptozocin with 5-fluorouracil, streptozocin with doxorubicin, and single-agent chlorozotocin, with doxorubicin/streptozocin demonstrating superiority. Nearly half of all patients in that study could be classified as responders based on biochemical criteria. However, both PFS and overall survival were significantly improved with the combination (P<.005 for both endpoints and both comparators).[4] These studies established the standard therapy for pNETs until 2011, although notably, later evaluation in the modern era of cross-sectional imaging would suggest that the radiographic response rate of pNETs to streptozocin-based doublet chemotherapy is actually less than 10%.[5,6] Importantly, these studies highlight some of the key study design issues that continue to arise in the field. Multi-institutional cooperation was required to achieve even modest accrual of a homogeneous group of patients and intermediate endpoints, such as objective radiographic response rate, were used due to feasibility. Also of note, given the challenges of patient accrual, the time lapse between each of these studies was approximately 10 years.

The development of octreotide, an octopeptide somatostatin analogue, was similar in its style and limitations. Following separately reported assessments in 25 carcinoid[7] patients and 22 patients with pNET,[8] consistent evidence of biochemical control was observed, and it became the standard therapy for patients with NETs of all primary sites for control of hormonal syndromes. Octreotide's development was prescient in its separation of NETs by primary site, but in turn hindered by small sample sizes. No evidence of tumor regression was observed, and no claim of improved PFS or overall survival was made in these early studies. It was not until the Prospective, Randomized Study on the Effect of Octreotide LAR in the Control of Tumor Growth in Patients With Metastatic Neuroendocrine Midgut Tumors (PROMID) study[9] that there was evidence from 85 randomized patients that a somatostatin analogue could delay time to progression in patients with midgut NETs. Most patients had minimal liver involvement, and there was no formal assessment of whether patients had progression before enrollment, although half of the enrolled patients were less than 4.3 months from diagnosis. Notably, the PROMID study used standard radiographic criteria to evaluate response and progression, and incorporated blinded central radiology review to determine progression.

Therefore, in considering the critical studies between 1970 and 2010, a steady march of progress is apparent. Themes of attempting to achieve patient population homogeneity through primary site stratification and selection, as well as collaborative adherence to standardized response criteria run throughout. Meanwhile, the evolution of the radiology field allowed for the use of standardized imaging criteria for response and blinded centralized radiology review.

PATIENT SELECTION

The primary issue in selecting patients with NET for clinical trials is ensuring the relevant homogeneity of the population under study. This is a challenging goal in NETs, as a homogeneous population of patients is required to address a focused research question, but defining eligible patients too narrowly could easily render accrual too slow to answer the question while it is still relevant to clinical practice. A homogeneous population may represent a selected group that is felt to be most likely to benefit from a given therapy, but may also represent a group with uniform prognosis, such that therapeutic impact can be more readily detected. Stratified randomization can allow for a heterogeneous population of patients with distinct prognoses to be balanced with respect to the primary endpoint. This strategy can permit larger studies to be completed without a completely homogeneous population, but allows limited interpretation of subgroup analyses, as the subgroups need not be balanced with respect to the stratification variables.

We have learned much about the biologically relevant heterogeneity of patients with NET in the past several years, as novel agents have been investigated in heterogeneous populations of patients with NET. In phase II studies of everolimus,[10] sunitinib,[11] and pazopanib,[12] clear differences in response rates between pNETs and extrapancreatic NETs were observed, suggesting that different primary sites have distinct biology and should be studied separately. The exact biological reasons for these differential responses remain obscure, but the introduction of next-generation sequencing to the neuroendocrine field has demonstrated clear genomic differences between well-differentiated pancreatic, small bowel, and pulmonary NETs. Although frequent lesions in MEN1, DAXX, ATRX, and the mammalian target of rapamycin pathway were observed in pNETs,[13] only occasional alterations of CDKN1B have been observed in small bowel NETs,[14] whereas ARID1A, EIF1AX, and MEN1 are most commonly altered in pulmonary NETs.[15] However, it remains unclear whether further splitting these tumors by molecular phenotype will be required to achieve biologically relevant homogeneity, and whether these genetic alterations beget similar pathophysiology in the context of different primary sites and histologies.

At present, our thinking is that separating NETs for clinical study by primary site is an appropriate approach when feasible. This is especially important in single-arm studies in which the comparison is against a historical control. In randomized studies, stratification may also be appropriate when primary site is prognostic, but there is reason to believe treatment may benefit a wider study population. In our view, primary site and histology are relevant proxies for unmeasurable biological variables, and as such are useful variables for achieving biologically relevant patient homogeneity in study design and execution.

The strategy of separating NETs by primary site is further supported by recent work in our group about the predictive value of phase II studies.[16] In that work, we conclude that drugs tested in different tumors have measurably distinct odds of eventual approval, in turn suggesting that different phase II designs may be required to reduce the frequency of advancing drugs to phase III studies based on false-positive phase II results. Although it remains to be demonstrated whether NETs of varied primary sites have distinct odds of therapeutic efficacy, the differences observed in the activity of sunitinib and streptozocin argue that pNETs should be considered separately from other NETs, as the prior probability of success is likely to be different.

In addition to grouping patients by primary site, the importance of progressive disease on study entry also has become apparent. Studying this population of patients serves 3 purposes. First, it studies the population of patients in greatest need of therapy, as indolent disease can often be observed without additional therapy in many patients. Second, it studies a more homogeneous population by excluding that fraction of patients who will have stable disease on study regardless of therapy. Finally, by selecting patients with more aggressive disease, it increases the event rate, thereby shortening the necessary follow-up time and accrual requirements. These properties allow for the more rapid completion of studies asking the most relevant questions about the population most in need of therapy. As a result, the field has moved toward including only patients with progressive disease within the 12 months before study enrollment, using that entry criterion in the pivotal studies of everolimus[17] and sunitinib.[18] In these studies, which included only patients with progressive pNETs, the median PFS was reassuringly similar, at 4.6 and 5.5 months, respectively.

ENDPOINT SELECTION

In the United States, drugs are presently approved for patient use based on randomized studies showing self-evident benefit, namely overall survival or patient quality of life. Given the extended duration of illness in patients with NET and the frequently heterogeneous postprogression course, which can include surgery, hepatic arterial therapy, and/or clinical trials, PFS is considered an acceptable surrogate endpoint in randomized phase III studies. PFS has been successfully used as a surrogate endpoint in the pivotal trials of everolimus,[17] sunitinib,[18] and lanreotide.[19] Quality of life has presented a greater challenge in patients with NET, as only recently have validated instruments been developed to measure the symptom burden of patients with functional NET.[20] As with therapies designed to prolong patient life, the ability to detect improved quality of life is a product of the measurement instrument, patient population, and treatment under investigation. Hopefully, with the advent of validated instruments, therapies aiming to ameliorate the symptom burden of refractory carcinoid syndrome will have a more direct path to approval.

In phase II studies, the optimal surrogate endpoints for ultimate benefit remain unclear. Classically, objective response rate as measured by the Response Evaluation Criteria in Solid Tumors (RECIST) has been used in phase II studies. However, recent studies have illuminated issues with that approach. Fundamentally, radiographic response in the population of patients enrolled in phase II studies has not been consistently predictive of radiologic response in the broader population assessed in phase III testing. In the case of everolimus, phase II studies estimated the objective response rate to be 10% to 20%[10,21] in patients with pNET, whereas the objective response rate observed in the randomized phase III was only 5%, as compared with 2% in the placebo arm.[17] Similarly, phase II estimation of response rate of pNETs to sunitinib was also more than 15%,[11] but the observed response rate in the randomized study was less than 10%.[18] This phenomenon has been previously described in the context of disconnected benefit as drugs and regimens advance from successful phase II studies to negative phase III trials,[22] but in the case of NETs, the lower response rate in phase III does not necessarily mean there is no antitumor activity or PFS benefit. Nonetheless, PFS may be a superior endpoint to objective response rate for phase II studies; however, randomization is necessary in most situations to interpret PFS results.

ENDPOINT ASSESSMENT

Investigators must not only determine which patients will be evaluated and what endpoints should be assessed, but also what methods should be used to standardize the measurements. In the case of NET clinical trials, PFS by modern RECIST criteria is considered adequate for pivotal phase III studies. However, we have recently discovered the perils of asynchronous centralized radiology review in our field.

In the RADIANT-2 (RAD001 In Advanced Neuroendocrine Tumors) study, octreotide with everolimus was compared with octreotide with placebo in the treatment of patients with advanced NETs and carcinoid syndrome, with PFS by central radiology review as the primary endpoint. That study had an important discordance between the investigator and central radiology assessments. The median PFS in the everolimus plus octreotide group was 16.4 months (95% confidence interval [CI] 13.7–21.2) by central review and 12 months (95% CI 10.6–16.1) by investigator review. However, more important than this quantitative difference is the influence of informative censoring, which effectively biased the study toward the null.

To understand the impact of informative censoring, one must consider the effect of different types of discordance between central and investigator review as patients' tumors grow. When the investigator measures progression but the central reviewer later measures stable disease, the investigator has already taken the patient off the protocol therapy, and the patient must be censored. Unfortunately, this censoring event violates an underlying principle of Kaplan-Meier analysis.[23] Patients censored for this reason are likely to have a different course than other patients who continue to be treated for the same time but there is no suspicion of progression. That is, the censoring has failed to be noninformative. Conversely, if the investigator measures stable disease but the central reviewer measures progression, the patient is categorized as having a progression event on the date of scan. Therefore, the observed event rate is reduced by those occasions when the central reviewer classifies patients as stable and the investigator has classified them as having progressive disease. Although this phenomenon would merely diminish the power of the study by reducing the event rate uniformly if these disagreements were distributed evenly between the 2 arms, they will not necessarily be distributed evenly. Rather, the censoring will happen more frequently in the arm with more progression events. In other words, if the experimental therapy is more effective than the control therapy, one would expect more informative censoring events to occur in the control arm, artificially inflating the PFS in that arm. This PFS inflation biases the study against observing a difference between the treatment arms[24–26] and may be more prominent in controlled studies in which there may be investigator desire to cross progressive patients over to the experimental arm.

In all, assessment of study endpoints has evolved significantly since the original studies of chemotherapies in NETs were performed. The field has moved from basing reports on physical examination findings to standardized radiology measurements to gauge response and progression. Blinded centralized radiology review adds another layer of rigor that is meant to reduce bias, but its retrospective use inadvertently trades one bias for another. Therefore, we would submit that real-time blinded central radiology review is an optimal strategy for minimizing bias in randomized studies using PFS as the primary endpoint when logistics allow.

STATISTICAL CONSIDERATIONS

In phase III registration studies, statistical designs are frequently created in collaboration with regulatory agencies, such as the US Food and Drug Administration. The design of phase II studies, however, is largely the province of clinical investigators. As such, there is significant variability in their designs, which is reasonable given the varied questions under study.

In some situations, single-arm phase II studies can still yield potentially useful information. However, as the design is dependent on differentiating the performance of a therapy from a historical control, the weakness of this design is the precision with which the clinical course of a relevant historical sample of patients can be estimated. Particularly as we enroll patients who have been heavily pretreated with multiple lines of targeted agents and have more narrowly defined diseases, historical PFS is extremely difficult to estimate. Most populations can be expected to have a minimal rate of spontaneous regression, so objective radiographic response (ORR) can still be used in single-arm studies. However, given the earlier discussion of response rate as compared with PFS, we would recommend that ORR be selected only in cases in which tumor shrinkage is felt to be more likely based on the therapy's mechanism of action.

For most new therapies, which historical precedent suggests would be more likely to benefit patients with NET with respect to PFS than ORR, we would favor randomized phase II designs as a method for limiting reliance on an inherently imprecise estimate of the historical control.

Beyond basic design issues, we would suggest that clinical investigators ought to consider the importance of the type I and type II error rates in determining the positive predictive value of a given phase II study. We have recently reported an analysis in which investigators can conceptualize phase II studies as predictive tests like any other in clinical medicine.[16] As such, studies can be considered to have predictive value for patient benefit and regulatory approval, in addition to their set sensitivity and specificity (or type I and type II error). Akin to the Bayesian reasoning that is familiar to clinical practitioners, the predictive value is dependent not only on the type I and type II error, but also the prior probability of patient benefit. Unfortunately, the prior probability of a drug truly being effective in any oncologic indication is quite low, with some sources estimating it to be 5% or less.[27] Although our estimate of the prior probability of drug efficacy in NETs is imprecise given the relative paucity of phase II studies in the reported sample set, we can impute that drugs in NET have a chance of success on the order of that observed in other gastrointestinal cancers, namely less than 40%. Such a prior probability makes the positive predictive value of a given phase II study particularly sensitive to changes in the type I error rate, whereas the negative predictive value has minimal sensitivity to changes in the type II error rate. These principles allow us to conclude that reducing the type I error rate in our phase II studies, with a compensatory acceptable increase in the type II error rate (ie, a reduction in power), can allow for improved positive predictive value without a meaningful sacrifice in negative predictive value, assuming the null and alternative hypotheses remained fixed. Such adjustments are conceptually similar to those required to "raise the bar" in phase II testing, which mechanically amount to increasing the difference between the null and alternative hypotheses while maintaining type I and type II error rates. The implications of either maneuver are to reduce the number of positive phase II studies, but increase the proportion of true positive results, meaning that more of the drugs deemed active in phase II testing would be expected to yield positive phase III studies and eventually attain regulatory approval.

SUMMARY

Taken together, we can take much inspiration and instruction from the significant clinical trial efforts in NETs over the past several decades. Our field continues to be dependent on our strong collegial spirit of collaboration, with even the largest NET centers needing to work together to complete randomized studies. This collaborative approach will be even more critical as we consider how narrowly to define the homogeneous patient population to be evaluated in any given study, and whether we will perform studies limited to molecularly defined subsets of anatomically restricted NET patients. Efforts to standardize assessment of tumor response and progression have continued, and have been aided by the advent of constant improvements in imaging technology and communications infrastructure. However, even with standardized assessments and blinded centralized radiology review, we have seen that biases can be inadvertently introduced. Finally, insights into the statistical properties of phase II studies empower us to make adjustments that avoid our inadvertent statistical bias toward false-positive phase II results.

What is the ideal design for a study in NET patients, given infinite resources? We would submit that once a meaningful scientific and clinical question has been identified, the first step is selecting the patient population. We would suggest that this population should include patients with a defined primary site(s) (pancreas, small bowel, or lung being the easiest to accrue). Molecular characterization should be considered, potentially with restriction to patients with a specific profile, if a biomarker has been validated in human studies to predict benefit or lack thereof. Progressive disease within 1 year before enrollment will further help define the population as the one with the greatest need and allow for a smaller study size. We would suggest that the most appropriate endpoint for most NET studies would be PFS; in the absence of a precise estimate of PFS historically in the same population, a randomized design is therefore optimal to observe an improvement over the alternative. Ideally, PFS in pivotal phase III studies would be determined by real-time blinded central radiology review to reduce the potential impact of informative censoring. Finally, we would suggest that careful constraint of the type I error rate, with a compensatory reduction in power, is a reasonable method for improving the yield of phase II studies so as to maximize the odds of success in phase III testing.

The future for clinical investigation in the NET field is quite bright. By continuing our collaborative efforts and adhering to rigorous trial design approaches, we have the ability to continue building on both our recent successes and our long history of strong clinical science.

REFERENCES

1. Broder LE, Carter SK. Pancreatic islet cell carcinoma. II. Results of therapy with streptozotocin in 52 patients. Ann Intern Med 1973;79:108–18.
2. Schein P, Kahn R, Gorden P, et al. Streptozotocin for malignant insulinomas and carcinoid tumor. Report of eight cases and review of the literature. Arch Intern Med 1973;132(4):555–61.
3. Moertel CG, Hanley JA, Johnson LA. Streptozocin alone compared with streptozocin plus fluorouracil in the treatment of advanced islet-cell carcinoma. N Engl J Med 1980;303:1189–94.
4. Moertel CG, Lefkopoulo M, Lipsitz S, et al. Streptozocin-doxorubicin, streptozocin-fluorouracil or chlorozotocin in the treatment of advanced islet-cell carcinoma. N Engl J Med 1992;326:519–23.
5. Cheng PN, Saltz LB. Failure to confirm major objective antitumor activity for streptozocin and doxorubicin in the treatment of patients with advanced islet cell carcinoma. Cancer 1999;86:944–8.
6. McCollum AD, Kulke MH, Ryan DP, et al. Lack of efficacy of streptozocin and doxorubicin in patients with advanced pancreatic endocrine tumors. Am J Clin Oncol 2004;27(5):485–8.
7. Kvols LK, Moertel CG, O'Connell MJ, et al. Treatment of the malignant carcinoid syndrome. Evaluation of a long-acting somatostatin analogue. N Engl J Med 1986;315(11):663–6.
8. Kvols LK, Buck M, Moertel CG, et al. Treatment of metastatic islet cell carcinoma with a somatostatin analogue (SMS 201-995). Ann Intern Med 1987;107:162–8.
9. Rinke A, Muller HH, Schade-Brittinger C, et al. Placebo-controlled, double-blind, prospective, randomized study on the effect of octreotide LAR in the control of tumor growth in patients with metastatic neuroendocrine midgut tumors: a report from the PROMID Study Group. J Clin Oncol 2009;27(28):4656–63.
10. Yao JC, Phan AT, Chang DZ, et al. Efficacy of RAD001 (everolimus) and octreotide LAR in advanced low- to intermediate-grade neuroendocrine tumors: results of a phase II study. J Clin Oncol 2008;26:4311–8.
11. Kulke MH, Lenz H-J, Meropol NJ, et al. Activity of sunitinib in patients with advanced neuroendocrine tumors. J Clin Oncol 2008;26:3403–10.
12. Phan AT, Halperin DM, Chan JA, et al. Pazopanib and depot octreotide in advanced, well-differentiated neuroendocrine tumours: a multicentre, single-group, phase 2 study. Lancet Oncol 2015;16(6):695–703.
13. Jiao Y, Shi C, Edil BH, et al. DAXX/ATRX, MEN1, and mTOR pathway genes are frequently altered in pancreatic neuroendocrine tumors. Science 2011; 331(6021):1199–203.
14. Francis JM, Kiezun A, Ramos AH, et al. Somatic mutation of CDKN1B in small intestine neuroendocrine tumors. Nat Genet 2013;45(12):1483–6.
15. Fernandez-Cuesta L, Peifer M, Lu X, et al. Frequent mutations in chromatin-remodelling genes in pulmonary carcinoids. Nat Commun 2014;5:3518.
16. Halperin DM, Lee JJ, Dagohoy CG, et al. The rational clinical experiment: assessing prior probability and its impact on the success of phase II clinical trials. J Clin Oncol 2015;33(26):2914–9.

17. Yao JC, Shah MH, Ito T, et al. Everolimus for advanced pancreatic neuroendocrine tumors. N Engl J Med 2011;364(6):514–23.
18. Raymond E, Dahan L, Raoul J-L, et al. Sunitinib malate for the treatment of pancreatic neuroendocrine tumors. N Engl J Med 2011;364:501–13.
19. Caplin ME, Pavel M, Cwikla JB, et al. Lanreotide in metastatic enteropancreatic neuroendocrine tumors. N Engl J Med 2014;371(3):224–33.
20. Yadegarfar G, Friend L, Jones L, et al. Validation of the EORTC QLQ-GINET21 questionnaire for assessing quality of life of patients with gastrointestinal neuroendocrine tumours. Br J Cancer 2013;108(2):301–10.
21. Yao JC, Lombard-Bohas C, Baudin E, et al. Daily oral everolimus activity in patients with metastatic pancreatic neuroendocrine tumors after failure of cytotoxic chemotherapy: a phase II trial. J Clin Oncol 2010;28:69–76.
22. Zia MI, Siu LL, Pond GR, et al. Comparison of outcomes of phase II studies and subsequent randomized control studies using identical chemotherapeutic regimens. J Clin Oncol 2005;23(28):6982–91.
23. Campigotto F, Weller E. Impact of informative censoring on the Kaplan-Meier estimate of progression-free survival in phase II clinical trials. J Clin Oncol 2014; 32(27):3068–74.
24. Dodd LE, Korn EL, Freidlin B, et al. Blinded independent central review of progression-free survival in phase III clinical trials: important design element or unnecessary expense? J Clin Oncol 2008;26(22):3791–6.
25. Fleming TR, Rothmann MD, Lu HL. Issues in using progression-free survival when evaluating oncology products. J Clin Oncol 2009;27(17):2874–80.
26. Fleischer F, Gaschler-Markefski B, Bluhmki E. How is retrospective independent review influenced by investigator-introduced informative censoring: a quantitative approach. Stat Med 2011;30(29):3373–86.
27. Kola I, Landis J. Can the pharmaceutical industry reduce attrition rates? Nat Rev Drug Discov 2004;3(8):711–5.

Index

Note: Page numbers of article titles are in **boldface** type.

A

Adjuvant therapy, of stage I, II, and III bronchial carcinoids, 90–91
Atypical carcinoids, bronchial and thymic, **83–102**

B

Bevcizumab, in experimental regimens for advanced pancreatic neuroendocrine
  tumors, 128–129
Biomarkers, of neuroendocrine tumors, gene studies as, in gastroenteropancreatic
  tumors, 35
    potential diagnostic, 26–29
      chromogranin A, 26–27
      pancreastatin, 28–29
      plasma 5-HIAA, 28
      urinary 5-HIAA, 27–28
    useful in follow-up, neurokinin A, 29
      neuron-specific enolase, 29
      pancreastatin, 28–29
Biopsies, challenges of small, in bronchial and thymic carcinoids, 86
  in bronchial and thymic carcinoids, 88
    challenges of small, 86
Bone metastases, from neuroendocrine tumors, markers for, 41
Bronchial carcinoid tumors, **83–102**
  challenge of small biopsies, 86
  diagnosis, 88–89
  incidence, etiology, and predisposing genetic factors, 84–85
  pathology, 85–86
  staging and prognosis, 89
  symptoms, 86–87
  treatment, 90–95
    locally advanced unresectable, 91
    stage IV, 91–96
      cytotoxic therapy, 93
      etoposide-platinum regimens, 93–94
      mTOR inhibitors, 94
      peptide receptor radionuclide therapy, 92
      somatostatin analogues, 92
      temozolomide-based therapies, 94
      vascular endothelial growth factor receptor inhibitors, 95
    stages I, II, and III, 90–91
      adjuvant therapy, 90–91
      radiation therapy, 91

Hematol Oncol Clin N Am 30 (2016) 219–232
http://dx.doi.org/10.1016/S0889-8588(15)00178-1
0889-8588/16/$ – see front matter © 2016 Elsevier Inc. All rights reserved.

Moving?

Make sure your subscription moves with you!

To notify us of your new address, find your **Clinics Account Number** (located on your mailing label above your name), and contact customer service at:

Email: journalscustomerservice-usa@elsevier.com

800-654-2452 (subscribers in the U.S. & Canada)
314-447-8871 (subscribers outside of the U.S. & Canada)

Fax number: 314-447-8029

Elsevier Health Sciences Division
Subscription Customer Service
3251 Riverport Lane
Maryland Heights, MO 63043